Outline of Fractures

INCLUDING JOINT INJURIES

D1079893

Outline of Fractures

INCLUDING JOINT INJURIES

John Crawford Adams

M.D.(London), M.S.(London), F.R.C.S.(England)
Consultant Orthopaedic Surgeon, St Mary's Hospital, London;
Civil Consultant in Orthopaedic Surgery, Royal Air Force;
Production Editor, Journal of Bone and Joint Surgery.

SEVENTH EDITION

WITHDRAWN
FROM STOCK

CHURCHILL LIVINGSTONE
EDINBURGH LONDON AND NEW YORK 1978

CHURCHILL LIVINGSTONE
Medical Division of Longman Group Limited

Distributed in the United States of America by
Longman Inc., 19 West 44th Street, New York,
N.Y. 10036 and by associated companies,
branches and representatives throughout
the world.

© LONGMAN GROUP LIMITED, 1978

First Edition 1957
Second Edition 1958
Third Edition 1960
   Reprinted 1962
Fourth Edition 1964
   Reprinted 1965
Fifth Edition 1968
   Reprinted 1969
   Reprinted 1970
Sixth Edition 1972
   Reprinted 1974
   Reprinted 1975
   Reprinted 1976
Seventh Edition 1978
ELBS Edition first published 1978

ISBN 0 443 01632 1 (Cased)
ISBN 0 443 01633 X (Limp)

British Library Cataloguing in Publication Data

Adams, John Crawford
   Outline of fractures—7th ed
   1. Fractures
   I. Title
   617'.15   RD101   77–30525

*Printed in Great Britain by William Clowes and Sons Ltd.,
London, Colchester and Beccles*

Preface

The publication of this seventh edition of *Outline of Fractures* is something of a landmark in the history of the book. Not only has it reached maturity (1978 marks the twenty-first anniversary of its first publication); but the opportunity has also been taken to reset the text throughout in more modern format, and to renew all the illustrations. To gain the fullest advantage from this, the book has been extensively revised and brought up to date, but with care not to increase the overall length.

The book is still intended—as it was originally—mainly for medical students, Fellowship students, physiotherapists and orthopaedic nurses, and as a reference source for general practitioners.

The continuing expansion of the medical curriculum has persuaded me to set out those sections of the material that are not important to the undergraduate in smaller type, so that the harassed student may omit them from his reading if he so desires. (This policy has already proved popular in the companion volume *Outline of Orthopaedics*.) The space thus gained has been used to bring in further detail in the small-print sections and to introduce text references, for the benefit of those studying for the higher examinations.

I appreciate that there is often more than one way of treating a fracture successfully, and with certain fractures there must always be a divergence of opinion on what is the best method. Some surgeons will always tend towards a conservative approach, whereas others will turn more readily to operative methods. The policy that I have favoured has been to lean towards the conservative school, but to advocate operation without hesitation when it seems to offer positive advantages that outweigh its hazards.

I have omitted reference to fractures of the face and jaw and to fractures of the skull, because these come more properly within the spheres of the facio-maxillary surgeon and of the neurosurgeon respectively.

Once again I extend my thanks to the staff of the Publishers, Messrs Churchill Livingstone, for their ready help and close cooperation at all stages.

London
1978

J. C. ADAMS

NOTE ON TERMINOLOGY

The anatomical nomenclature used in this book conforms to that recommended by the International Anatomical Nomenclature Committee and approved at the Eighth International Congress of Anatomists at Wiesbaden in 1965. This nomenclature, which differs only in minor respects from the earlier Birmingham revision of the Basle nomenclature, has been adopted at most schools of anatomy, and it is to be hoped that it will become the standard terminology acceptable alike to anatomists and surgeons.

The recommended method of recording and expressing joint movement conforms to that laid down by the American Academy of Orthopaedic Surgeons in the booklet published by the Academy in 1965 and approved by most of the Orthopaedic Associations of the English-speaking world. The guiding principle of the method is that for any joint the extended 'anatomical position' is regarded as zero degrees, and movement at the joint is measured from this starting position. For example, in the knee the straight position is described as zero degrees and the fully flexed position is expressed as (say) 145 degrees of flexion.

Contents

Introduction

The treatment of fractures on a precise scientific basis has been possible only since adequate radiographic techniques became available. Although Roentgen announced his discovery of X-rays in 1895, several years elapsed before the necessary apparatus was developed for clinical use. So it may be said that modern fracture treatment began to develop at about the beginning of the present century. Before that time surgeons had to rely entirely upon a knowledge of dissected specimens and upon clinical evidence in determining the nature of an injury. It is evident, therefore, that they must have worked largely 'in the dark' (Figs. 1–3).

It was at about the beginning of the century, too, that surgeons began to think more in terms of open operations in the treatment of difficult fractures. Antiseptic surgery (introduced by Lister in 1867), and its offspring aseptic surgery, were relatively recent innovations, and before their introduction open operations upon bone were virtually prohibited by the risk of infection.

Even when the advantages of an aseptic technique and of radiography became available, operative fracture surgery was still severely handicapped by the lack of inert metals with which to fix the bones in apposition. Internal appliances of iron, mild steel or silver corroded and partly dissolved away in the tissues, causing a local reaction which often hindered union. This problem was not overcome until the period between the first and second world wars, when metallurgists developed alloys that could remain indefinitely in the tissues without corrosion.

In recent years the trend in fracture treatment has been towards the exercise of sound judgement and common sense rather than a slavish adherence to rigid precepts. No longer is it accepted automatically that because the bone fragments are not in exact apposition manipulation must be carried out: some fractures do not require reduction. Likewise it is no longer held that because a bone is fractured it must necessarily be rigidly immobilised until the fragments are united: some fractures do not need immobilisation. But above

References, page 291.

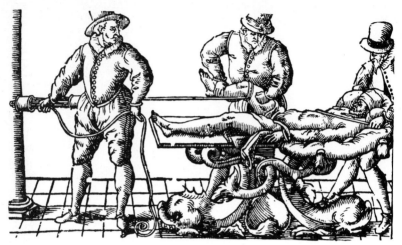

Fig. 1

An early illustration showing manipulation of the hip for 'dislocation'. Since X-rays were then unknown, the surgeon must often have been ignorant of whether he was dealing with a dislocation or with a fracture. (From the English translation of Ambroise Paré's *Treatise on Injuries*, 1678.)

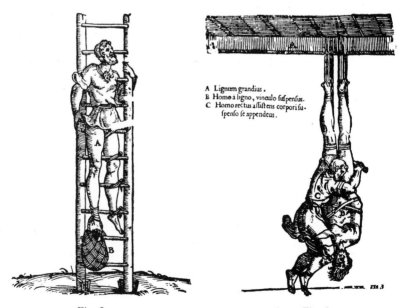

A Lignum grandius.
B Homo à ligno, vinculo suspensus.
C Homo rectus assistens corpori suspenso se appendens.

Fig. 2   Fig. 3

Two methods of applying powerful traction to reduce a dislocated hip, as described by Galen (*Opera*, 1625).

all has come the realisation that in the treatment of a fracture it is not the bone alone that matters. Attention must be paid to the soft tissues, and especially to the muscles, whose function must be preserved by active use within the limits imposed by necessary splintage, and redeveloped by graduated activity when the splintage is removed.

Those who wish to study further the history and development of orthopaedic and fracture surgery are referred to the papers by Mayer, by Platt and by Osmond-Clarke published in 1950, and by Rocyn Jones published in 1956.

References and bibliography, page 291.

CHAPTER 1

Pathology of fractures and fracture healing

A fracture may be a complete break in the continuity of a bone or it may be an incomplete break or crack.

Classification
Fractures may be subdivided, according to their aetiology, into three groups: 1) fractures caused solely by sudden injury; 2) fatigue or stress fractures; and 3) pathological fractures.

Fractures caused solely by sudden injury. These fractures form by far the largest group. They occur through bone that was previously free from disease. Such a fracture may be caused by *direct violence*—as when a metatarsal bone is fractured by a heavy weight dropped on the foot; or by *indirect violence* transmitted along the bone—as when the head of the radius or the clavicle is fractured in a fall on the outstretched hand.

So great is the preponderance of this group over the other two that the term 'fracture', if unqualified, is generally taken to signify this type of injury.

Fatigue fractures. Fatigue or stress fractures occur not from a single violent injury but from oft-repeated stress. Why they should occur—in bones that show no evidence of disease—has not been determined precisely. They have been likened to the fractures that occur in certain metals when 'fatigued' by repeated stress. With few exceptions fatigue or stress fractures are confined to the bones of the lower limb. The great majority occur in the metatarsals, but other well recognised sites are the shaft of the fibula, the shaft of the tibia, and the neck of the femur.

Pathological fractures. The term 'pathological' is applied to a fracture through a bone already weakened by disease. Often the bone gives way from trivial violence, or even spontaneously. The causes of pathological fractures will be considered later (p. 18).

OPEN AND CLOSED FRACTURES

A fracture is closed or simple when there is no communication between the site of fracture and the exterior of the body (Fig. 4). A fracture is open or compound when there is a wound of the skin surface leading down to the site of fracture (Fig. 5). It must be

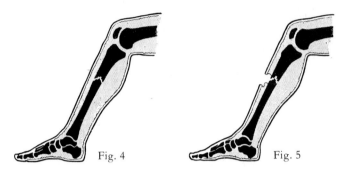

Fig. 4   Fig. 5

Figure 4—Closed or simple fracture. There is no communication between the fractured bone and the body surface. Figure 5—Open or compound fracture. There is a wound leading down to the site of fracture. Organisms may gain access through the wound and infect the bone.

stressed that the presence of a wound of the skin in association with a fracture does not necessarily mean that the fracture is an open fracture: it is classed as open or compound only when a direct communication exists between the body surface and the fractured bone ends.

The distinction between closed and open fractures is important because an open fracture is liable to be contaminated by organisms introduced from without, whereas a closed fracture is free from that risk.

PATTERNS OF FRACTURE

Fractures are often designated by descriptive terms denoting the shape or pattern of the fracture surfaces (Fig. 6). The following terms are in general use: transverse fractures; oblique fractures; spiral fractures; comminuted fractures (with more than two fragments); compression or crush fractures; greenstick fractures (incomplete breaks occurring only in the resilient bones of children). Impacted fractures are those in which the bone fragments are driven so firmly together that they become interlocked and there is no movement between them.

The pattern of fracture is of more than academic interest. It may indicate the nature of the causative violence and may thus give a clue to the easiest method of reduction. For instance, a fracture occurring transversely through a long bone has almost certainly been

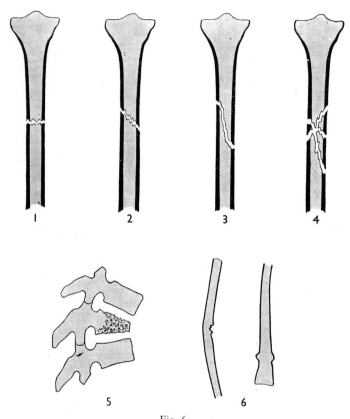

Fig. 6

Common patterns of fracture. 1. Transverse fracture. 2. Oblique fracture. 3. Spiral fracture. 4. Comminuted fracture. 5. Compression fracture. 6. Greenstick fractures.

caused by an angulation force rather than a twisting force, whereas a spiral fracture has equally surely been caused by a twisting strain.[1]

The pattern of fracture also gives an indication of the likely stability of the fragments. Thus a transverse fracture is unlikely to

[1] In its behaviour to violence an adult long bone may be compared with a stick of chalk. A simple experiment will show that the chalk is broken transversely if an angulatory force is applied, whereas it breaks spirally if a twisting force is used.

become redisplaced after reduction, whereas an oblique or spiral fracture is prone to redisplacement unless projecting spikes of bone can be locked into notches in the opposing surface (Fig. 7). A com-

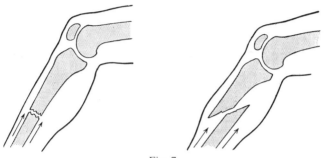

Fig. 7

A transverse fracture is stable against redisplacement whereas an oblique or spiral fracture tends to be redisplaced by the elastic pull of the muscles.

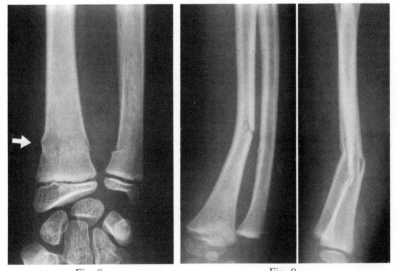

Fig. 8   Fig. 9

Radiographs of typical greenstick fractures in children. The fractures shown in Figure 8 were caused by a longitudinal compression force, and those in Figure 9 by an angulation force.

pression fracture does not lend itself well to anatomical reduction, because the spongy bone substance is crushed almost to powder and cannot be restored fully to its original trabecular form. Thus in cases of compression fracture—for instance of a vertebral body or of the calcaneus—it may be wise to accept the altered shape of the bone as permanent and to concentrate upon restoring function, rather than to attempt to restore the bone to its original form.

Greenstick fractures are peculiar to children, whose bones, especially before the age of ten, are springy and resilient like a freshly cut sapling. Bone of this type can be 'crumpled' like a concertina by a longitudinal compression force (Fig. 8). An angulation force tends to bend the bone at one cortex and to buckle or break it at the other, thus producing an incomplete fracture (Fig. 9). Although with severe violence children's bones often suffer complete fracture, incomplete fractures of the greenstick type are more common, especially in young children.

HEALING OF FRACTURES

A fracture begins to heal as soon as the bone is broken, and provided the conditions are favourable healing proceeds through a number of stages until the bone is consolidated.

The histological features of fracture repair at various intervals after injury have been well described by Ham and Harris (1956). Their description applies mainly to rib fractures in the rabbit, but the evidence suggests that the repair process is similar in man, at any rate when the conditions are comparable. Nevertheless it must be appreciated that the pattern of healing is not constant for all bones and in all circumstances. The repair of a tubular bone shows striking differences from the repair of a cancellous bone; and the pattern of healing in a given bone is probably influenced by such factors as the rigidity of fixation of the fragments and the closeness of their coaptation.

Repair of tubular bone

For purposes of simplicity the process of healing of a fractured tubular bone may be considered as occurring in five stages: 1) stage of haematoma; 2) stage of subperiosteal and endosteal cellular proliferation; 3) stage of callus; 4) stage of consolidation; 5) remodelling. It must be emphasised, however, that these stages are not sharply demarcated and that two or more stages of healing may be seen at the same time in different parts of the bone. The process of healing of a tubular bone is illustrated diagrammatically in Figure 10.

Stage of haematoma. When a bone is fractured blood seeps out through torn vessels and forms a haematoma between and around the fracture surfaces. The haematoma is contained by the surround-

References and bibliography, page 291.

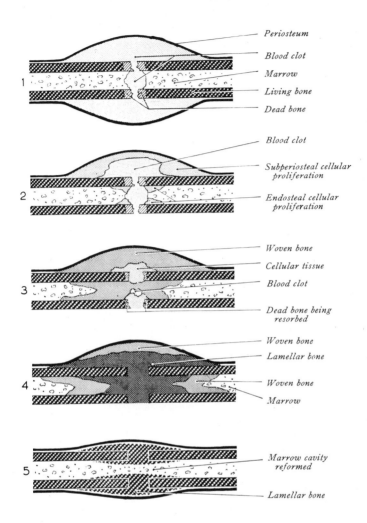

Periosteum
Blood clot
Marrow
Living bone
Dead bone

Blood clot
Subperiosteal cellular proliferation
Endosteal cellular proliferation

Woven bone
Cellular tissue
Blood clot
Dead bone being resorbed

Woven bone
Lamellar bone
Woven bone
Marrow

Marrow cavity reformed
Lamellar bone

Fig. 10

Stages in the healing of a fracture. 1. Stage of haematoma, with necrosis of bone immediately adjacent to the fracture. 2. Stage of subperiosteal and endosteal cellular proliferation. The cellular tissue, which may contain islands of cartilage, pushes forward from each side of the fracture at the expense of the blood clot, which is absorbed and takes little or no part in the actual repair. 3. Stage of callus. The proliferating cells give rise to osteoblasts, which lay down intercellular substance; this becomes calcified, to form woven bone or callus. 4. Stage of consolidation. Osteoblasts continue the process of repair, laying down lamellar bone at the expense of the woven bone. 5. Remodelling. Bone is strengthened in the lines of stress and resorbed elsewhere. The bone is thus restored more or less to its original form.

ing soft tissues—periosteum and muscles—which may be stripped up from the bone ends to a variable extent.

The fracture inevitably divides most of the capillaries that run longitudinally in the compact bone, and the ring of bone immediately adjacent to each side of the fracture becomes ischaemic over a variable length, usually a few millimetres. Deprived of their blood supply, the osteocytes near the fracture surfaces die.

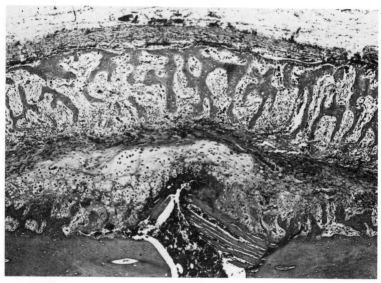

Fig. 11

Section showing healing fracture of human rib three weeks after injury. The fracture is seen in the lower part of the section. In the limited area shown the original bone fragments are dead, as indicated by the empty lacunae. Between the fragments is nothing more than old blood clot: union is occurring mainly around the periphery of the fracture. Next to the bone (near bottom left) is a thin layer of woven bone. Above this, near the middle of the section, is young fibrous tissue, bounded above by the old periosteum. Outside this is a thicker layer of typical woven bone, and outside this again is the new periosteum. (Haematoxylin and eosin, × 40.)

Stage of subperiosteal and endosteal cellular proliferation. The most prominent feature in the early stages of repair is proliferation of cells from the deep surface of the periosteum close to the fracture. These cells are the precursors of osteoblasts, which will later lay down the intercellular substance. They form a collar of active tissue that surrounds each fragment and grows out towards the other fragment. It should be noted that this cellular tissue is not formed by organisation of the clotted fracture haematoma. In fact the blood clot takes little or no part in the repair: it is pushed aside by the proliferating tissue and is eventually absorbed.

Simultaneously with the subperiosteal proliferation there is cellular activity within the medullary canal, where the proliferating cells appear to be derived from the endosteum and from the marrow tissue of each fragment. This tissue, too, grows forward to meet and blend with similar tissue growing from the other fragment.

Within the cellular tissue that grows forward outside and inside the bone to bridge the fracture there may be seen islands of cartilage. The cartilage is variable in amount: sometimes it is profuse but it may be absent. Evidently it is not an essential element in the process of healing.

Stage of callus. As the cellular tissue that has grown out from each fragment matures the basic cells give origin to osteoblasts, and in places to chondroblasts which form the cartilage already referred to. The osteoblasts lay down an intercellular matrix of collagen and polysaccharide which soon becomes impregnated with calcium salts to form the immature bone of fracture callus. This, from its texture, has been termed 'woven' bone (Fig. 11). The formation of this bridge of woven bone imparts obvious rigidity to the fracture, and when the injured bone is a superficial one the callus may be felt as a hard mass surrounding the fracture. The mass of callus or woven bone is also visible in radiographs and gives the first radiological indication that the fracture is uniting.

Stage of consolidation. The woven bone that forms the primary callus is gradually transformed by the activity of osteoblasts into more mature bone with a typical lamellar structure.

Stage of remodelling. When union is complete the newly formed bone often forms a bulbous collar which surrounds the bone and obliterates the medullary canal (Fig. 10(4)). The size of the mass varies from case to case. It tends to be large when there has been much periosteal stripping, when the fracture-haematoma has been large, and when there is marked displacement of the fragments. It is usually small when the bone fragments are in exact anatomical apposition, and especially when the fragments are rigidly fixed in close apposition by a metal plate with screws or by an intramedullary nail (Batten 1969). Callus is usually profuse in children, because the periosteum is easily stripped from the bone by extravasated blood.

In the months that follow union the bone is gradually strengthened along the lines of stress at the expense of the surplus bone outside the lines of stress, which is slowly removed. This process of remodelling is going on constantly, but inconspicuously, in every bone throughout life, but it becomes especially obvious after a fracture.

In children remodelling after a fracture is usually so perfect that eventually the site of the fracture becomes indistinguishable in

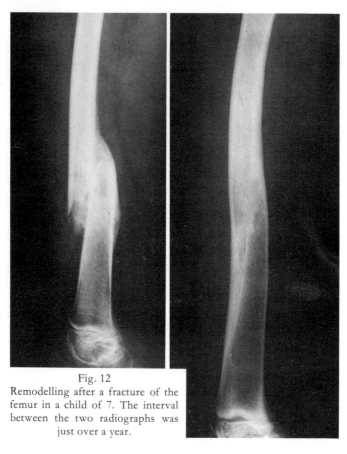

Fig. 12
Remodelling after a fracture of the femur in a child of 7. The interval between the two radiographs was just over a year.

radiographs (Fig. 12). In adults remodelling generally falls short of this ideal, and the site of a fracture is usually permanently marked by an area of thickening or sclerosis.

Repair of cancellous bone
Healing of a fractured cancellous bone follows a different pattern from that of a tubular bone. Because the bone is of a uniform spongy texture and has no medullary canal there is relatively a much broader

area of contact between the fragments than in the case of a tubular bone, and the open meshwork of trabeculae allows easier penetration by bone-forming tissue. Union can occur directly between the bone surfaces and it does not have to take place through the medium of external callus and endosteal callus as in a tubular bone.

The first stage of healing is the formation of a haematoma, into which new blood vessels and proliferating osteogenic cells from the fracture surfaces penetrate until they meet and fuse with similar tissue growing out from the opposing fragment. Osteoblasts then lay down the intercellular matrix, which becomes calcified to form woven bone.

Origin and activation of bone-forming cells. The foregoing is no more than a basic sketch of the processes concerned in the repair of a fracture. There has been much research into the complex biological processes by which repair is initiated and carried through to its completion, but many of the details are still not fully understood. In recent years some of the problems have been studied afresh with the aid of the electron microscope.

It is clear that the actual laying down of bone is a function of osteoblasts. But it is not yet agreed where they come from or what stimulates their activity. It has been thought that the deep surface of the periosteum contains 'resting' osteoblasts which are capable of activation and proliferation under the appropriate stimulus. Similar 'resting' osteoblasts are believed to exist in the endosteum, the thin layer that lines the medullary canal of the long bones. Whatever may be the contribution of these sources, there is abundant evidence that osteoblasts may be newly formed from cells in the bone marrow. The precise nature of these precursor cells is uncertain, but it seems probable that they belong to the reticulo-endothelial group (Danis 1957; Burwell 1964). The mechanism by which these cells are stimulated to differentiate into osteoblasts is unknown. It is widely believed that the stimulus may be a chemical one, dependent upon a specific substance liberated in the region of the fracture, possibly by necrotic cells (Urist and McLean 1952; Bridges and Pritchard 1958). This hypothetical substance has been termed an inductor.

The work of Trueta (1963), embodying studies with the electron microscope, has helped to elucidate some of these problems and has lent support to the view that osteoblasts may be derived from certain cells within the marrow, belonging to the reticulo-endothelial group. Trueta emphasised the important part played by the small blood vessels— capillaries and sinusoids—in the repair of a fracture. His studies led him to the belief that new blood vessels are attracted centripetally towards the fracture from the surrounding area, possibly under the stimulus of a chemical inductor substance liberated by sick or dead osteocytes in the

References and bibliography, page 291.

ischaemic bone adjacent to the fracture. He produced convincing evidence that the endothelial cells that line these new blood vessels can divide to form migratory 'intermediate' cells that are the precursors of osteoblasts. Moreover, he showed that these osteoblasts retain a direct cytoplasmic connection, through their filamentous processes, with the ancestral endothelial cells, whence presumably they derive their blood-borne nutriment. And when these osteoblasts finally surround themselves with intercellular substance and become osteocytes, locked each in its own lacuna, the fine cytoplasmic filaments still persist within the canaliculi of the Haversian systems. Trueta claimed further that under the influence of different stimuli, the nature of which is uncertain, the small blood vessels of bone are important agents in bone resorption, a fundamental part of the process of remodelling. First the mineral deposit, apatite, is washed away, possibly by a substance formed by degenerating osteocytes. Thereupon congregations of osteocytes, osteoblasts or intermediate cells coalesce to form multinucleated osteoclasts. These may themselves aid in the process of bone resorption, though the possibility must be recognised that osteoclasts may be merely the residue, not the agents, of bone removal.

Rate of union

The time taken for a fracture to unite is so variable that hard and fast rules cannot be laid down. In young children union is nearly always rapid, callus often being visible radiologically within two weeks and the bone being consolidated in four or six weeks (Figs. 13–14). In older children union occurs a little less rapidly. When adult life is reached age has little effect upon the rate of union.

In adults the time usually required for consolidation of a fractured long bone, in favourable conditions, is about three months, though in many cases it extends to four or even five months, especially in the case of a large bone such as the femur.

Fractures through cancellous bone unite in a somewhat shorter time than fractures through hard cortical bone.

Factors that influence the speed of union

There are a number of factors, apart from the age of the patient and the type of bone (cortical or cancellous), that may influence the speed of union. Favourable factors are a plentiful supply of blood to the bone fragments and, important in some fractures, immobility. Conversely, union may be hindered or even prevented by impairment of the blood supply even to one of the fragments, or by movement between the fragments. That is not to say, however, that movement is always harmful: many fractures unite readily despite almost constant movement between the fragments — for instance, fractures of the ribs, of the clavicle or of the shaft of the femur. In these instances movement is angulatory and does not damage the flexible granulations that bridge the fracture from an early stage. Movement that is harmful is usually rotatory or shearing movement, which may sever the delicate capillaries in the bridging tissue: such movement is liable to occur particularly in fractures of the forearm bones, of the scaphoid bone and of the neck of the femur, if the fragments are not perfectly immobilised. Other factors that may hinder union are infection

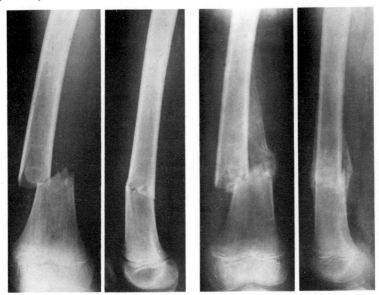

Fig. 13   Fig. 14

Radiographs illustrating the speed with which fractures unite in young children. Figure 13—Initial radiographs of a fractured femur in a child of 8. Figure 14—Three weeks later, showing advanced callus formation. A similar fracture in an adult would be expected to take at least three months to reach the same stage of union.

of the bone, interposition of soft tissue, or involvement of the bone by a tumour. A fracture within a joint may be more liable than most other fractures to non-union, possibly because the presence of synovial fluid about the site of fracture hinders the formation of granulation tissue across the fracture gap. These matters are considered further in the section on delayed union and non-union of fractures (p. 54).

Recently, attempts have been made to stimulate union in recalcitrant fractures by electrical impulses. This work is still mainly experimental and in a stage of development, but encouraging results in clinical cases have already been claimed (Bassett, Pilla and Pawluk, 1976).

FATIGUE OR STRESS FRACTURES

Fatigue fractures in metal are well known to engineers. In consequence of repeated stress there is a gradual rearrangement of molecular structure which weakens the metal and permits a crack to occur. It may be that there is a similar molecular change in human bones: but whether this is so or not, the analogy between fatigue fractures in metal and those seen clinically in man is apt so far as the

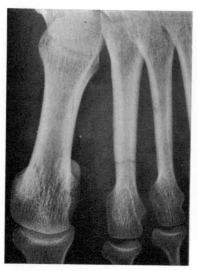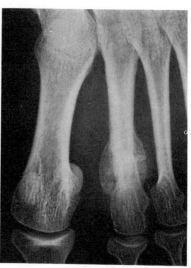

Fig. 15

Fatigue or stress fracture of the second metatarsal bone, often termed a march fracture. This is the commonest site for fatigue fractures. In the first radiograph (left), taken soon after the onset of symptoms, the fracture is hardly visible: it can just be seen as a hairline crack. Two weeks later (right) the radiograph is much more striking, the fracture now being surrounded by a mass of callus.

predisposing cause is concerned. In most cases of fatigue fracture of bone there is a history of oft-repeated minor stresses preceding the onset of pain: prolonged walking or marching in the case of fractures of the metatarsal bones, and repeated running or dancing in the case of fractures of the fibula or tibia. These three bones—metatarsal, fibula and tibia—are the commonest sites of fatigue fracture in that order, but the femur and occasionally other bones may be affected.

The great difference between a fatigue fracture and an ordinary 'traumatic' fracture is that there is no single specific causative injury in cases of fatigue fracture. The onset of pain in the affected bone is gradual or insidious, seldom abrupt. The pain is increased by continued activity and relieved by rest. Examination reveals well marked local tenderness over the affected bone. Soon afterwards there is swelling, with perhaps some local thickening, over the site of fracture. It is important to remember that radiologically nothing abnormal may be seen at first: it is only after two, three or four weeks that radiographic changes appear (Figs. 15–17). Even then

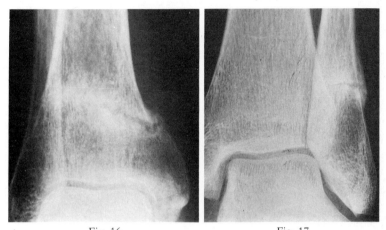

Fig. 16   Fig. 17

Figure 16—Fatigue fracture of lower end of tibia. Figure 17—Healing fatigue fracture of lower end of fibula.

the fracture itself may show only as a faint hairline crack, usually more or less transverse in direction: only rarely is there any displacement of the fragments. More striking than the fracture is the zone of callus that surrounds it. Faint at first—seen only as a haze near the bone—this new bone may eventually form a dense fusiform mass about the site of fracture. It has occasionally been mistaken for a bone sarcoma, an error that should not occur if the features of fatigue fracture are properly understood.

PATHOLOGICAL FRACTURES

A pathological fracture occurs through a bone that is already weakened by disease. Often the bone gives way from trivial violence, or even spontaneously. In many cases the patient, when directly questioned, will admit to having suffered pain or discomfort in the region of the affected bone for some time before the fracture. The underlying disease of the bone may be local and circumscribed, or it may be a generalised disorder affecting several bones or the whole skeleton.

Table I. The more important causes of pathological fracture.

LOCAL DISEASE OF BONE

Infections
Pyogenic osteomyelitis (usually in chronic form)
Syphilitic infection (osteolytic form)

Benign tumours
Chondroma (enchondroma)
Giant-cell tumour (osteoclastoma)

Malignant tumours
Osteosarcoma (osteogenic sarcoma)
Ewing's tumour
Metastatic carcinoma (especially from lung, breast,
    prostate, thyroid and kidney)
Metastatic sarcoma (from primary in another bone)

Miscellaneous
Simple bone cyst
Monostotic fibrous dysplasia
Eosinophilic granuloma
Bone atrophy in paralytic conditions such as poliomyelitis
Tabes dorsalis
Brittle state after irradiation

GENERAL AFFECTIONS OF THE SKELETON

Congenital disorders
Osteogenesis imperfecta (fragilitas ossium)

Diffuse rarefaction of bone
Senile osteoporosis
Parathyroid osteodystrophy
Cushing's syndrome
Infantile rickets
Coeliac rickets
Renal rickets (renal osteodystrophy)
Tubular rickets (Fanconi syndrome and related disorders)
Nutritional osteomalacia
Idiopathic steatorrhoea

Disseminated tumours
Multiple myeloma (myelomatosis)
Diffuse metastatic carcinoma

Miscellaneous
Osteitis deformans (Paget's disease)
Polyostotic fibrous dysplasia
Gaucher's disease
Hand-Schüller-Christian disease

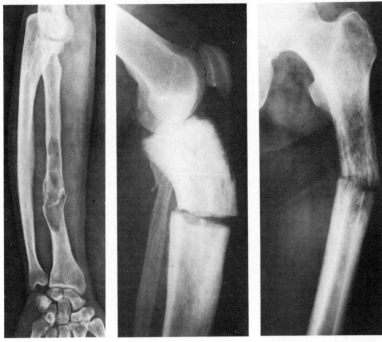

Fig. 18   Fig. 19   Fig. 20

Examples of pathological fractures. Figure 18—Fracture through a bone cyst in
the radius. Figure 19—Fracture through a tibia affected by osteitis deformans
(Paget's disease). Figure 20—Fracture at the site of a carcinomatous metastasis
in the upper half of the femoral shaft.

Causes. The causes of pathological fractures are shown classified
in Table I, and illustrative radiographs are shown in Figures 18–24.
When a local or circumscribed lesion of bone is responsible the
commonest cause is metastatic carcinoma, usually from the lung,
breast, prostate, thyroid or kidney. Such fractures occur most
frequently in the vertebral bodies (especially of the thoracic or
lumbar region) (Fig. 22), in the proximal half of the femoral shaft
(Fig. 20) and in the proximal half of the humerus (Fig. 23); but no
bone is immune. Another common cause is a bone cyst, usually in
a long bone (Fig. 18). In cases of pathological fracture from diffuse
or generalised affections of the skeleton the commonest cause is
osteoporosis of the senile type, and the bones most often affected
are the thoracic or lumbar vertebral bodies (Fig. 21) and the neck
or trochanteric region of the femur. Another common cause is
osteitis deformans (Paget's disease of bone), with fracture usually
of the shaft of the tibia or femur (Fig. 19).

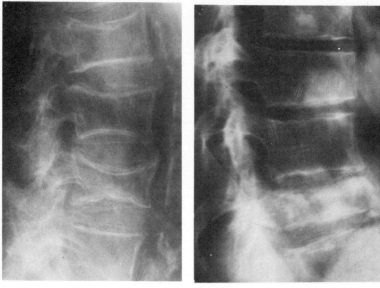

Fig. 21   Fig. 22

Further examples of pathological fractures. Figure 21—Vertebral fractures from generalised osteoporosis. Note the partial collapse of several vertebral bodies, with marked ballooning of the discs at the expense of the vertebral end plates. Figure 22—Vertebral fracture from carcinomatous metastasis. A single vertebral body is affected.

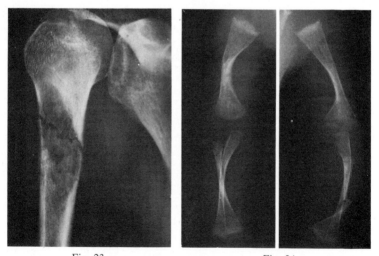

Fig. 23   Fig. 24

Figure 23—Pathological fracture from carcinomatous metastasis near upper end of humerus. Figure 24—Recent and old fractures of the bones of the upper limbs in an infant with osteogenesis imperfecta (fragilitas ossium).

Will the fracture unite? Whether or not a pathological fracture will unite depends largely upon the nature of the underlying disorder of the bone. When this is a generalised affection such as osteogenesis imperfecta, osteitis deformans (Paget's disease), or one of the diffuse rarefying diseases of bone (Table I), the fracture may be expected to unite, often in about the usual time. A fracture at the site of a bone cyst or a benign tumour will also generally unite, though there may be some delay. On the other hand, in fractures through a bone weakened by infection union is often seriously delayed or may fail altogether unless the infection is eradicated. Fractures through the site of a malignant tumour often remain un-united, but union may sometimes occur, especially after appropriate treatment by irradiation or hormones.

References and bibliography, page 291.

CHAPTER 2

Clinical and radiological features of fractures

The presence of a fracture can nearly always be inferred from the history and the clinical findings alone, but radiographs are necessary to establish its precise nature.

HISTORY

A statement that the patient is unable to stand or walk after an injury, or to use the injured part, must always arouse suspicion of a fracture. A history of visible bruising appearing a day or so after an accident is also suggestive. In many cases, however, the history does not provide reliable evidence on which to distinguish between a fracture and a simple strain or contusion.

Although in most fractures there is a distinct history of injury it should be remembered that in cases of fatigue fracture and of pathological fracture there may be a spontaneous onset of pain and disability without any causative injury.

Caution. The doctor is sometimes misled into believing that no fracture exists by the fact that the patient has retained the use of the painful limb. But in certain cases reasonable function is often preserved despite a fracture. The types of fracture that may be overlooked in this way include impacted fractures, fatigue fractures, fractures of small bones especially in the wrist, and, in children, minor greenstick fractures. If the common sites of these types of fracture are borne in mind mistakes in diagnosis should be avoided. *Impacted fractures:* The commonest sites are the neck of the humerus, the lower end of the radius, and the neck of the femur. *Fatigue fractures:* The commonest sites are the second and third metatarsal bones, and the shaft of the tibia or fibula. *Fractures of carpal bones:* Fractures of the scaphoid bone are particularly liable to be overlooked. *Greenstick fractures:* These are common in the forearm bones of children.

CLINICAL EXAMINATION

The objective signs of fracture are so well known that only a brief summary is required here. The following features, though not in themselves diagnostic, are fairly constant and should always arouse suspicion of a fracture: 1) visible or palpable deformity; 2) local swelling; 3) visible bruising (ecchymosis); 4) marked local tenderness over bone; 5) marked impairment of function. The following features give unmistakable evidence of fracture: 1) abnormal mobility (that is, demonstrable movement between the fragments); and 2) crepitus or grating when the injured part is moved.

Clinical evidence of fracture must always be confirmed or refuted by radiographic examination.

ADDITIONAL CLINICAL INVESTIGATIONS

When a diagnosis of fracture has been made the surgeon should continue his examination to determine the answers to the following four questions: 1) Is there a wound communicating with the fracture? 2) Is there any impairment of the circulation distal to the fracture? 3) Is there any evidence of nerve injury? 4) Is there any evidence of visceral injury? These facts should always be ascertained before treatment is begun. The presence of a wound communicating with the fracture, or of damage to a major blood vessel or viscus, makes the case an urgent surgical emergency, and may influence greatly the treatment of the fracture itself. And although a nerve injury does not necessarily affect the treatment of the fracture it is important that it be discovered at the first examination, lest the surgeon be accused later of having caused it by his treatment.

Skin wound. The presence of a skin laceration does not necessarily mean that the fracture is an open (compound) one. In some cases a laceration is incidental to the fracture and does not communicate with it. With careful examination there is seldom difficulty in deciding, from the position and nature of the wound, whether or not it communicates with the bone.

State of the circulation. The part of the limb distal to the fracture must be examined for evidence of circulatory impairment. The examination should be repeated frequently in the first forty-eight hours after a fresh fracture that has been immobilised in plaster or that has been operated upon: severe pain within the plaster, or marked swelling of the digits, should arouse suspicion that all is not well. The following tests, taken together, will always give the required information.

Colour. A pink colour is reassuring. A blue, grey or white colour should arouse suspicion but in itself it does not necessarily signify circulatory impairment.

Warmth. Warm digits suggest a circulatory flow, though it may be sluggish. Cold digits do not necessarily bode ill, especially if the limb is encased in a fresh plaster that is still damp.

Arterial pulses. The pulses, if available for palpation, are a reliable guide to the state of the circulation, but when the limb is encased in plaster they are not readily accessible. If necessary, the plaster should be trimmed sufficiently to allow access to the pulses.

Capillary return. When the digital pulp or a nail bed is compressed with a finger nail an area of blanching can be seen around the point of pressure. If on release of the pressure the blood flows back briskly into the blanched area in a pink flush the circulation is adequate. If the return is sluggish or absent, obstruction of the circulation should be suspected. This test should be interpreted with caution, because a capillary flush (albeit less brisk than normal and dusky in colour) may be observed even when the arterial circulation is occluded, if the venous return is also obstructed. Only when the returning flush is as rapid as in the sound limb, and pink, does it testify to the integrity of the circulation.

Nerve conductivity. An ischaemic nerve quickly loses its ability to transmit impulses—a fact that can be put to advantage when examining the state of the circulation. Loss of sensibility in the digits, in the absence of physical injury to the nerves, suggests ischaemia. In deciding whether sensory impairment is caused by physical trauma to a nerve or by ischaemia it should be remembered that in ischaemic lesions all the nerve trunks in the limb are likely to be affected, whereas it is unusual for all the trunks to be involved in an injury (except in brachial plexus injuries and cauda equina injuries). Total insensibility of a hand or foot therefore suggests ischaemia, whereas insensibility in the territory of a single nerve denotes mechanical injury. Motor tests of nerve conductivity are less reliable than tests of sensibility because the long flexors and extensors of the digits are innervated high up in the forearm and leg and may therefore continue to move the digits despite complete ischaemia in the distal part of the limb.

State of the spinal cord and peripheral nerves. Simple tests of sensibility, motor function, and sweating are sufficient to indicate whether or not there has been an injury to the nervous system. Bladder function must also be investigated in suspected injuries of the spinal cord or cauda equina.

State of the viscera. Visceral injuries will give characteristic symptoms and signs which must be looked for in accordance with general surgical principles. It is particularly important to investigate the state of the bladder and urethra in every fracture involving the anterior part of the pelvis.

RADIOGRAPHIC EXAMINATION

Radiographic examination must always be insisted upon when there is any suspicion of a fracture. Although in a high proportion of cases the findings will be negative the cost is one that must be paid for the assurance that a fracture is not overlooked. Not only is the failure to diagnose a fracture a serious matter for the patient; it is also important from the medico-legal point of view.

Radiographic technique. The standard technique is to take two projections in planes at right angles to one another—usually antero-posterior and lateral. The films should always include a good length of bone above and below the site of suspected injury, including the adjacent joint.

In special situations additional oblique or tangential projections may be required. These are helpful particularly at sites where a fracture is notoriously difficult to detect, such as the head of the radius and the scaphoid bone. There is an occasional place for tomography, mainly in the study of complex regions such as the spine.

Many examples could be given to illustrate the danger of relying

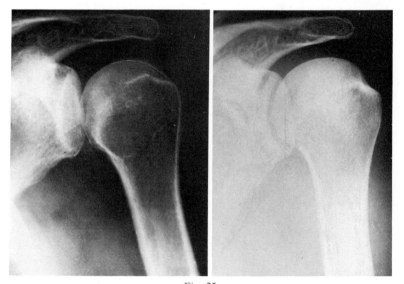

Fig. 25

The routine antero-posterior radiograph (left) might be thought to show the head of the humerus normally situated in the glenoid fossa. In fact it is dislocated posteriorly. (A clue is that the arm is held in medial rotation.) Compare with the reduced position shown on the right. This case exemplifies the need to obtain radiographs in two planes before the possibility of displacement can be discounted.

only on a single radiograph. If the radiographic examination is inadequate the diagnosis of fracture or dislocation may easily be missed. For instance, in a case of posterior dislocation of the shoulder the radiograph may appear virtually normal if only an antero-posterior projection is made. This is because the humeral head, though displaced backwards out of the socket, may still cast a radiographic shadow that superimposes fairly accurately upon that of the glenoid cavity (Fig. 25). Only in a lateral view is it evident that the humeral head has in fact lost all contact with the glenoid cavity.

When radiographs show evidence of a fracture or dislocation the examination should not end there. The films must be further scrutinised, and if necessary further films must be obtained, to provide answers to the following questions. 1) Is the fracture an ordinary traumatic fracture, a fatigue fracture or a pathological fracture? 2) Are the fragments displaced, and if so in what direction? 3) Are the fragments in satisfactory alignment? 4) Does the fracture appear to be a recent one, and if it it does not appear to be recent, is there any evidence of union? 5) Is there evidence of any associated injury, for instance of the adjacent joint or of a neighbouring bone?

TESTS OF UNION

At a certain stage in the treatment of a fracture it is necessary to ascertain whether or not sound union has occurred. The decision is made from a combination of clinical and radiological evidence.

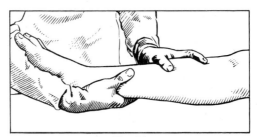

Fig. 26
Testing for union after a fracture of the tibia. The clinical signs of union are: 1) absence of movement at the fracture site; 2) absence of tenderness on palpation over the bone; and 3) absence of pain at the fracture site when stress is applied.

Clinical tests of union. There are three clinical tests of union: 1) absence of mobility between the fragments; 2) absence of tender-ness on firm palpation over the site of fracture; and 3) absence of pain when angulation stress is applied at the site of fracture (Fig. 26). These tests together are reliable, but they should always be confirmed by radiological studies.

Radiological criteria of union. There are two radiological features that indicate union: 1) visible callus bridging the fracture and blending with both fragments (Fig. 27); and 2) continuity

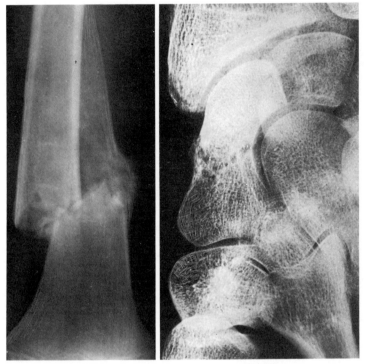

Fig. 27   Fig. 28

Radiological criteria of union. Figure 27—Bridging of the fracture by callus. Figure 28—Continuity of bone trabeculae across a fracture of the scaphoid bone.

of bone trabeculae across the fracture (Fig. 28). Of these, visible callus is generally the earlier and the more reliable sign. Trabecular continuity across the fracture is evidence of mature union, but over-lapping of the radiographic shadows of the two fragments may give a false impression of trabecular continuity when in fact it does not exist.

CHAPTER 3

Principles of fracture treatment

This chapter is concerned with broad principles rather than with details, but the principles can be applied, with suitable modifications, to any fracture.

INITIAL MANAGEMENT

Before definitive treatment of a fracture is undertaken attention must be directed to first aid treatment, to the clinical assessment of the patient with special reference to the possibility of associated injuries or complications, and to resuscitation.

First aid

The doctor who chances to be at the scene of an accident should seldom attempt more than to ensure that the airway is clear, to cover any wound with a clean dressing, to provide some form of immobilisation for a fractured limb, and to make the patient comfortable while awaiting the arrival of the ambulance.

In the moving of a patient with a fractured limb it will be found that pain is lessened if traction is applied to the limb while it is being moved. If it is suspected that there may be a fracture of the spinal column special care is necessary in transport, lest injury to the spinal cord or cauda equina be caused or aggravated. It is most important to avoid flexing the spine, because flexion may cause or increase vertebral displacement, jeopardising the spinal cord. In certain types of fracture extension is also potentially dangerous to the cord. Accordingly the patient should be lifted bodily on to a firm surface, with care to avoid both flexion and extension.

Temporary immobilisation for the long bones of the lower limb is conveniently arranged by bandaging the two limbs together so that the sound limb forms a splint for the injured one. In the upper limb support may be provided by bandaging the arm to the chest, or, in the case of the forearm, by improvising a sling.

Haemorrhage hardly ever demands a tourniquet for its control. All ordinary bleeding can be controlled adequately by firm bandaging over a pad. Only if profuse pulsatile (arterial) bleeding persists despite firm pressure over the wound, with the patient recumbent, does the need for a tourniquet arise. Pending its application, firm manual pressure over the main artery at the root of the limb may be applied to control the bleeding.

If morphia or a similar drug is given at the scene of the accident a note to that effect should be sent with the patient when he is admitted to hospital.

Clinical assessment

It must be emphasised again that an immediate assessment is required to determine 1) whether there is a wound communicating with the fracture; 2) whether there is evidence of a vascular injury; 3) whether there is evidence of a nerve injury; and 4) whether there is evidence of visceral injury.

Resuscitation

Many patients with severe or multiple fractures are shocked on arrival at hospital. Time must be spent on resuscitation before definitive treatment for the fracture is begun. The mainstays of anti-shock treatment are immediate replenishment of the circulating blood to restore a normal blood volume, and early adjustment of the electrolyte balance. Emphasis must also be placed on maintenance of a clear airway and of adequate pulmonary ventilation.

TREATMENT OF UNCOMPLICATED CLOSED FRACTURES

The three fundamental principles of fracture treatment—reduction, immobilisation, and preservation of function—are well known, and there is still no better way of discussing the treatment of a fracture than under these three headings.

REDUCTION

This first principle must be qualified by the words 'if necessary'. In many fractures reduction is unnecessary, either because there is no displacement or because the displacement is immaterial to the final result (Figs. 29–30). A considerable experience of fractures is needed before one can say with confidence whether or not reduction is advisable in a given case. If it is judged that perfect function can be restored without undue loss of time despite some uncorrected displacement of the fragments there is clearly no object in striving for perfect anatomical reduction. Indeed, meddlesome intervention may sometimes be detrimental, especially if it entails open operation. To take a simple example, there is no object in striving to replace perfectly the broken fragments of a child's clavicle, because normal function and appearance will be restored without any intervention

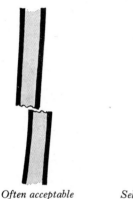 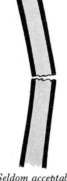

Often acceptable   *Seldom acceptable*

Fig. 29
Imperfect apposition may often be accepted, whereas mal-alignment of more than a few degrees must usually be corrected.

whatever; and the same applies to most fractures of the clavicle in adults. Likewise there is nothing to be gained in striving for perfect reduction of a fracture of the neck of the humerus in an old person—an ideal that may demand open operation for its attainment—when results that are as good or better may be expected from conservative treatment despite imperfect reduction.

In general, it may be said that imperfect apposition of the fragments can be accepted much more readily than imperfect alignment (Figs. 29–30). For example, in the shaft of the femur a loss of contact of half a diameter might be acceptable whereas an angular deformity of twenty degrees would usually demand an attempt at improvement. When a joint surface is involved in a fracture the articular fragments must always be restored as nearly as possible to normal, to lessen the risk of subsequent osteoarthritis.

METHODS OF REDUCTION

When reduction is decided upon it may be carried out in three ways: 1) by closed manipulation; 2) by mechanical traction with or without manipulation; or 3) by open operation.

Manipulative reduction

Closed manipulation is the standard initial method of reducing most of the common fractures. It is usually carried out under general anaesthesia, but local or regional anaesthesia is sometimes appropriate. The technique is simply to grasp the fragments through the soft tissues, to disimpact them if necessary, and then to adjust them as nearly as possible to their correct position.

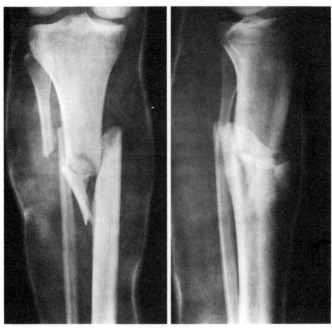

Fig. 30

In the case of this fracture it proved impossible to restore perfect apposition of the fragments by manipulation. Nevertheless the alignment was good and the clinical deformity was slight. The position was accepted. Four months later the function of the limb was virtually normal. Operative reduction might have been undertaken here but the subsequent course showed that it was unnecessary.

Reduction by mechanical traction

When the contraction of large muscles exerts a strong displacing force some mechanical aid may be necessary to draw the fragments out to the normal length of the bone. This applies particularly to fractures of the shaft of the femur, and to certain types of fracture or displacement of the cervical spine.

Traction may be applied either by weights or by a screw device; and the aim may be to gain full reduction rapidly at one sitting with anaesthesia, or to rely upon gradual reduction by prolonged traction without anaesthesia.

Operative reduction

When other methods fail—and occasionally as a method of choice— the fragments are reduced under direct vision at open operation. When operative reduction is resorted to, the opportunity should always be taken to fix the fragments internally to ensure that the position is maintained (see p. 41).

IMMOBILISATION

Like reduction, this second great principle of fracture treatment must be qualified by the words 'if necessary'. Whereas some fractures must be splinted rigidly, there are many that do not require immobilisation to ensure union, and there are some in which excessive immobilisation is actually harmful (Figs. 31–34).

INDICATIONS FOR IMMOBILISATION

There are only three reasons for immobilising a fracture: 1) to prevent displacement or angulation of the fragments; 2) to prevent movement that might interfere with union; or 3) to relieve pain. If in a given fracture none of these indications applies, there is no need for immobilisation. It follows from the first of these criteria, however, that if reduction has been necessary immobilisation will also be required.

Prevention of displacement or angulation. As a general rule the broken fragments will not become displaced more severely than they were at the time of the original injury. Therefore if the original position is acceptable immobilisation to prevent further displacement is often unnecessary. In fractures of the shafts of the major long bones, however, immobilisation is usually necessary in order to maintain correct alignment.

Prevention of movement. As has been mentioned already, absolute immobility is not always essential to union of a fracture. It is only when movement might shear the delicate capillaries bridging the fracture that it is undesirable, and theoretically rotation movements are worst in this respect. There are three fractures that constantly demand rigid immobilisation to ensure their union—namely, those of the scaphoid bone, of the shaft of the ulna, and of the neck of the femur.

Examples of fractures that heal well without immobilisation are those of the ribs, clavicle and scapula, certain fractures of the

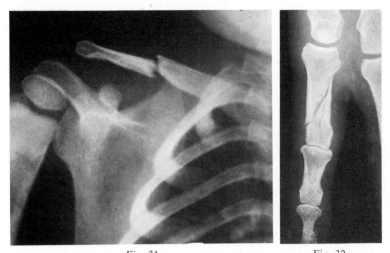

Fig. 31   Fig. 32

Two examples of fractures for which immobilisation is unnecessary. Figure 31—
Fracture of the clavicle. Figure 32—Undisplaced fracture of a phalanx of a finger.

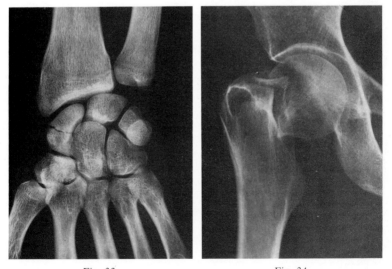

Fig. 33   Fig. 34

Two examples of fractures that require rigid immobilisation. Figure 33—Fracture
of the scaphoid bone. Figure 34—Fracture of the neck of the femur.

humerus and femur, and fractures of the metacarpals, metatarsals, and phalanges. In some fractures excessive immobilisation may do more harm than good. The injured hand in particular tolerates prolonged immobilisation badly. Whereas the wrist may be immobilised for many weeks or even months with impunity, to immobilise injured fingers for a long time is to court disaster in the form of permanent joint stiffness.

Relief of pain. Probably in about half of all the cases in which a fracture is immobilised the main reason for immobilisation is to relieve pain. With the limb thus made comfortable, it can be used much more effectively than would otherwise be possible.

METHODS OF IMMOBILISATION

When immobilisation is deemed necessary there are three methods by which it may be effected: 1) by a plaster of Paris cast or other external splint; 2) by continuous traction; or 3) by internal fixation.

Immobilisation by plaster or splint

For most fractures the standard method of immobilisation is by a plaster of Paris cast. But for some fractures a splint made from metal, wood or plastic is more appropriate—for example, the Thomas's splint for fractures of the shaft of the femur, or a plastic collar for certain injuries of the cervical spine.

Plaster technique. Plaster of Paris is hemihydrated calcium sulphate. It reacts with water to form hydrated calcium sulphate. The reaction is exothermic, a fact that is evidenced by noticeable warming of the plaster during setting.

Plaster bandages may be prepared by impregnating rolls of book muslin with the dry powdered plaster, but most hospitals now use ready-made proprietary bandages. These are best used with cold water because setting is too rapid with warm water; 'home-made' bandages, however, set more slowly and should be used with warm water.

Most surgeons use a thin lining of stockinet or cellulose bandage to prevent the plaster from sticking to the hairs and skin (Fig. 35). The use of a lining is certainly recommended because it adds greatly to the comfort of the plaster. If marked swelling is expected, as after an operation upon the limb, a more bulky padding of surgical cotton wool should be used.

The plaster bandages are applied in two forms: round-and-round bandages, and longitudinal strips or 'slabs' to reinforce a particular area. Round-and-round bandages must be applied smoothly without tension, the material being drawn out to its full width at each turn. Slabs are prepared by unrolling a bandage to and fro upon a table: an average

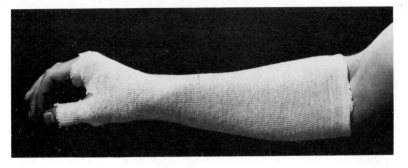

Fig. 35

A layer of stockinet forms a comfortable lining which prevents the plaster from sticking to the hairs. An alternative is to use a single thickness of cellulose bandage. The hand is shown in a position of function, with slight dorsiflexion at the wrist and the thumb opposed.

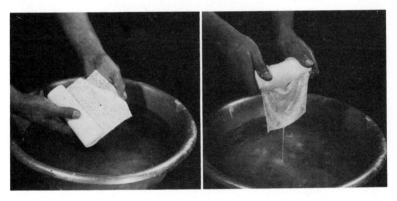

Fig. 36

Technique of soaking a plaster bandage. *Left*—The end is unwound for a few centimetres so that it will be found easily when the bandage is wet. *Right*—The wet bandage is squeezed lightly from the ends but is not wrung out.

slab consists of about twelve thicknesses. The slabs are placed at points of weakness or stress and are held in place by further turns of plaster bandage.

A plaster is best dried simply by exposure to the air: artificial heating is unnecessary. A plaster will not dry satisfactorily if it is kept covered by clothing or bed-linen.

Removing a plaster. There is still no better instrument for removing a plaster than the plaster shears. These act on the principle of a punch, not of scissors. There are two essential points to remember in the operation of plaster shears: 1) The line of cut should be over soft tissues and concavities and should avoid the bony prominences (Figs. 37 and 38).

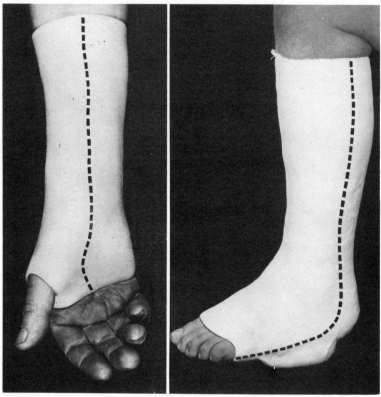

Fig. 37   Fig. 38

Correct lines of cut for removal of plasters with the hand shears. In the case of
the forearm plaster (Fig. 37) the cut should be made in the midline of the anterior
surface, crossing the wrist in the hollow between the tuberosity of the scaphoid
bone and the pisiform bone. Only one cut is required, because the plaster is thin
enough to be opened out without difficulty when it has been cut through. In the
case of the leg plaster (Fig. 38) two cuts should be made. The first cut should be
made along the lateral surface and should pass behind the lateral malleolus, in
the hollow between the malleolus and the heel. Thence it should extend along
the lateral border of the sole of the foot. The second cut should be made along
a corresponding line at the medial side of the plaster, passing behind the medial
malleolus.

2) The point of the shears should be slid along in the plane immediately
deep to the plaster—in the case of a cotton-lined plaster, between the
plaster and the lining. It will be found that if only one handle of the
shears is oscillated—namely the handle that is farther away from the
plaster—the point of the blade will be directed constantly away from
the skin towards the inside of the plaster, and will remain automatically
in the correct plane (Fig. 39).

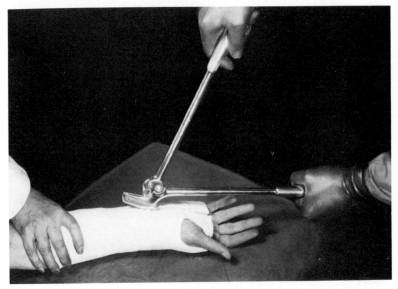

Fig. 39

To show the technique of operating the plaster shears. Only the handle away from the plaster (in this case the one in the surgeon's right hand) is oscillated: the other handle is held steady, parallel to the surface of the plaster. In this way the point of the blade is always directed outwards against the inside of the plaster, away from the patient's skin.

If the use of the shears is properly mastered there is hardly any need for other instruments such as saws or knives. The electric oscillating saw is valuable for dealing with very thick plasters and for cutting 'windows' through a plaster, but most surgeons find that it is noisy and rather frightening for the patient; moreover it creates an unpleasant amount of dust. In its present form it is unlikely to supersede the ordinary hand shears for daily routine use.

The plaster spreader is a useful instrument with which to open up a plaster cast that has been split down one side.

Other external splints. Apart from plaster of Paris, splints that are in general use are mostly those for the thigh and leg (Figs. 40–42) and for the fingers (Fig. 43). Individual splints may also be made from malleable strips of aluminium, from wire (Fig. 43), or from heat-mouldable plastic materials such as polyethylene foam (Fig. 44).

Precautions in the use of plaster and splints. When a plaster has been applied over a fresh fracture, or after operation upon a limb, careful watch must always be kept for possible impairment of the circulation. Undue swelling within a closely fitting plaster or splint may be sufficient to impede the arterial flow to the distal

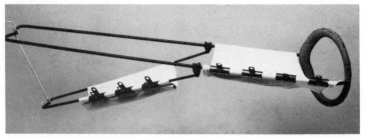

Fig. 40

Thomas's splint with Pearson knee flexion attachment, used mainly for fractures of the shaft of the femur. Note the canvas strips slung between the two bars to support the limb.

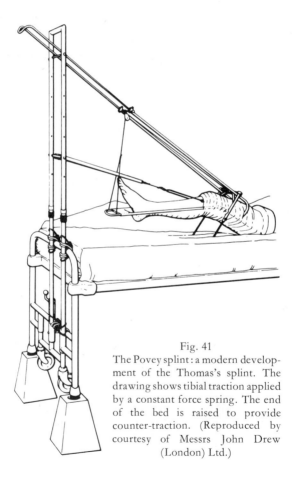

Fig. 41

The Povey splint: a modern development of the Thomas's splint. The drawing shows tibial traction applied by a constant force spring. The end of the bed is raised to provide counter-traction. (Reproduced by courtesy of Messrs John Drew (London) Ltd.)

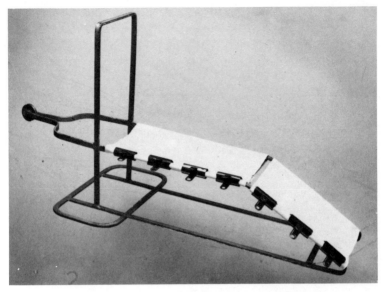

Fig. 42

Braun's frame. Though no longer widely used, it is still a convenient splint when traction upon the lower end of the tibia is required, or when the foot and lower leg are to be elevated to combat oedema.

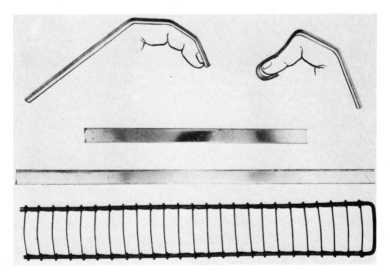

Fig. 43

Finger splints made from malleable aluminium strip, also shown unmoulded; and Cramer malleable wire, from which various splints may be improvised.

part of the limb. The period of greatest danger is between twelve and thirty-six hours after the injury or operation. Severe pain within the plaster, and marked swelling of the digits, are warning signs that should call for a careful reassessment of the state of the peripheral circulation. The clinical tests to be applied were described on page 23.

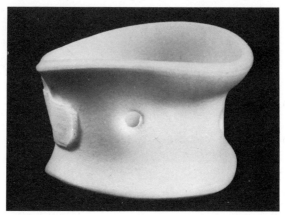

Fig. 44
Cervical collar constructed from
polyethylene foam ('Plastozote').

It should be noted that after operations upon the limbs a coagulated blood-soaked dressing may act in exactly the same way as a tight plaster and may seriously obstruct the circulation.

If a plaster has to be split for threatened circulatory arrest it is important that it be split *throughout its length*. Dressings and bandage under the plaster should also be divided right down to the skin, and the plaster should be opened up thoroughly from top to bottom. Nothing less than this can be regarded as adequate when the consequences of half-hearted measures may be catastrophic.

Immobilisation by continuous traction
In some fractures—notably those of the shaft of the femur and certain fractures of the shaft of the tibia—it may be difficult or impossible to hold the fragments in proper position by a plaster or external splint alone. This is particularly so when the plane of the fracture is oblique or spiral, because the elastic pull of the muscles

then tends to draw the distal fragment proximally so that it overlaps the proximal fragment. In such a case the pull of the muscles must be balanced by continuous traction upon the distal fragment, either by a weight or by some other mechanical device (Fig. 45). Continuous traction of this type is usually combined with some form

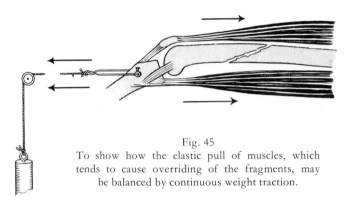

Fig. 45

To show how the elastic pull of muscles, which tends to cause overriding of the fragments, may be balanced by continuous weight traction.

of splintage to give support to the limb against angular deformity —usually a Thomas's splint in the case of a femoral shaft fracture or a Braun's splint in the case of the tibia. The 'gallows' or Bryant method of traction for femoral shaft fractures in young children employs the principle of immobilisation by traction without any additional splintage (Fig. 236, p. 223). Also in this category is traction upon the skull for cervical spine injuries.

Immobilisation by internal fixation

Operative or internal fixation should be undertaken in the following circumstances: 1) if it is impossible to maintain an acceptable position by splintage alone or in combination with traction; 2) when it has been necessary to operate upon a fracture to secure adequate reduction; and 3) as a method of choice in certain fractures, to secure rigid immobilisation and to allow earlier mobility of the patient. Opinion differs among surgeons on how freely this third indication for operation should be interpreted (see p. 44).

Methods of internal fixation. The following are the methods in general use (Fig. 46): 1) metal plate held by screws; 2) bone graft held by screws; 3) intramedullary nail; 4) nail-plate (combined nail and plate); 5) transfixion screws; 6) circumferential wires or bands; 7) suture through attached soft tissues. The choice of method depends upon the site and pattern of the fracture.

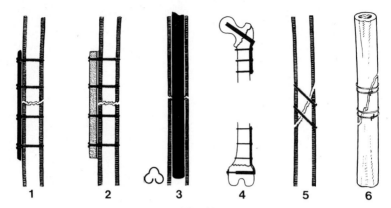

Fig. 46

Six methods of internal fixation for fractures. 1. Plate and screws. 2. Cortical bone graft and screws. 3. Intramedullary nail. 4. Nail-plate and screws. 5. Oblique transfixion screws (for spiral or oblique fractures). 6. Circumferential wire or band (for spiral or oblique fractures).

Metal plate and screws. This method is applicable to long bones. Usually a single four-hole plate suffices, but a six-hole plate may be preferred for the femur, and occasionally there is a place for double plates, one on each side of the bone.

Fixation by ordinary plates has the disadvantage that the bone fragments are not forcibly pressed into close contact: indeed if there is any absorption of the fracture surfaces the plate tends to hold the fragments apart, and this may sometimes be a factor in the causation of delayed union. In order to counter this disadvantage of simple plates and to improve coaptation at the time of plating, special compression devices are available by which the fragments are forced together before the plate is finally screwed home. It is not yet proved, however, that these compression plates are in fact more effective than ordinary plates.

Bone graft and screws. This method entails the sacrifice of bone from another part of the body or the use of stored bone. It is a satisfactory method but in fresh fractures success can often be attained by simpler means. Thus it finds a place mainly for fractures with delayed union or non-union (see p. 56).

Intramedullary nail. This technique is excellent for many fractures of the long bones, especially when the fracture is near the middle of the shaft. It is being used increasingly for fractures of the femur, tibia, humerus and ulna. It is also used routinely for fractures of the neck of the femur. The commonly used Kuntscher-type nail is hollow and of clover-leaf section (Fig. 46). but other types are also available, notably the nail of rounder section used by the Swiss (A.O.[1]) school. In some situations it may be more appropriate to use a stiff wire or a screw instead of the conventional nail.

Combined nail and plate. The nail-plate is a standard method of fixation for fractures of the trochanteric region of the femur (Fig. 225). It is also used commonly for fractures of the supracondylar region of the femur (Fig. 241). The nail-plate is usually in one piece, but it sometimes consists of separate nail and plate components held together rigidly by a bolt. As a general rule a one-piece nail-plate is to be preferred to a two-piece device because there is always a risk that loosening may occur between the nail and the plate component of a two-piece nail-plate.

Transfixion screws. The use of a transfixion screw has wide application in the fixation of small detached fragments—for instance the capitulum of the humerus, the olecranon process of the ulna or the medial malleolus of the tibia. A single screw usually suffices. Transfixion screws directed obliquely as in Figure 46(5) are also appropriate for the fixation of long oblique or spiral fractures of the shaft of a long bone—especially the tibia. In this case at least two screws should be inserted to ensure rigid fixation.

Circumferential wires or bands. These are applicable to the same types of case as oblique transfixion screws. They afford good fixation in appropriate cases, but they have not gained much favour because it is feared that they may strangle blood vessels in the periosteum and thus possibly hinder union.

Suture through soft tissues. In the case of avulsion of certain bony prominences—particularly the medial epicondyle of the humerus—exact anatomical reposition is not essential and it may be sufficient to anchor the detached fragment by sutures of catgut or wire through the attached soft tissues and periosteum.

Metals for internal fixation

Metals used for internal fixation of fractures or for internal prostheses must be resistant to corrosion in the tissues: silver, iron, ordinary steel, and nickel-plated steel are all unsuitable. A special stainless steel containing chromium, nickel and molybdenum and known as 18/8 Mo steel has been, and still is, widely used; but a non-ferrous alloy containing chromium, cobalt and molybdenum (produced under various trade names such as Vitallium, Vinertia, Coballoy, Alivium) has even better resistance to corrosion in the body and is

[1] Association for osteosynthesis.

being used as the metal of choice for all types of internal appliance except wire, for which it is technically unsuitable. The metallic element titanium has also proved resistant to corrosion in the body, but it is used far less widely than the chromium-cobalt alloys.

Discussion on the place of operative fixation

In recent years there has been a tendency at many centres to resort much more freely than in the past to operation in the treatment of limb fractures, often as a deliberate first choice. As will be seen in a later chapter, operative fixation is already accepted on substantial evidence as the best routine method of treating fractures of the neck of the femur and most fractures of the trochanteric region. But hitherto most fractures of the shafts of the long bones have been treated conservatively—generally with excellent results although often at the cost of rather a long time in hospital or away from work. Now, many surgeons would have us extend the more radical policy of routine operative fixation—particularly by intramedullary nailing or by rigid plating—to include most fractures of the shaft of the femur or of the tibia, and many fractures of the upper limb as well. This trend must be examined.

The reasons for advocating surgical intervention for fractures that were formerly managed conservatively are threefold. Firstly, there may be a substantial reduction in the time that the patient must spend in hospital and away from work. Secondly, in a favourable case function of the limb—and particularly of the joints—may be restored earlier because the need for plaster or other external splintage can often be eliminated. And thirdly, it is hoped that by providing rigid fixation of the fracture complications such as delayed union and non-union will be reduced. In themselves, these objectives are unexceptionable; but there are arguments on the other side. The chief of these is that operative fixation, especially when combined with open reduction, entails risks that are absent or minimal with conservative treatment. Occasional fatalities—for instance from pulmonary embolism—are probably unavoidable, and major wound infection is by no means uncommon after lengthy open operations for reduction and internal fixation. Extensive stripping of soft tissues from the bone may also lead to adhesions that restrict joint movement, and may jeopardise the blood supply to the bone fragments, thereby hindering union. Thus the objects of the operation may sometimes be defeated.

It is often difficult to strike a fair balance between these conflicting arguments, and it is important to weigh up all the factors in every case: the age of the patient, the site and nature of the fracture, problems of employment, and economic circumstances. Advanced age should always weigh heavily in favour of an operation that will enable the patient to get out of bed sooner, whereas anything that might favour infection, such as an open wound or a pressure blister, should weigh heavily against open operation. In general, it is probably fair to say that whereas the scope of operative fixation of fractures is undoubtedly much wider now than it was a decade ago, nevertheless a cautionary attitude should still be maintained in the case of fractures that are known to do well with conservative treatment: in the absence of definite indications, operation should be avoided in such a case, even though it may mean that recovery of function may take a little longer.

Yet the situation is not static. Advances in surgery and in the ancillary services constantly make for greater reliability and safety, and it may be expected that gradually the scope of operation in fracture treatment will be widened further. Already the technique of intramedullary fixation has been simplified by improved reamers and nails, and the risk of infection has been reduced by closed suction-drainage of the wound by vacuum bottles. Furthermore we now have available the radiographic image intensifier with television monitor. This equipment allows closed fractures to be manipulated with instantaneous radiographic control in normal light and without appreciable risk of harmful radiation to patient or surgeon.[1] With its aid, it is possible in the case of many fractures to reduce the fragments into anatomical position without exposing the site of fracture, and to guide a long nail down the length of the medullary cavity through no more than a 'stab' incision at the end of the bone.

REHABILITATION

Improved results in the treatment of fractures owe much to rehabilitation, perhaps the most important of the three great principles of fracture treatment. Reduction is often unnecessary; immobilisation is often unnecessary; rehabilitation is always essential. In Britain, much of the credit for early enlightenment on the principles of rehabilitation must go to Watson-Jones (1940).

Rehabilitation should begin as soon as the fracture comes under definitive treatment. Its purpose is twofold: 1) to preserve function so far as possible while the fracture is uniting; and 2) to restore function to normal when the fracture is united. This purpose is achieved not so much by any passive treatment as by encouraging the patient to help himself.

The two essential methods of rehabilitation are active use and active exercises. Except in cases of minor injury the patient should be under the close supervision of a physiotherapist throughout the whole duration of treatment.

Active use

This implies that the patient must continue to use the injured part as naturally as possible within the limitations imposed by necessary

---

[1] A clear distinction must be made between this remote-control technique and *direct* radiographic screening. Direct screening of fractures, even with the image-intensifier, is still to be condemned because of the radiation hazard.

treatment (Fig. 47). The degree of function that can be retained depends upon the nature of the fracture, the risk of redisplacement of the fragments, and the extent of any necessary splintage. Although in some injuries rest may be necessary in the early days or weeks there should be a graduated return to activity as soon as it can be allowed without risk.

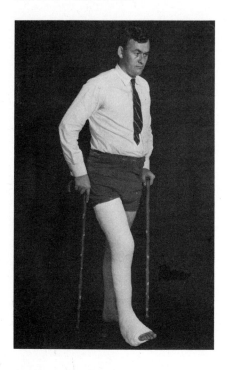

Fig. 47
Rehabilitation. Active use of
the injured limb.

Active exercises

These comprise exercises for the muscles and exercises for the joints. They should be encouraged from an early stage. While a limb is immobilised in a plaster or splint, exercises must be directed mainly to the preservation of muscle function by static contractions. The ability to contract a muscle without moving a joint is soon acquired under proper supervision.

When restrictive splints are no longer required exercises should be directed to mobilising the joints and building up the power of the muscles. Finally, when the fracture is soundly united treatment can be intensified, movements being carried out against gradually increased resistance until normal power is regained (Fig. 48).

Although every adult patient with a major fracture should

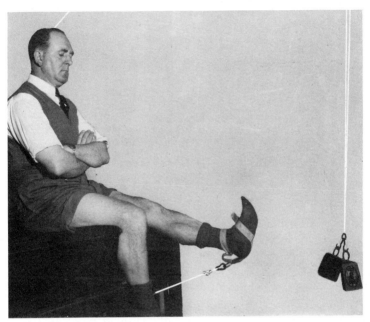

Fig. 48
Rehabilitation. Muscle strengthening by resistance exercises.

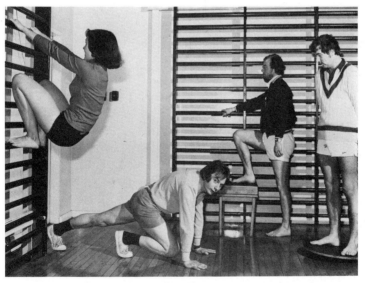

Fig. 49
Rehabilitation. Class exercises.

attend for supervised exercises as often as possible, it should be impressed upon him that this organised treatment plays only a part in his rehabilitation, and that much depends upon his continuing his normal activities so far as possible when he is away from the department. Physiotherapy is often enormously helpful, but it should supplement, not supplant, the patient's independent efforts (Fig. 49).

So far as children are concerned, supervised exercises are relatively unimportant, and in most cases the child may safely be left to his own endeavours, aided when necessary by encouragement from the parents, who should always be fully informed of the programme of treatment and the likely course of events.

The full importance of rehabilitation has been widely recognised only within the last thirty years or so. Previously, there was a tendency to insist upon rigid splintage and prolonged rest for an injured limb or spine. Disuse favoured the collection of oedema fluid about the fracture and in the limb as a whole. Muscles wasted, and joints became stiff. Recovery was a very slow process and often there was severe permanent disability. Memories of such an outcome, once only too common, serve as a reminder that rehabilitation, now taken so much for granted, is indeed an essential principle of fracture treatment.

TREATMENT OF OPEN FRACTURES

An open (compound) fracture always demands urgent attention in a properly equipped operation theatre. The sooner the wound can be dealt with adequately the smaller is the risk of infection arising from contaminating organisms.

Principles of treatment

The object is to clean the wound and whenever necessary to remove all dead and devitalised tissue and all extraneous material, leaving healthy well vascularised tissues that are able to ward off infection from the organisms that must inevitably remain even after the most meticulous cleansing.

The extent of the operation required depends upon the size and nature of the wound. The simplest type of case is that in which there is merely a small puncture wound caused by a sharp spike of bone forcing its way through the skin. In such a case it is often clear, when the wound is carefully inspected, that there is no serious contamination, and it may be unnecessary to do more than to clean the area with water or a mild detergent solution and to suture the skin edges. At the other extreme is the grossly contaminated wound of a gunshot injury, with severe tearing and bruising of the soft tissues over a wide area, and often with much comminution of the bone. Then the only hope of preventing serious infection lies in a most painstaking cleansing of the wound and in the avoidance of immediate skin closure.

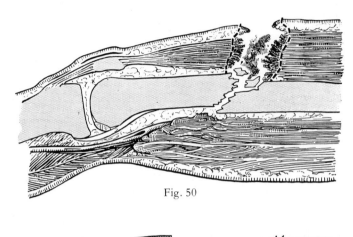

Fig. 50

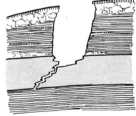
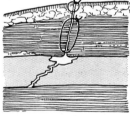

Fig. 51   Fig. 52

Diagrams illustrating the principles of operation for open fracture. The aim is to clean away all dirt and foreign matter and to remove dead and devitalised muscle and small loose fragments of bone, leaving the wound surfaces clean and viable. Figure 50—Margin of necrotic tissue to be removed is shown. Figure 51—After excision and cleansing. Figure 52—Freshened edges of wound sutured. In certain circumstances—particularly after gunshot wounds—the wound is left open rather than sutured. (For details see text.)

Technique of operation for major wounds

The operation is begun by enlarging the skin wound if this is necessary to display clearly the extent of the underlying damage. The whole wound is then flushed with copious quantities of water or saline to remove as completely as possible all contaminating dirt: at the same time any pieces of foreign matter such as shreds of clothing are picked out with forceps. In general, the emphasis should be on thorough cleaning of the tissues rather than on drastic excision: nevertheless tissue that is obviously dead should be excised (Figs. 50–52), and it is particularly important that dead or devascularised muscle be removed in order to reduce the risk of infection by gas-forming organisms (gas gangrene). Bone fragments that are small and completely detached may be removed, but large fragments, which usually retain some soft-tissue attachments, should be preserved. Damage to a major blood vessel is dealt with, according to circumstances, by ligation, suture, or grafting. The ends of severed nerve trunks may be tacked lightly together with one or two sutures, to facilitate later definitive repair.

The question of skin closure

At the conclusion of the operation a decision must be made whether or not it is safe to close the wound. The decision should rest on two factors: 1) the time since the injury; and 2) the degree of contamination. If the operation is done within a few hours of the injury, and if contamination has been slight, the wound should be closed primarily, either by direct suture or by immediate skin grafting, as appropriate (see below).

On the other hand, if more than eight or ten hours have elapsed since the injury, or if contamination has been severe, infection must be regarded as almost inevitable if the wound is sutured, and it should therefore be left open and dressed with sterile gauze. In such a case delayed closure may be undertaken as soon as it is clear that infection has been aborted or overcome—often a matter of no more than a few days. This technique of delayed primary suture has become standard practice in the management of gunshot wounds, which are always heavily contaminated, and the temptation to suture such a wound immediately should always be resisted.

Methods of skin closure. Whether skin closure is undertaken primarily or after an interval, the ideal method is by direct suture of the skin edges. But this is not always feasible. Whether it is practicable or not depends upon the amount of skin destroyed and lost in the injury. If the skin loss is negligible and the skin edges can be brought together without tension direct suture should be carried out. But if the skin edges will not come together easily the wound should be closed by a free split-skin graft.

Treatment of the fracture

Once the wound has been dealt with the treatment of the fracture itself should follow the general principles already suggested for closed fractures. The only difference is that in open fractures there should be a greater reluctance to resort to operative methods of fixation, especially if there seems to be a serious risk of infection; and if it is decided that metallic internal fixation must be employed the metal should be placed well away from the suture line.

Supplementary treatment in cases of open fracture

Prophylaxis against tetanus. A patient who has previously been immunised against tetanus by tetanus toxoid should be given a booster dose of toxoid. If the patient has not previously been immunised it is wise to begin immunisation with a standard dose of toxoid and to follow this up with a second dose six weeks later.

Antibiotics. A course of treatment by ampicillin, cloxacillin and fucidic acid or by other appropriate antibiotics should be begun immediately and continued until the danger of infection is past.

Anti-gas-gangrene serum. It is now believed that anti-gas-gangrene serum is ineffective as a prophylactic agent and its routine use is not recommended. Reliance should be placed rather upon meticulous cleansing of the wound with excision of all devitalised muscle, and upon appropriate antibiotics.

Precautions

In severe open fractures, with perhaps considerable loss of blood, there is a greater liability to shock than there is in closed fractures, and appropriate measures of resuscitation are often required.

Patients treated for open fractures must be watched closely for signs that may indicate infection. The temperature chart should always be noted: any large sustained rise of temperature should be taken as an indication to inspect the wound. When there has been much contusion of muscle the possible development of gas gangrene must always be borne in mind.

References and bibliography, page 291.

CHAPTER 4

Complications of fractures

In the great majority of fractures union proceeds according to expectation, function of the injured part is gradually restored, and little if any permanent disability remains. But not quite every fracture has this happy outcome. Complications inevitably occur in a proportion of them—some slight, some severe, a few catastrophic. These complications may be considered in two groups: 1) those that are concerned with the fracture itself; and 2) those that are attributable to associated injury involving other tissues. They may be listed as in the following table (Table II).

Table II. Twelve complications of fractures classified into intrinsic and extrinsic groups

Complications related to the fracture itself	Complications attributable to associated injury
Infection	Injury to major blood vessels
Delayed union	Injury to nerves
Non-union	Injury to viscera
Avascular necrosis	Injury to tendons
Mal-union	Injuries and post-traumatic
Shortening	affections of joints
	Fat embolism

INFECTION

Infection is virtually confined to open (compound) fractures, in which the wound is contaminated by organisms carried in from outside the body. Exceptionally a closed (simple) fracture may become infected when it is converted into an open fracture by operative intervention.

Wound infection occasionally remains superficial and the bone escapes, but more often the infection extends to the bone, giving rise to osteomyelitis. This is a serious complication, because once a bone is infected with pyogenic organisms the infection tends to become chronic (Fig. 53). Part of the bone may die through impairment of its blood supply, forming a sequestrum which may lie loose within a cavity in the bone for an indefinite period unless it is removed surgically. In such a case there is nearly always a persistent discharge of pus from a sinus. Infection is a potent factor in delaying or preventing union (Fig. 54).

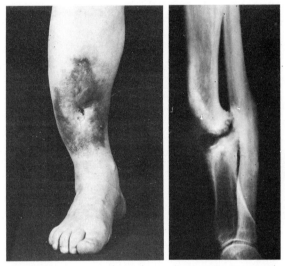

Fig. 53   Fig. 54

Osteomyelitis with purulent discharge persisting twenty years after a fracture of the tibia. The radiograph (Fig. 54) shows that the fracture is still ununited. The fibula is hypertrophied because it has been supporting most of the body weight.

Prevention. Every effort must be made to prevent infection in cases of open (compound) fracture by prompt and meticulous excision of all dead and contaminated tissue, in the manner already described (p. 48).

Treatment. *Acute recent infection.* In cases of established infection in the acute stage the main essential of treatment is to provide adequate drainage. The wound is left open and potential pockets in which pus might collect are eliminated by appropriate incision or excision of tissue. Dressings need not be frequent. Between dressings the limb is often best immobilised in plaster of Paris. In a favourable case the infection is gradually overcome: indications of its quiescence are that the discharge of pus ceases and the wound becomes lined by healthy granulations. At this stage closure may be attempted either by secondary suture, if practicable, or by grafting with split skin.

Chronic infection. If the infection of the bone passes into a persistent stage (chronic osteomyelitis) pus continues to discharge and fragments of the bone may die and separate as sequestra. At this stage a more radical operation is required if permanent healing is to be obtained. All sequestra must be removed, and bone that is honeycombed with small pus-containing cavities must be chiselled away. Large cavities in the bone are de-roofed and 'saucerised', and they may be finally obliterated either by filling with a pedicled muscle flap or, in the case of a superficial bone such as the tibia, by lining the saucerised cavity with a split-skin graft applied direct to the raw bone. Occasionally it may be wise to excise widely the entire block of infected bone and to replace it by a cancellous bone graft from the ilium (Nicoll 1960).

DELAYED UNION

There is no absolute time beyond which a fracture is in a state of delayed union: the border-line is arbitrary, and it depends to some extent upon the bone affected. But as a general rule union is deemed to be delayed if the fragments are still freely mobile three or four months after the injury. If a state of delayed union persists for many months it eventually passes into a state of non-union. The distinction between the two states is clear: whereas in delayed union there is nothing in the condition of the bones to indicate that union will fail altogether, in non-union characteristic changes are observed radiologically which suggest that union will never occur (Figs. 55–56).

Causes. The causes of delayed union are like those of non-union, but acting in less degree (see p. 55).

Treatment. In most cases of delayed union treatment is expectant at first, for one hopes that the fracture will eventually unite satisfactorily without surgical intervention. Usually patience is rewarded. But there may come a time—perhaps six months or so after the beginning of treatment—when, if union does not appear to be progressing, surgical treatment must be considered. In most such cases some form of bone grafting operation offers the best prospect of promoting union (see p. 56).

NON-UNION

If a fracture remains ununited for many months distinctive radiological changes take place which indicate a likely permanent state of non-union. The bone ends at the site of fracture become dense and rounded, so that in contrast the fracture line itself appears increasingly clear-cut (Figs. 54 and 56). Pathologically, the process of healing appears to have come to an end, and there is no attempt to bridge the fracture with callus. Instead, the gap between the bones

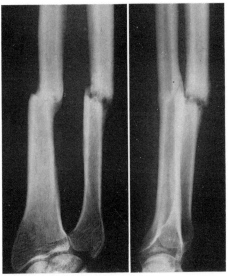
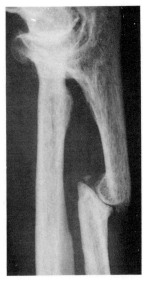

Fig. 55   Fig. 56

Radiographs illustrating the distinction between delayed union (shown in the ulnar fracture in Figure 55) and non-union (Fig. 56). In delayed union there is no radiographic feature to suggest that union will not occur, whereas in non-union the fractured ends of the bone are sclerotic and rounded, and there may be signs of the attempted formation of a false joint. (Another example of non-union is shown in Figure 178, page 177.)

is filled with fibrous tissue. In some cases a cavity may form in this fibrous bridge, suggesting an attempt to form a false joint (pseud-arthrosis).

Causes. Eight factors are believed to favour non-union: 1) infection of the bone; 2) inadequate blood supply to one or both fragments; 3) excessive shearing movement between the fragments; 4) interposition of soft tissue between the fragments; 5) loss of apposition between the fragments (including over-distraction by traction apparatus); 6) dissolution of the fracture haematoma by synovial fluid (in fractures within joints); 7) the presence of corroding metal in the immediate vicinity of the fracture; 8) destruction of bone, as by a tumour (in pathological fractures). Sometimes two or more of these factors may act together. Acting in slighter degree, these same factors may be responsible for delayed union.

Treatment. The treatment of non-union depends upon the site of the fracture and the degree of the disability. In some cases the condition may cause only slight disability and is best left untreated—as, for instance, in certain fractures of the scaphoid bone. More often, however, non-union of a fracture is disabling and surgical treatment is desirable. Most ununited fractures of the long bones lend themselves well to treatment by bone grafting, which is usually successful in promoting union. In certain circumstances—especially when the fracture is within or near a joint—other operations may be more appropriate, such as excision of one of the fragments or its replacement by a prosthesis.

Bone grafting for delayed union and non-union

Bone grafts are usually obtained from another part of the patient's body (autogenous grafts). If it is impracticable or undesirable to take bone from the patient's own body, grafts obtained from another human subject may be used (allografts; homogenous grafts). They are generally stored frozen or chemically preserved in a 'bone bank' until required. Grafts obtained from animals (heterogenous grafts) have been used on a limited scale in recent years. Such grafts are now prepared commercially in sterile packages after elimination of their antigenic properties by deproteinisation. They have the advantage of convenience, and the discomfort to the patient entailed in taking an autogenous graft is avoided. Nevertheless such grafts often fail to promote union of the fracture, and consequently they are little used. Autogenous grafting is much more reliable, and is the method of choice.

Bone transferred as a graft from one site to another does not survive in a living state. Even in a fresh graft the bone cells die, though in the case of an autogenous graft a few cells that are near the surface may possibly survive. The purpose of the graft is mainly to serve as a scaffolding or temporary bridge upon which new bone is laid down. Thus the whole of a graft is eventually replaced by new living bone. This process of replacement is dependent upon adequate revascularisation of the graft; so a graft that lies in a highly vascular bed is more likely to succeed than one that is surrounded by relatively ischaemic tissue.

Technique. Bone for grafting may be obtained as a solid slab, or it may be used in the form of multiple slivers or of small chips.

Slab grafts. A slab graft is usually obtained from strong cortical bone: the subcutaneous part of the tibia is a common site. The graft is fixed to the freshened recipient bone either by screws or by inlaying. Such a graft serves as an internal splint as well as a framework for the growth of new bone (Fig. 57).

Sliver grafts. Sliver or strip grafts are generally obtained from spongy cancellous bone—especially from the ilium. They are laid about the fracture, usually deep to the periosteum, and are held in place by suture of the soft tissues over them (Fig. 58). The simplicity of this method of grafting was emphasised by Phemister (1947).

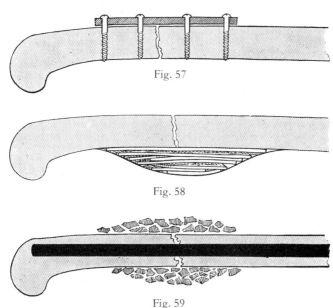

Fig. 57

Fig. 58

Fig. 59

Examples of bone grafting techniques. Figure 57—Cortical slab graft held by four screws. Figure 58—Sliver grafts of cancellous bone laid deep to the periosteum and held in place by the overlying soft tissues. Figure 59—Cancellous chip grafts used in conjunction with an intramedullary nail.

Chip grafts. These also are preferably obtained from cancellous bone. The chips are packed firmly around the site of fracture in the same way as sliver grafts (Fig. 59). Chip grafts are often used to reinforce slab grafts or sliver grafts, and to fill cavities.

Bone grafting may be combined with internal fixation by a metal plate or nail, and usually the limb is further protected by plaster until the fracture is united.

AVASCULAR NECROSIS

Avascular necrosis (death of bone from deficient blood supply) may have serious consequences. Not only is it sometimes a cause of intractable non-union; it also leads in many cases to disabling osteoarthritis or to total disorganisation of a joint.

Pathology. Avascular necrosis occurs when the blood supply to a bone or part of a bone is interrupted by an injury (or, rarely, by disease). It usually occurs as a complication of a fracture near the articular end of a bone, especially where the terminal fragment is

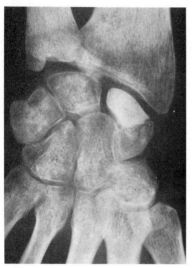 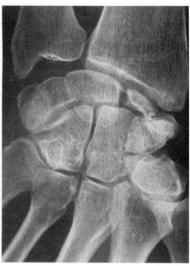

Fig. 60   Fig. 61

Avascular necrosis of proximal half of scaphoid bone. Figure 60—Two months after the fracture the dead fragment appears relatively dense because it has not shared in the osteoporosis from disuse that has affected the surrounding bones. Figure 61—At a later stage the dead fragment is seen collapsed into an irregular mass. Osteoarthritis is inevitable.

devoid of vascular soft-tissue attachments and depends for its nutrition almost entirely upon the intra-osseous vessels, which may be torn at the time of the injury. It may also occur after a dislocation if vital blood vessels supplying the bone are torn or occluded. In either case the immediate consequence of the ischaemia is that the bone cells die, and if the affected part of the bone lies mainly within a joint cavity (as it usually does) there is little chance that it will be revascularised from the surrounding tissues before irreversible changes of structure and form have taken place. The avascular bone gradually loses its rigid trabecular structure and becomes granular or 'gritty'. In this state the bone crumbles easily, and under the stress imposed by muscle tone or body weight it may eventually collapse into an irregular mass (Fig. 61). This process of disintegration and collapse may sometimes be very slow: it may occur within a year of the injury but on the other hand it may take as long as three or even four years. Meanwhile the overlying articular cartilage usually also dies, because its basal layers, normally nourished through vessels in the subchondral bone, are devitalised. Thus in most cases a joint whose surface suffers avascular necrosis is doomed to crippling osteoarthritis whether or not the causative fracture eventually unites. Only in a few instances (usually in children) does the cartilage receive enough nourishment from the synovial fluid to enable its deeper layers to survive until the underlying bone is revascularised.

Sites. The sites at which avascular necrosis occurs most frequently are the head of the femur after fracture of the femoral neck (p. 203) or after dislocation of the hip (p. 194), the proximal half of the scaphoid bone after a fracture through the waist of the bone (p. 173), and the body of the talus after a fracture through the neck of the talus (p. 274). Sometimes an entire bone may suffer avascular necrosis after a dislocation—notably the lunate bone (p. 171).

Diagnosis. In many cases, though not in all, avascular necrosis may be recognised from radiographs about one to three months after the injury. Because it has no blood supply, the avascular fragment is unable to share in the general osteoporosis from disuse that affects the surrounding bones, and it stands out in sharp contrast by virtue of its relatively greater density (Fig. 60). In the later stages, when collapse has occurred, the radiographic findings are characteristic. The bone, or the affected part of it, has lost its normal height and has a shrunken, crumbled appearance (Fig. 61).

Treatment. Because of the likelihood of disorganisation of the adjacent joint, avascular necrosis often demands early operation. In many cases it is wise to excise the avascular fragment, and if necessary to reconstruct the joint by some form of arthroplasty or to stabilise it by arthrodesis.

MAL-UNION

Mal-union implies union of the fragments in an imperfect position. In slight degree it occurs in a great many fractures, but in practice the term is reserved for cases in which the resulting deformity is of clinical significance. Examples are shown in Figures 62, 64 and 75.

Mal-union should usually be avoided by competent initial treatment of the fracture, but there are occasions when some impairment of position must be accepted as inevitable despite the greatest care.

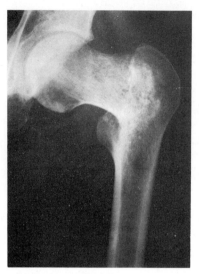
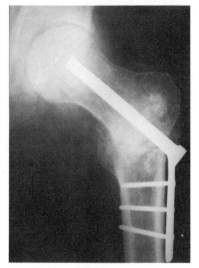

Fig. 62   Fig. 63

Figure 62—Mal-union of a trochanteric fracture in a young man. Note that the neck-shaft angle, normally 130 degrees, has been reduced to about 90 degrees. Figure 63—After corrective osteotomy and fixation by nail-plate. (In old persons, who are the usual victims of this injury, a deformity such as this would usually be accepted.)

Treatment. Each case must be considered on its merits. In some cases the disability is slight and can be accepted without treatment. In others it is desirable to correct the deformity by refracturing or dividing the bone and, after correction has been gained, fixing the fragments by the appropriate means (Fig. 63).

SHORTENING

Shortening of a bone after fracture may arise from three causes (Figs. 64–66): 1) mal-union, the fragments being united with overlap or with marked angulation; 2) crushing or actual loss of bone, as in severely comminuted compression fractures or in gun-shot wounds when a piece of bone is shot away; and 3) in children, interference with the growing epiphysial cartilage. As a rule epiphysial growth is more likely to be impaired by a crushing injury involving the epiphysial plate than by an avulsion injury with fracture-separation of the epiphysis.

Shortening is important only in the lower limb. Shortening of up to two centimetres is not significant and is hardly noticed. If it is more than two centimetres it should be corrected by appropriate raising of the shoe, or occasionally by a leg shortening operation on the longer side. Uncorrected shortening may cause aching in the back from tilting of the pelvis and consequent scoliosis.

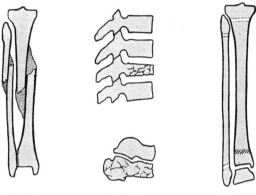

Fig. 64   Fig. 65   Fig. 66

Three causes of bone shortening after a fracture. Figure 64—Mal-union (with overlap or angulation). Figure 65 —Crushing of bone. Figure 66—Arrest of epiphysial growth (in this case affecting the tibia alone).

INJURY TO MAJOR BLOOD VESSELS

Every fracture causes damage to adjacent soft tissues in some degree— especially to muscles, fascia, and minor blood vessels—but in most cases the damage is repaired spontaneously along with the healing of the fracture. Occasionally an important artery is damaged, either by the agent causing the fracture (for instance, a bullet) or by the sharp edge of a bone fragment displaced at the time of the injury or subsequently. This complication may have serious consequences— indeed it may lead to loss of the limb—but fortunately it is uncommon. The vessel may be torn across, it may be contused and occluded by thrombosis, or it may merely be temporarily sealed by spasm. The effect may be: 1) a traumatic aneurysm; or 2) impairment of blood supply in the territory of the damaged vessel with consequent gangrene, ischaemic paralysis of nerves, or ischaemic contracture of muscles. It is important to remember that an equally calamitous vascular occlusion may be caused by an over-tight plaster or bandage, especially in the first two days after an injury or operation, when swelling reaches its peak.

The most important examples of arterial injury complicating fractures are shown in Figure 67.

Treatment. When a limb fracture is complicated by damage to a main blood-vessel the case must be handled as an urgent emergency, because the effects of ischaemia quickly become irreversible. The treatment depends upon whether the occlusion is primary (signs of ischaemia present when the patient is first received) or secondary (ischaemia becoming apparent after reduction and immobilisation of the fracture).

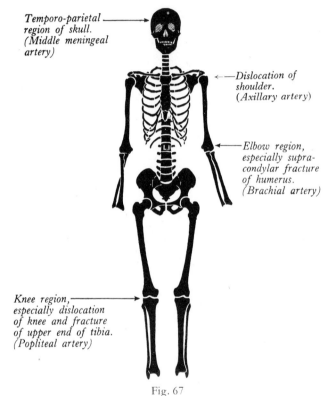

Temporo-parietal region of skull. (Middle meningeal artery)

←—*Dislocation of shoulder. (Axillary artery)*

←——*Elbow region, especially supra-condylar fracture of humerus. (Brachial artery)*

Knee region, especially dislocation of knee and fracture of upper end of tibia. (Popliteal artery)

Fig. 67

Some sites at which fractures are liable to be complicated by damage to important blood vessels. (The skull injury is included only for completeness; its treatment falls within the sphere of the neurosurgeon.)

If the arterial injury is evident when the patient is first received it must be assumed that the vessel has been occluded by direct injury. The following action must be taken *First step:* Any external splint or bandage that might be causing constriction is removed, and gross displacement of the fragments, if not already reduced, is corrected so far as possible by gentle manipulation. If these measures fail to bring about a return of adequate circulation within half an hour the next step is taken. *Second step:* At operation the damaged artery is exposed and the nature of the injury determined. If the occlusion is due to kinking or spasm of the artery an attempt is made to relieve it by freeing the vessel and painting the adventitia with a solution of papaverine. If the vessel is found to be divided or punctured it may be possible to restore patency by direct suture of the freshened ends, and when there is extensive occlusion by thrombosis this may be combined with endarterectomy. Or it may be practicable to excise the damaged segment and to effect repair with a vein graft. When the artery has been dealt with the fracture should usually be fixed internally to prevent the possibility of further vascular damage from recurrent displacement.

If vascular occlusion becomes evident only after the fracture has been reduced and immobilised in plaster arterial spasm is the probable cause. No time should be lost before splitting the plaster and the underlying dressings *throughout their length*, and opening up the plaster thoroughly right down to the skin. If this fails to restore the circulation within half an hour the affected artery should be explored and dealt with as outlined above.

INJURY TO NERVES

Peripheral nerves are injured by fractures much more often than major arteries. Well recognised sites at which a nerve is liable to be damaged are shown in Figure 68.

Nerve injuries were classified by Seddon (1942) into three types— neurapraxia, axonotmesis, and neurotmesis. In *neurapraxia* the damage is slight and it causes only a transient physiological block. Recovery occurs spontaneously within a few weeks. In *axonotmesis* the internal architecture of the nerve is preserved, but the axons are so badly damaged that peripheral degeneration occurs. Recovery can occur spontaneously, but it depends upon regeneration of the axons and may take many months (two or three centimetres a month is the usual speed of regeneration). In *neurotmesis* the structure of the nerve is destroyed by actual division or by severe scarring. Recovery is possible only after excision of the damaged section, with end-to-end suture of the stumps or bridging by a nerve graft (Seddon 1976).

In closed injuries the nerve is usually contused by the sharp edge of a bone fragment but retains its continuity. The lesion may be a neurapraxia or an axonotmesis, and spontaneous recovery is to be

References and bibliography, page 291.

expected. Occasionally the nerve is severed (neurotmesis). In open fractures—especially those caused by penetrating injuries—the nerve is more often severed by the agent causing the fracture than by the bone edge itself.

Treatment. In closed injuries it may usually be assumed that the nerve is in continuity, and spontaneous recovery may be awaited with

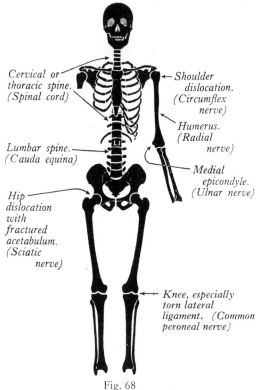

Fig. 68

The sites at which fractures or dislocations are most commonly complicated by nerve injuries.

reasonable confidence. If the first signs of recovery are not observed within the expected time (calculated from the site of injury and length to be regenerated, on the assumption that a regenerating nerve fibre will grow at the rate of two or three centimetres a month) exploration is advised so that, if the nerve is found divided or badly scarred, it may be repaired.

In open fractures caused by a transfixion or piercing injury it should be assumed that the nerve is severed. The wound should be explored and the nerve identified. If it is severed, the ends should be tacked together lightly with one or two sutures but definitive repair of the nerve should be postponed until the wound is healed. (The divided ends are seldom sufficiently cleanly cut to permit primary repair.) The best time for secondary nerve repair is three or four weeks after the injury. At that time the extent of the scarring, and consequently the length of nerve to be resected, can be determined accurately, and thickening of the nerve sheath makes suture technically easier.

The treatment of injuries of the spinal cord and cauda equina is considered on page 106.

INJURY TO VISCERA
Like arteries and nerves, viscera may be damaged either by the agent causing the fracture or by impalement upon a sharp fragment of bone. Examples are: laceration of pleura or lung complicating fractures of the ribs; and rupture of the bladder or urethra, or penetration of the colon or rectum, complicating fractures of the pelvis.

Treatment. The treatment of visceral injuries complicating fractures should follow general surgical principles. Because of the risk to life that attends such injuries, their treatment must take precedence over the treatment of the fracture.

INJURY TO TENDONS
In open fractures tendons may be severed by the agent causing the fracture. Treatment is by surgical reconstruction. Delayed rupture of the tendon of extensor pollicis longus is a well known complication of fracture of the lower end of the radius (p. 167).

INJURIES TO JOINTS
Acute joint injuries such as dislocation, subluxation, or ligamentous strain are common complications of fractures. These injuries will be considered separately in Chapter 6.

INTRA-ARTICULAR AND PERI-ARTICULAR ADHESIONS
Joint stiffness from adhesions is common after fractures, especially those that are near a joint. Some joints are much more vulnerable in this respect than others. Thus the knee, the elbow, and the finger joints stiffen easily and often suffer permanent impairment, whereas the hip and the wrist usually regain their full mobility without difficulty.

Intra-articular adhesions occur chiefly after a fracture that has involved the articular surface of a bone. Blood is poured out into the joint (haemarthrosis), and although such an effusion can be absorbed completely without causing ill effect, it may leave residual strands of fibrin which later become organised into fibrous adhesions between opposing folds of synovial membrane.

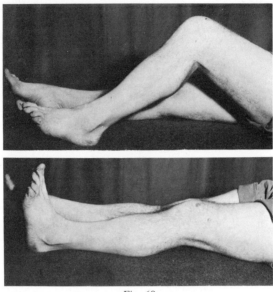

Fig. 69

Impaired range of knee movement six months after a fracture of the shaft of the femur. Stiffness is caused more often by peri-articular and intramuscular adhesions, or by adhesion of muscle to the underlying bone, than by adhesions within the joint itself.

Peri-articular changes are a more frequent cause of joint stiffness than intra-articular adhesions (Fig. 69). In consequence of the injury itself, and of possibly prolonged immobilisation, oedema fluid collects in the tissues, binding together the connective tissue fibres. This leads to loss of resilience of the peri-articular tissues such as joint capsule and ligaments, and in the case of muscles it impairs the free gliding of the fibres one upon another. A further common factor in the causation of stiffness is direct adhesion of muscle to the underlying bone at the site of fracture.

Treatment. Joint stiffness from the causes mentioned will nearly always respond well to active exercises, preferably carried out under the supervision of a physiotherapist. The exercises may have to be continued for a long time—even for a year or more—before the greatest restoration of movement is gained.

Manipulation. In the occasional case in which steady improvement is not being gained by exercises and active use, manipulation under anaesthesia may be considered. In general, manipulation is more likely to be successful in overcoming stiffness from intra-articular adhesions (that is, after direct injury or operation upon the joint) than in cases of peri-articular or muscular rigidity. Manipulation should seldom be recommended until active exercises have had a thorough trial for at least two months, and usually longer.

Caution. Manipulation for joint stiffness should be carried out with extreme care. A bone may easily be fractured if excessive force is used, especially in an elderly patient. The patella in particular is easily broken during manipulation for stiffness of the knee, and the humerus during manipulation of the shoulder. Great force should never be used: it is better to gain slight improvement by repeated gentle manipulation than to rely upon a single forcible movement.

Operation. Rarely, joint stiffness is so severe and so resistant to prolonged conservative treatment that an attempt to free the joint by operation may have to be considered. This applies particularly to intractable stiffness of the knee from adhesions in and about the quadriceps muscle after fracture of the shaft of the femur (p. 226).

POST-TRAUMATIC OSSIFICATION

Post-traumatic ossification—sometimes called myositis ossificans[1]— is a rare cause of joint stiffness after a fracture or dislocation. It occurs only in cases of severe injury to a joint, and especially when the capsule and periosteum have been stripped from the bones by violent displacement of the fragments. Blood collects under the stripped soft tissues, forming a large haematoma about the joint. Instead of being absorbed, the haematoma is invaded by osteoblasts and becomes ossified (Fig. 70). If a large mass of bone is formed the restriction of joint movement may be severe.

This complication is encountered most commonly in the elbow after fracture-dislocation. There is a greater risk of its occurrence in children than in adults because in children the periosteum is only loosely attached to the long bones and is easily stripped from them. There is also a relatively high incidence in patients with prolonged or permanent brain damage from head injury, and in patients' with paraplegia from spinal injuries.

[1] The use of the term myositis ossificans to denote post-traumatic ossification about a joint should be avoided. Ossification occurs deep to the muscles and is not associated with an inflammatory lesion of the muscles, as the name implies.

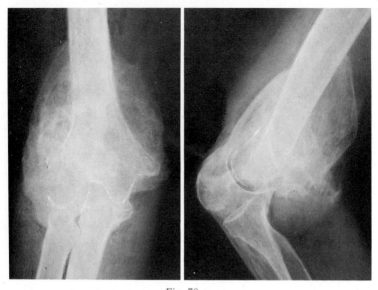

Fig. 70

Post-traumatic ossification about the elbow after a severe fracture-dislocation. The ossification has occurred in the haematoma beneath the stripped-up periosteum and capsule.

Treatment. After a severe injury of a joint—and especially of the elbow in children—the risk of the formation of a large haematoma should be minimised by enforcing complete rest for the joint, preferably in a plaster, for three or four weeks. In an established case of para-articular ossification with limitation of joint movement treatment at first should consist only of gentle active exercises, with avoidance of strains that might provoke further bleeding beneath the soft tissues. After several months it may be justifiable to excise a mass of bone that is blocking movement, but the operation is not always successful and it must be approached with caution. In joint stiffness from this cause manipulation is likely to do more harm than good and it should be avoided.

SUDECK'S POST-TRAUMATIC OSTEODYSTROPHY
(Sudeck's atrophy)

Sudeck's osteodystrophy,[1] atrophy, or post-traumatic painful osteoporosis, is an occasional cause of prolonged disability after fractures

---

[1] Paul Hermann Sudeck, a German surgeon, described a type of acute bone atrophy in 1900. In fact, however, he was referring to acute inflammatory bone atrophy rather than to post-traumatic atrophy.

or other injuries of the limbs. It is characterised by pain, swelling, and marked joint stiffness in the hand or foot of the injured limb. The cause and the exact nature of the condition are unknown. Some surgeons believe that it is no more than an exaggerated form of the bone atrophy or osteoporosis that accompanies disuse, but most regard it as a distinct entity.

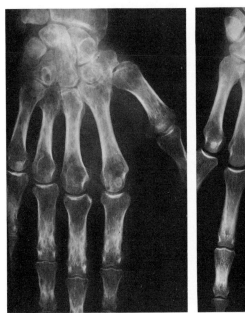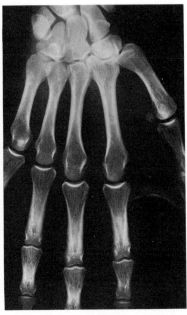

Fig. 71   Fig. 72

Figure 71—Sudeck's atrophy affecting the hand after a Colles's fracture. A normal hand is shown for comparison (Fig. 72). The osteoporosis comes on more rapidly and is more extreme than the osteoporosis of disuse, and the bone changes are accompanied by oedema, glazing of the skin, and marked stiffness of the joints.

The symptoms are noticed about two months after the injury, or when the plaster is removed. The function of the limb is not regained as it should be with active use and exercises. Instead, the patient complains of severe pain in the affected hand or foot when he attempts to use it. On examination the extremity is swollen and hyperaemic. The skin creases are obliterated, giving the surface a glossy appearance. The nails and the hair of the hand or foot are atrophic. The palmar aponeurosis may be thickened. Joint movements are severely impaired, especially the metacarpo-phalangeal and interphalangeal joints in the case of the hand ('frozen hand'). Radiographs show spotty osteoporosis, often of severe degree (Figs. 71–72).

Diagnosis. Sudeck's atrophy has features that distinguish it from the osteoporosis that is commonly seen in limbs immobilised for a long time. In particular, the marked swelling, the glossy stretched appearance of the skin, and the marked stiffness of the joints, are characteristic. In addition, the rarefaction of the bones—often with a spotty texture—is more extreme.

Treatment. Most cases respond slowly but surely to efficient conservative treatment. The mainstay of treatment is active exercise, with active use of the limb so far as the pain will allow. These measures may be aided by periods of elevation and local heat in the form of paraffin wax baths. Much patience and encouragement are required, and the patient should be under the care of a skilled physiotherapist. With conservative treatment on these lines adequate recovery is usually gained in two to four months.

In obstinate cases success has been claimed for repeated sympathetic block or for permanent sympathetic denervation by ganglionectomy.

OSTEOARTHRITIS
(Osteoarthrosis[1])

Any roughening or irregularity of a joint surface will accelerate the wear-and-tear changes that form the basis of osteoarthritis. Osteoarthritis, therefore, is likely to develop sooner or later after any displaced fracture which involves an articular surface unless the fragments can be replaced so perfectly in position that the smooth contour of the joint surface is unimpaired (Figs. 73–74). Even a slight step between the fragments may lead to serious subsequent disability from arthritis, especially in a weight-bearing joint.

Avascular necrosis as a cause of severe osteoarthritis or of total disorganisation of a joint was mentioned on page 57.

In fractures that do not directly involve a joint surface there is a risk of later osteoarthritis if the fragments unite with angular deformity, throwing the joint out of its correct alignment, because mal-alignment of joint surfaces causes excessive stress at one part of the joint and consequently accelerates wear-and-tear changes. An example of osteoarthritis developing in these circumstances is osteoarthritis of the knee due to bow-leg deformity after a mal-united fracture of the femoral shaft (Figs. 75–76).

---

[1] The term *arthrosis* is sometimes used to denote a degenerative lesion of a joint, but without valid etymological grounds. Ever since the Greek era *arthritis* has had the connotation 'disease of a joint'. In Greek the word meant simply 'of the joint', νοσος (disease) being understood or sometimes stated. The suffix '-itis' was similarly added to other parts of the body to imply disease of that part. Only more recently has '-itis' been misapplied to denote inflammatory disease. It is therefore still correct to use 'arthritis' as a generic term to cover all types of joint disease, including degenerative disease. The suffix '-osis', also derived from the Greek, had a meaning quite unrelated to disease. It implied a process or activity, as in hypnosis or metamorphosis. Its use to imply degenerative disease is a comparatively recent extension which cannot be justified etymologically.

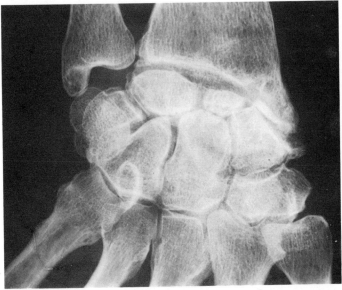

Fig. 73

Osteoarthritis of the wrist complicating an ununited fracture of the scaphoid bone. Note the spurring of the margins of the radio-scaphoid joint, and narrowing of articular cartilage.

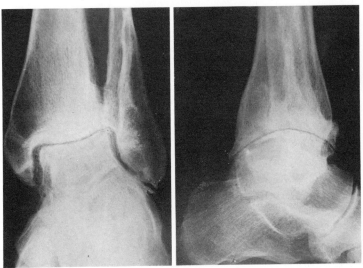

Fig. 74

Osteoarthritis of the ankle after a fracture-subluxation with incongruity of the joint surfaces. Note the marked narrowing of the joint space, indicating loss of articular cartilage.

As would be expected, the risk of osteoarthritis after a fracture varies according to the severity of the residual damage to the joint, and it is much greater in the weight-bearing joints of the lower limb than in the relatively lightly stressed joints of the upper limb.

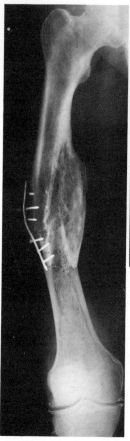

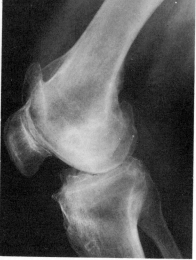

Fig. 76

Figure 75—Old fracture of femoral shaft which united with excessive lateral bowing. (The old-time plate and screws were evidently of unsuitable metal, for they have partly disintegrated.) Figure 76—Corresponding knee of the same patient twenty years after the fracture, showing advanced osteoarthritis. There is always a liability to osteoarthritis when the line of weight transmission through a hinge joint is shifted laterally or medially.

Fig. 75

The interval between the fracture and the development of osteoarthritis also varies widely. After severe damage to a joint osteoarthritis may become clinically evident within six or nine months of the injury, whereas in cases of slight damage or malalignment it may not become apparent for fifteen or twenty years or more.

FAT EMBOLISM

Fat embolism, though uncommon, is one of the most serious complications of fractures, and despite recent improvements in management it is still often fatal. The essential feature is occlusion of small blood vessels by fat globules.[1]

Pathology. Occlusion of small vessels has its most significant effects in the lungs and in the brain. In the lungs there are oedema and haemorrhages in the alveoli, so that transfer of oxygen from alveoli to arterioles is impaired. This leads to hypoxaemia, which may be severe. In the brain there may be multiple petechial haemorrhages. Petechial haemorrhages occur also in other organs and in the skin.

Clinical features. Fat embolism occurs mainly after severe fractures in the lower limbs, particularly those of the femur and tibia. The onset is usually within two days of injury, but it is notable that there is a symptom-free period between injury and onset—an important point of distinction from cerebral contusion. The presenting feature is usually cerebral disturbance in the form of marked restlessness, confusion, drowsiness or coma. These cerebral symptoms may be caused partly by petechial haemorrhages in the brain, but in large measure they are probably secondary to hypoxia from occlusion of small vessels in the lungs. Associated features are tachypnoea and dyspnoea. The other common clinical manifestation is a petechial rash, usually on the front of the neck, anterior axillary folds or chest, or in the conjunctivae. The finding of such a rash strongly supports a diagnosis of fat embolism. *Investigations:* The most useful investigation is arterial blood gas analysis. This may show reduction of the partial pressure of oxygen in the blood (PO_2) well below the normal 100 millimetres of mercury and often below the critical level of 60 millimetres of mercury at which respiratory failure is likely.

Treatment. Fat embolism is spontaneously reversible if the patient can be tided over the dangerous period of hypoxia. This may usually be corrected by the administration of 100 per cent oxygen, if necessary with positive pressure respiration. The oxygen requirement should be controlled by repeated blood gas analysis.

---

[1] There is histological evidence that fat embolism occurs in minor degree very commonly after fractures: usually it does not cause symptoms. Here the term fat embolism is used only for those cases in which clinical features are evident, presumably from small vessel occlusion on a massive scale.

References and bibliography, page 291.

CHAPTER 5

Special features of fractures in children

It has been mentioned already that in some respects fractures behave differently in children and in adults. The differences are mostly not fundamental but are rather differences of degree.

PATHOLOGY

The most obvious difference between the bones of children and those of adults is the presence in childhood of cartilaginous growth plates at each end of the major long bones but usually at only one end of the 'short' long bones (metacarpals and metatarsals). Here it may be recalled that the greater proportion of the growth of the bone, and later closure of the growth plate, occurs in the humerus at the proximal end, in the radius and ulna at the distal end, in the femur at the distal end, and in the tibia and fibula at the proximal end. In other words, the most growth occurs 'away from the elbow and towards the knee'.

The growth plate is a potentially weak point in the bone, and at certain sites the epiphysis may be avulsed, usually taking with it a fragment of the metaphysis. A further important point about the cartilaginous plate is that in certain types of fracture growth at the plate may be arrested.

In childhood the long bones also differ from the adult state in that they are more resilient and springy, withstanding greater deflection without fracture. This accounts for the frequency—in young children a predominance—of incomplete fractures of the greenstick type (p. 5). Such fractures do not occur in adults.

Another striking feature of children's bones is that the periosteum is attached only loosely to the diaphysis, and in consequence it is easily stripped from the bone over a considerable part of its length by blood collecting beneath it. This subperiosteal haematoma is soon replaced by callus, which therefore is often seen to extend a long way up and down the shaft, even when there has been little displacement of the fragments.

In the matter of sites of fracture, children present similarities to, and differences from, adults. In both children and adults fractures of the lower forearm, of the clavicle, and of the tibia and fibula are among the commonest injuries. But in children, unlike adults, fractures of the scaphoid bone and of the neck and trochanteric region of the femur are uncommon. On the other hand, serious fractures of the elbow region (especially supracondylar fractures and fractures of the capitulum of the humerus) are relatively common, and indeed they present some of the most difficult problems of all childhood injuries.

Healing of childhood fractures is nearly always rapid, and the younger the child the more rapid the healing. In infancy a fracture may be soundly united in two or three weeks. In later childhood the average time required for union gradually increases, and after growth has ceased age has little effect upon the rate of union.

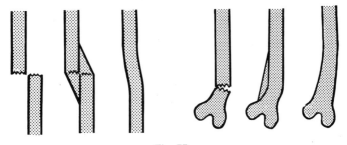

Fig. 77

Although remodelling of bone in a child can efface a fracture completely (*left*), it cannot fully correct tilting of a joint surface (*right*).

Similarly, remodelling is very active and complete in early childhood: so much so that all evidence of a past fracture may be obliterated within a matter of months (Fig. 12, p. 12). It must be remembered, however, that remodelling can never fully restore a joint surface to its normal alignment if it has been tilted sideways by angulation at the site of fracture (Fig. 77).

Injuries of the growth plate. After a fracture of a long bone in a child growth is often accelerated for a time, perhaps from hyperaemia of the epiphysial cartilages; but any consequent discrepancy of length is slight and of no clinical significance (Edvardsen and Syversen 1976). On the other hand, growth may be seriously disturbed if the growth plate (epiphysial cartilage) is damaged in such a way that a bony bridge is formed across the plate between epiphysis and diaphysis, leading to premature epiphysial fusion. If the whole area of the growth plate is fused all growth ceases at that particular site, and the degree of consequent shortening of the bone will depend upon the age at which premature fusion occurs: the younger the patient the greater the eventual shortening. If, however, premature fusion occurs in only a part of the epiphysial plate, further growth will be prevented at that

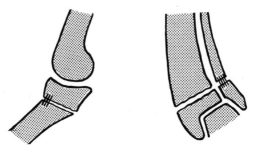

Fig. 78

Premature fusion at one part of the growth plate, with continuation of growth elsewhere, leads to angular deformity. Bowing will also occur if epiphysial arrest occurs in only one bone of a pair (*right*).

point but will continue in the undamaged part of the plate, thus leading to angulation deformity (Fig. 78). Angulation will also occur if there is premature arrest in one bone of a pair, as in the forearm or lower leg. Thus, for instance, if growth is arrested at the lower epiphysis of the fibula but continues in the corresponding epiphysis of the tibia, the ankle region will be bowed into valgus.

In general, fractures that damage the growth plate in such a way as to cause premature fusion tend to be of the crushing type: avulsion injuries are less likely to have this effect.

DIAGNOSIS

Recognition of a fracture may be more difficult in a child than in an adult. As a rule complete fractures do not present any special difficulty, but an incomplete fracture is sometimes overlooked because the more dramatic signs of fracture are often absent. Thus there may be no deformity, no abnormal mobility, no crepitus. Moreover, a history of injury is not always forthcoming, especially in a young child who is unable to speak for himself. Sometimes, indeed, the parents attempt deliberately to conceal the fact that an infant has been injured, especially when there has been ill-treatment ('battered baby syndrome'). Recognition of the true nature of the case may then be difficult, even with the aid of radiographs, for these infantile fractures often affect the metaphysial regions of the long bones, they are often multiple, and they may produce abundant callus: the radiographic appearance may thus be atypical, and confusion may arise with such conditions as scurvy, syphilis, osteomyelitis or bone tumours. Irrespective of the history, the possibility of injury should always be considered when marked loss of function or unwillingness to use a limb is associated with local pain and tenderness.

COMPLICATIONS

Complications of fractures in children are broadly similar to those that occur in adults, though the incidence is different. Failure of union is very unusual in children, except in fractures at one particular site, namely the capitulum of the humerus. In general, other complications are also less frequent than in adults, but two that are important and relatively common require special mention: injury to the brachial artery complicating supracondylar fracture of the humerus, and post-traumatic ossification about the elbow after a displaced fracture or dislocation. This latter complication may lead to severe restriction of movement at the affected joint.

An important complication that is peculiar to children is disturbance of growth after injuries involving the growth plate. The effects of such injuries have already been discussed (p. 75).

References and bibliography, page 291.

CHAPTER 6

Joint injuries

In order of decreasing severity, joint injuries may be classed as dislocation, subluxation, strain, or contusion.

Before these are described individually it is necessary to consider briefly certain aspects of the normal anatomy of a joint.

The stability of joints. Joint surfaces are held in contact by the shape of the articulating surfaces, by the ligaments, by the surrounding muscles, and by atmospheric pressure. The importance of each of these factors varies with different joints. Thus in the hip the deep socket and the almost spherical femoral head in themselves afford great security against displacement, and in the elbow also the shape of the bones makes for reasonable intrinsic stability. On the other hand the joints of the fingers and the knee depend for their stability mainly on the ligaments; and the shoulder depends largely on the surrounding muscles.

The function of ligaments. The purpose of a ligament is to prevent abnormal movement at a joint. For this it does not always depend entirely on its intrinsic strength; it may rely largely upon the action of the supporting muscles, which contract reflexly to protect the ligament when it comes under harmful stress. Some ligaments are better protected by muscles than others. For example, the ligaments of the shoulder, the wrist and the hip are well protected by muscles, whereas the collateral ligaments of the finger joints and of the knee, and the inferior tibio-fibular ligament, are poorly protected. In general, it is found that a ligament that is not well guarded by muscles is intrinsically stronger than one that is well protected.

DISLOCATION AND SUBLUXATION

A joint is dislocated or luxated when its articular surfaces are wholly displaced one from the other, so that all apposition between them is lost (Figs. 81 and 83). A joint is subluxated when its articular surfaces are partly displaced but retain some contact one with the other (Fig. 80).

Dislocation or subluxation of a joint may be congenital, spontaneous (pathological), traumatic, or recurrent. It is only with traumatic and with recurrent dislocation or subluxation that we are concerned here.

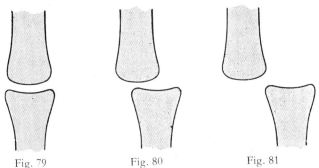

Fig. 79   Fig. 80   Fig. 81

To show the difference between subluxation and dislocation of a joint. Figure 79—The normal state: joint surfaces congruous. Figure 80—Subluxation: incomplete loss of contact between the joint surfaces. Figure 81—Dislocation: total loss of contact between the joint surfaces.

TRAUMATIC DISLOCATION OR SUBLUXATION

Injury is by far the commonest cause of dislocation and subluxation. Any joint may be affected, but those most commonly dislocated are the shoulder, elbow, hip, ankle, and interphalangeal joints. In many cases dislocation or subluxation is associated with a fracture of one or both of the opposing bones: when this occurs the injury is termed a fracture-dislocation or fracture-subluxation.

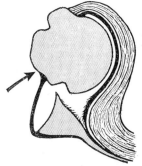

Fig. 82

Intracapsular dislocation of the gleno-humeral joint. The capsule and periosteum have been stripped from the front of the neck of the scapula. This is the typical state of affairs in recurrent dislocation of the shoulder.

Dislocation cannot occur without some damage to the protective ligaments and joint capsule. Usually the capsule and one or more of the reinforcing ligaments are torn, permitting the articular end of one of the bones to escape through the rent. Sometimes the capsule is not torn in its substance but is stripped from one of its bony attachments (Fig. 82). Or, if the ligament withstands the force of the injury, a fragment of bone at one or other attachment of the ligament may be avulsed. It is not always that one of the bone ends protrudes outside the joint capsule: sometimes the joint surfaces may be completely dislocated and yet both remain within the capsule (intracapsular dislocation, Fig. 82).

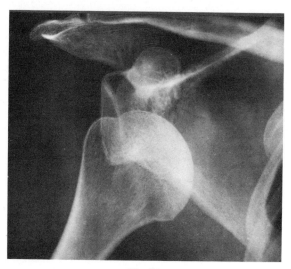

Fig. 83
A typical anterior (subcoracoid) dislocation of the shoulder.

In joints that depend for their stability mainly upon the surrounding muscles, dislocation will occur most easily when the muscles are off their guard. This probably explains the high incidence of shoulder dislocations in patients suffering epileptic fits.

Diagnosis. In most cases of dislocation the clinical features are sufficiently striking to make the diagnosis obvious. Nevertheless it not infrequently happens that a dislocation is overlooked, especially when the bony landmarks are obscured by severe swelling or by obesity. Certain dislocations are more liable to be overlooked than others: posterior dislocation of the shoulder is particularly notorious in this respect (Fig. 25), and rather surprisingly posterior dislocation of the hip is occasionally overlooked when there is a co-existing fracture of the shaft of the femur on the same side (Helal and Skevis 1967).

In doubtful cases the diagnosis must depend finally on adequate radiographic examination. It must be emphasised that radiographs should always be taken in two planes at right angles to one another, because a dislocation may not be apparent in a single projection (Fig. 25, p. 25). When a dislocation has been reduced, further radiographs should always be obtained, in order both to confirm the reduction and to determine whether or not there is an associated fracture.

In cases of subluxation the clinical features alone are seldom diagnostic, and reliance must be placed mainly on the radiographic evidence.

Complications. For the most part the complications that may follow a dislocation are the same as those of a fracture near a joint. They may be summarised as follows: 1) infection (after open dislocation); 2) injury to important soft-tissue structure (artery; nerve); 3) avascular necrosis of one of the articulating bone ends from damage to the vessels supplying it; 4) persistent instability leading to recurrent dislocation or subluxation; 5) joint stiffness from intra-articular or peri-articular adhesions, from Sudeck's atrophy, or from post-traumatic ossification about the joint ('myositis ossificans'); 6) osteoarthritis from damage to the articular cartilage or from persistent incongruity of the joint surfaces.

Treatment. Clearly the first principle of treatment of a dislocation or a subluxation is to reduce the displacement. This is usually achieved by closed manipulation, but sometimes operation may be required.

Treatment of the ligamentous injury. When the displacement has been corrected the next problem is how to deal with the injury of the soft tissues, and especially of the ligaments. In a few instances a ruptured ligament may be best repaired by operation (for example, a complete rupture of the medial ligament of the knee), but in most cases it may safely be allowed to heal spontaneously. In that case the only remaining question is whether the joint should be immobilised during the stage of healing, or whether movement should be allowed.

It has been found that, in general, normal function is restored most rapidly when movement of the injured joint is encouraged from the beginning, or at the latest within a few days of the injury. Accordingly a policy of early mobilisation should be adopted unless special indications for immobilisation exist. Three such indications are: 1) rupture of an important ligament which is largely responsible for the stability of the joint (for example, the conoid and trapezoid ligaments of the acromio-clavicular joint, the medial or lateral ligament of the knee, the lateral ligament of the ankle, and the inferior tibio-fibular ligament); 2) a serious risk of post-traumatic ossification or 'myositis ossificans' (in practice the elbow and possibly the hip are the only joints that need be immobilised on this account); and 3) severe pain.

Treatment of fracture-dislocations. When a dislocation or subluxation is associated with a fracture the principles of treatment are to reduce the joint displacement first, and then to deal with the fracture on its merits.

RECURRENT DISLOCATION OR SUBLUXATION

Certain joints are liable to repeated dislocation or subluxation. Usually, but not always, there has been an initial violent dislocation which leaves the ligaments or the articular surfaces permanently damaged. The joints most often affected are the shoulder (p. 123), the sterno-clavicular joint (p. 117), the patello-femoral joint (p. 234), and the ankle (p. 270).

STRAIN

A strain is an incomplete rupture of a ligament. It may be acute or chronic.[1] An acute strain is caused by sudden injury, and there is usually macroscopic damage to the ligament. A chronic strain is

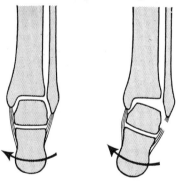

Fig. 84

Doubt about the integrity of a ligament is best resolved by radiographing the joint while the ligament is held under stress by manual force. If the joint space is not shown to be widened on the affected side the ligament is intact (*left*). Marked widening of the joint space with tilting of the joint surfaces away from one another indicates that the ligament is torn (*right*).

caused by long-continued stress (for example, foot-strain from prolonged standing), and the changes in the ligament are usually microscopic. We are concerned here only with acute strains.

The force that causes an acute strain is intermediate between one that the ligament can withstand without suffering injury and one that

[1] No sharp distinction is made here between a *strain* and a *sprain*. The term *strain* is preferred, because in technical language it has the meaning that we wish to express—namely structural damage resulting from excessive stress; whereas *sprain* is often used in a lay sense without a precise meaning. Some surgeons, however, restrict the term *strain* to a chronic strain caused by long-continued stress, and use the term *sprain* to denote an acute ligamentous injury.

is great enough to rupture the ligament completely. A strain of a ligament that is well protected by muscles may occur either because the force is too great for the muscles to withstand, or because the muscles are caught off their guard.

Clinical features. There is a history of injury such as would impose a stretching force upon the ligament involved. There are local pain and tenderness, with moderate swelling and sometimes a visible ecchymosis. Pain is aggravated when the joint is moved in a direction that tenses the injured ligament.

Diagnosis. Although a strain may be diagnosed with reasonable confidence from the clinical features, radiographs should always be obtained to exclude a fracture or subluxation. In distinguishing between a simple strain and a complete rupture of a ligament a reliable method is to obtain radiographs while stress is applied to the joint in the direction of the original force, the patient being anaesthetised if necessary. If the ligament is only strained the joint will remain stable, but if the ligament is torn it will be possible to subluxate the joint, separating the articular surfaces widely on the side of the injury (Figs. 84 and 247).

Treatment. The treatment of a strain depends upon the ligament affected and upon the severity of the pain and disability. As after a dislocation, the general principle should be to encourage early activity and to avoid cumbersome external splintage so far as possible. If pain and swelling are severe it may be wise to immobilise the joint in plaster for the sake of comfort, but immobilisation need never be prolonged for more than two or three weeks.

CONTUSION

Contusion of a joint may involve the capsule, the synovial membrane, and occasionally the articular cartilage. The injury sets up a local inflammatory reaction with swelling and serous exudate. *Clinically* there is a history of a direct blow over the joint. There are swelling and local tenderness on palpation. There may be an effusion of fluid in the joint, with slight restriction of movement. Radiographs should always be obtained to exclude the possibility of fracture. Healing occurs spontaneously and only symptomatic treatment is required.

Occasionally, severe contusion of articular cartilage, especially of the hip or of the metatarso-phalangeal joint of the big toe, has been followed after an interval of months or years by the development of osteoarthritis in the same joint, and a causal relationship must be accepted as probable.

References and bibliography, page 291.

CHAPTER 7

Cervical spine

Vertebral injuries are seen less commonly in the cervical spine than in the thoracic and lumbar regions. On the other hand they are often more serious, not only on account of a greater risk of injury to the spinal cord, but also because there is a greater liability to persistent disability from aching pain and stiffness of the neck. Moreover there is an increasing incidence of subluxations and strains in this area caused by sudden recoil of the head in rear-end automobile collisions—the so-called whip-lash injury. In most cases the effects are relatively minor from a structural point of view, but disability may nevertheless be prolonged.

In many cases violent injuries of the cervical spine cause death so quickly that the patient never reaches the surgeon; thus the cases seen clinically do not reflect the true total incidence of cervical spine injuries.

Classification
Injuries of the cervical spine may be classified as follows.
  Wedge compression fracture of vertebral body
  Burst fracture of vertebral body
  Extension subluxation
  Flexion subluxation
  Dislocation and fracture-dislocation
  Fracture of the atlas
  Fracture-dislocation of the atlanto-axial joint
  Intra-spinal displacement of soft tissue
  Fracture of spinous process

Diagnosis
Cervical injuries are often associated with head injuries, the effects of which may mask the spinal lesion and cause it to be overlooked. It thus behoves the surgeon to take careful note of the condition of the neck (preferably with the help of good radiographs) in every case of serious head injury. This point needs special emphasis.

Radiography. Much care is needed in the interpretation of radiographs of the neck. This is often difficult because the cervical vertebrae are so irregular in shape, and the shadows of their various processes may be confusing when superimposed. For this reason it is seldom sufficient to rely only upon antero-posterior and lateral radiographs: additional projections are required. Firstly, lateral radiographs with the head flexed and with the head extended may reveal instability that is not shown in the routine lateral film. Secondly, oblique views at 45 degrees are especially helpful in demonstrating the intervertebral foramina and the articular processes: they should be taken both from half-right and from half-left because it is not uncommon for subluxation or dislocation of a lateral intervertebral joint to occur on one side only. Thirdly, a special projection through the open mouth is used to obtain an antero-posterior radiograph of the atlas and axis. Finally, if doubt still exists, cineradiography with the image intensifier may be decisive.

Mechanism of injury

Major injuries of the cervical spine are usually caused by indirect violence, such as falls on to the head or other violent movements transmitted from the skull. The mechanism may be an excessive movement in any direction—flexion, extension, lateral flexion, or rotation—or a vertical compression force acting upon a straight spine; and the nature of the injury bears a fairly constant relationship to the mechanism of its causation (Roaf 1960). It should be appreciated, however, that many injuries are caused by a combination of forces rather than by violence acting in a single direction.

Flexion and flexion-rotation injuries are common: flexion alone tends to cause a wedge compression fracture (Fig. 85), whereas combined flexion and rotation causes subluxation (Fig. 86), dislocation (Fig. 87), or fracture-dislocation. A flexion or flexion-rotation force may also cause massive displacement of an intervertebral disc, without bone injury (Fig. 98).

A hyperextension force may fracture the neural arch, especially of the atlas or axis, or it may fracture the dens [odontoid process] of the axis. Alternatively, hyperextension may rupture the anterior longitudinal ligament and the annulus fibrosus, forcing the vertebral bodies apart anteriorly (extension subluxation) (Fig. 89). Hyperextension of an osteoarthritic cervical spine, in which the spinal canal is already narrowed by osteophytes, may lead to damage to the spinal cord through impingement upon it of infolded pieces of the tough ligamentum flavum (Fig. 99).

Vertical compression acting through the skull may cause a fracture of the atlas (Fig. 96) or a 'burst' fracture of a vertebral body (Fig. 88).

References and bibliography, page 291.

Stable and unstable injuries

Nicoll (1962) and Holdsworth (1970) have emphasised the importance of distinguishing fractures and dislocations that are stable by virtue of intact posterior ligaments from those that are unstable because the posterior ligaments have been torn, usually by a rotation force. A stable fracture or dislocation is not liable to displacement greater than that caused at the time of the injury, whereas an unstable fracture or dislocation is liable to further displacement, with grave peril to the spinal cord. It follows that external splintage or internal fixation may be unnecessary for stable injuries whereas it is essential for unstable injuries.

WEDGE COMPRESSION FRACTURE OF VERTEBRAL BODY

A severe flexion force may crush the cancellous bone of one or more of the vertebral bodies (Fig. 85). The compression is always most marked at the front of the vertebral body, which consequently

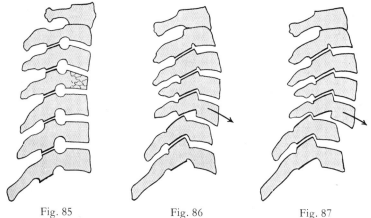

Fig. 85   Fig. 86   Fig. 87

Flexion and flexion-rotation injuries. Figure 85—Wedge compression fracture of a cervical vertebral body. Figure 86—Subluxation of the cervical spine at C. 5–6. The articular processes remain in contact over a small area. Displacement is often confined to one side. Reduction is possible simply by extending the spine. Figure 87—Dislocation of the cervical spine. The articular processes are interlocked. Manipulative reduction is impossible unless the articular processes are first disengaged by powerful traction.

becomes wedge-shaped. The posterior ligaments are intact; so the fracture is stable. This injury is not likely to be complicated by injury to the spinal cord.

Treatment. It is unnecessary to attempt reduction, and all that is required is to support the neck for two months in order to relieve pain. This may be achieved either by a collar of plaster of Paris extending from the chin to the mid-sternum, or by a plastic collar (usually of polythene) (Fig. 91), which has the advantage over plaster that it may be removed for washing and shaving. When the collar is discarded a course of mobilising and muscle-strengthening exercises should be arranged.

BURST FRACTURE OF VERTEBRAL BODY

A 'burst' fracture may be regarded as a variant of the wedge compression fracture. It is caused by a vertical compression force transmitted directly along the line of the vertebral bodies while the cervical spine is straight, whereas a wedge compression fracture is a consequence of similar violence acting upon a flexed spinal column. The force ruptures one of the vertebral end plates and the intervertebral disc is forced into the body of the

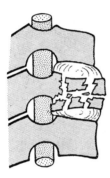

Fig. 88
Burst fracture of vertebral body caused by a vertical force acting upon a straight cervical column.

vertebra. The effect is to produce a comminuted compression fracture, the fragments of which appear to have burst out peripherally in all directions (Fig. 88). The spinal cord may escape injury, but often it is damaged by posterior fragments of the vertebral body which may be driven back into it. The burst fracture is thus more dangerous than the simple wedge compression fracture. But like the wedge compression fracture it is stable against further displacement because the ligaments are intact. It is uncommon.

Treatment. Provided there is no injury to the spinal cord treatment is simple. Reduction is not necessary, and external support is required only to relieve pain. It may be provided by a well fitted collar of plaster or of polythene (Fig. 91), as described for wedge compression fracture.

The management of patients with injury to the spinal cord is described in Chapter 9 (p. 106). Whenever possible, such injuries should be treated at a specially equipped centre for paraplegics.

EXTENSION SUBLUXATION

In this injury the anterior longitudinal ligament is ruptured by a severe extension force and the vertebral bodies are forced apart anteriorly (Fig. 89) (Barnes 1948; Taylor and Blackwood 1948). The spinal cord may or may not escape injury. The spine is unstable in extension but is stable while the neck is in the neutral position or in flexion.

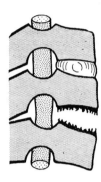

Fig. 89

Extension subluxation. The anterior longitudinal ligament is ruptured.

Treatment. The neck must be supported in the neutral position or in slight flexion, preferably by a plaster collar which should be retained for at least two months.

FLEXION SUBLUXATION

In flexion subluxation of the cervical spine there is forward displacement of one vertebra upon another, but the displacement is not sufficient to cause total overriding of the articular processes (Figs. 86 and 90). Often there is a rotational element in the causative violence, with the consequence that partial overriding of the articular processes occurs on one side only (Beatson 1963). The injury usually occurs in the lower half of the cervical column. Clinically, there is severe pain and the patient is unwilling to move the neck. Radiographs should confirm the diagnosis, but when the head is held erect the displacement may be corrected spontaneously, and the injury may be overlooked unless radiographs are taken with the spine flexed (Figs. 92 and 93). Since the posterior ligaments are damaged the injury must be regarded as unstable.

In cases of subluxation the spinal cord usually escapes serious injury, but if the spine is osteoarthritic even slight subluxation may be dangerous, for the spinal canal may already be narrowed by osteophytes.

Treatment. It is necessary first to reduce the subluxation by

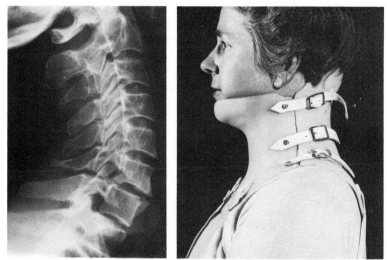

Fig. 90   Fig. 91

Figure 90—Persistent subluxation between sixth and seventh cervical vertebrae after an old injury. A buttress of new bone has formed in front of the body of C. 7. The spinal cord was not injured. Figure 91—Polythene collar as used for minor compression fractures and stable subluxations of the cervical spine.

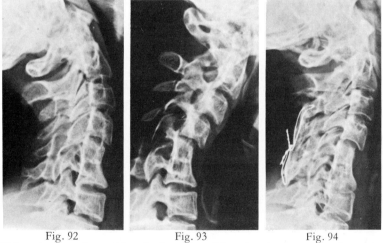

Fig. 92   Fig. 93   Fig. 94

This patient's neck was injured when a box fell on her head. Initial radiographs taken with the head erect (Fig. 92) did not show any vertebral displacement, though they did reveal a congenital anomaly in the form of fusion of the fifth and sixth vertebrae. Only when a lateral radiograph was taken with the neck flexed was forward subluxation of the fourth vertebra upon the fifth shown (Fig. 93). Because of persistent instability posterior vertebral fusion by bone grafts was undertaken (Fig. 94).

extending the cervical spine, and thereafter to prevent redisplacement by holding the neck extended, preferably in a plaster collar moulded well down over the sternum. The plaster should be worn for two months. The spine often becomes stabilised spontaneously by the formation of a buttress of bone anteriorly (Fig. 90). If follow-up radiographs show that the cervical spine continues to subluxate in flexion local fusion of the affected vertebrae should be advised (Fig. 94).

DISLOCATION AND FRACTURE-DISLOCATION

The articular surfaces are out of contact and there is overriding of the articular processes (Fig. 87). There may be associated compression fractures of the vertebral bodies or a fracture of the neural arch. This is a very unstable injury.

Damage to the spinal cord—often complete transection but sometimes an incomplete lesion—is a common complication of this injury. Nevertheless it is surprising what severe displacement may sometimes occur without injury to the spinal cord.

Treatment. Careful handling is necessary lest further displacement cause or aggravate an injury of the spinal cord. Reduction is best effected by skull traction under radiographic control. Traction is applied through skull calipers, the tips of which engage in small holes made low in each parietal region (Fig. 95). With this method traction of up to twenty pounds can be maintained without much discomfort to the patient, and this is often sufficient to disengage the overriding articular processes within a few hours. While this heavy traction is being applied it is important that a close watch be kept on the patient's neurological state, because it is possible to damage the spinal cord or the medulla by injudicious traction on an injured spine. When radiographs confirm that the articular processes have been disengaged reduction is completed by gradually extending the cervical spine. Light traction is then maintained. In the absence of paraplegia a well moulded collar of plaster-of-Paris or of polyethylene (Fig. 91) may be applied within a few days if the reduction is considered stable; but if there seems any risk of redisplacement it is better to continue with traction for three weeks before the collar is applied. The patient is then allowed up, and the subsequent treatment is like that of uncomplicated compression fracture.

Indications for operation. Operation may be required for: 1) irreducible locking of articular processes; and 2) persistent instability.

Irreducible locking of articular processes. If interlocked articular processes cannot be disengaged by traction, operative excision of the processes obstructing reduction may be necessary. This is most likely to be the case when attempted reduction has been delayed for more than a week. Operative reduction should be followed by fusion of the affected segments of the spine by means of bone grafts.

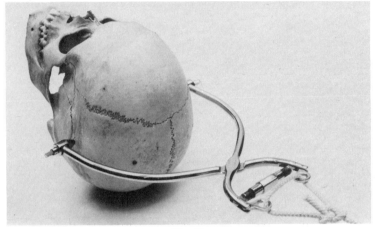

Fig. 95
Cone's (Barton's) traction calipers applied to a skull to
show the position of insertion of the points.

Persistent instability. If gradual redisplacement occurs after initial reduction and immobilisation it may be advisable to stabilise the affected region of the spine by operative fusion. The operation entails the placing of bone grafts to bridge the joint below the displaced vertebra. In posterior fusion the grafts are placed between the spinous processes and laminae: at the same time the spinous processes are wired together with stout stainless-steel wire to ensure fixation while the bone grafts become incorporated (Fig. 94). Alternatively, fusion may be secured anteriorly by laying a bone graft in a deep slot cut in the front of the bodies of the affected vertebrae.

Because of the frequency of late redisplacement after conservative treatment for cervical dislocations and fracture-dislocations, local fusion of the spine is advised more freely now than it was in the past. In fact it is becoming accepted that early local fusion should be advised in almost every case of major displacement as a safeguard against recurrence of the deformity with its risk to the spinal cord.

Spinal cord injury. The management of patients with tetraplegia or paraplegia is considered separately in Chapter 9 (p. 106).

FRACTURE OF THE ATLAS

The atlas may be fractured by a vertical force acting through the skull, the bony ring formed by the anterior arch and the posterior arch of the atlas being forced open by the impact of the occipital condyles (Fig. 96) (Jefferson 1920; Grogono 1954). It corresponds to the burst fracture

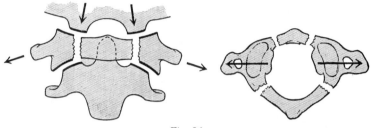

Fig. 96
Fracture of the atlas caused by a vertical compression force.

already described for the lower cervical vertebrae (p. 87). Displacement is seldom severe, and more often than not the spinal cord escapes serious injury.

Treatment. In the absence of injury to the spinal cord it is sufficient to support the injured region for three months by a plaster or plastic collar (Fig. 91).

FRACTURE-DISLOCATION OF THE ATLANTO-AXIAL JOINT
(Fracture of the dens of the axis)

The normal atlanto-axial joint depends for its stability upon the snug fit of the anterior arch and the transverse ligament of the atlas over the dens [odontoid process] of the axis. This stability may be lost if the transverse ligament is defective or if the dens is fractured. Forward displacement of the atlas from inflammatory softening of the transverse ligament is well recognised in cases of infection involving the throat or neck, but traumatic rupture of the ligament is seldom seen clinically. When the atlas is displaced by violence there is nearly always a fracture at the base of the dens, and the dens fragment is displaced together with the atlas. Displacement is for-wards in flexion injuries (Fig. 97), and backwards in extension injuries. Forward displacement is the more common. Sometimes there is a fracture of the dens without displacement.

It is difficult to assess the true incidence of injury to the spinal cord from fracture-dislocation of the atlanto-axial joint, because complete transection of the cord at this level would cause immediate death and the patient would not reach the surgeon. In the cases seen clinically, however, there is usually either no evidence of spinal cord damage or only slight dysfunction. Some-times there has been late paresis from secondary displacement of an ununited fracture.

Clinically, the patient is often seen supporting his head in his hands. Diagnosis depends upon radiological examination (p. 85).

Treatment. If there is no displacement it is sufficient to support the cervical spine and occiput for three months by a plaster or plastic collar. If

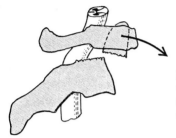

Fig. 97
Fracture of the base of the dens with anterior displacement of the dens with the atlas. The spinal cord often escapes serious damage.

displacement is present, reduction should be attempted by sustained weight traction through skull calipers (Fig. 95). Since the position may be unstable, traction should be maintained for four weeks before the patient is allowed up with a plaster or plastic support. Bony union does not always occur but close fibrous union is usually adequate. Occasionally, persistent instability demands local operative fusion between the atlas and axis.

INTRA-SPINAL DISPLACEMENT OF SOFT TISSUE
Rarely, cases of neck injury are encountered in which there has clearly been a severe injury to the spinal cord—as evidenced by partial or

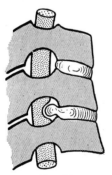
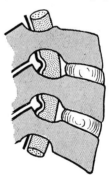

Fig. 98   Fig. 99
Possible causes of damage to the spinal cord in the absence of demonstrable bone injury or displacement. Figure 98—Massive prolapse of an intervertebral disc. Figure 99—Infolding of ligamentum flavum during forced hyperextension. Another possible cause is momentary subluxation with spontaneous reduction.

complete tetraplegia or paraplegia—and yet there is no radiographic sign of bone injury or displacement. In some such cases it is possible that the cord injury has been caused by momentary vertebral displacement that has become reduced spontaneously (Fig. 89). In other instances, however, it has been shown that forcible displacement of soft tissue into the spinal canal has been responsible. The soft tissue concerned may be 1) the nucleus pulposus of an intervertebral disc, or 2) a posterior fold of ligamentum flavum.

Displacement of intervertebral disc material

Massive prolapse of the nucleus pulposus of an intervertebral disc is a well recognised cause of spinal cord compression (Fig. 98) (Barnes 1951). When the prolapse occurs suddenly from injury a violent flexion-compression force is usually responsible. The displacement may be demonstrated by myelography, and if the cord is not irreparably damaged relief may follow operative removal of the displaced disc material.

Infolding of ligamentum flavum

It has been shown that in full extension of the cervical spine folds of the ligamentum flavum become invaginated into the spinal canal, and these indentations, if produced suddenly by a hyperextension injury, may be sufficient to damage the spinal cord (Fig. 99) (Barnes 1951; Taylor 1951). The risk of cord injury from this cause is greatly increased if the spinal canal is already narrowed by the encroachment of osteophytes in a patient with advanced osteoarthritis.

FRACTURE OF SPINOUS PROCESS

This injury usually affects either the seventh cervical or the first thoracic spine. It is caused by muscular action such as is entailed by heavy shovelling, and because of its occurrence among clay shovellers the injury has been termed 'clay-shovellers' fracture'. There are severe pain and tenderness localised to the affected spinous process.

Treatment. Treatment may be conservative or operative. Conservative treatment is by rest from heavy activities until the acute pain begins to subside, followed by a programme of special exercises. Operative treatment is by excision of the avulsed fragment of bone. There seems to be little to choose between the two methods; so conservative treatment should usually be advised. In these injuries ultimate restoration of normal function can be expected with confidence.

References and bibliography, page 291.

CHAPTER **8**

Spine and thorax

Fractures of the spine may involve the vertebral bodies or the posterior elements—transverse processes and spinous processes. Injuries of the vertebral bodies tend to occur from compression, flexion or twisting forces, whereas the posterior elements are more likely to be damaged by direct violence.

Many spinal injuries are benign and cause little or no permanent disability. The important exception, of course, is a major vertebral fracture or displacement in which the spinal cord or cauda equina is damaged. These are grave injuries, often resulting in permanent paralysis.

Fractures of the thoracic cage may be relatively minor injuries, as for instance when a single rib is fractured. But chest injuries must never be regarded lightly because complications are common and often serious. Indeed, a major crushing injury of the chest is one of the most lethal emergencies in the whole realm of accident surgery.

Classification
Injuries of the spine and thorax may be classified as follows.

> **Major fractures and displacements of the thoracic or lumbar vertebrae**
> Wedge compression fracture of vertebral body
> Burst fracture of vertebral body
> Dislocation and fracture-dislocation
>
> **Minor fractures of the spinal column**
> Fractures of transverse processes
> Fracture of the sacrum
> Fracture of the coccyx
>
> **Fractures of the thoracic cage**
> Fractures of the ribs
> Fractures of the sternum

MAJOR FRACTURES AND DISPLACEMENTS OF THE THORACIC AND LUMBAR VERTEBRAE

These are the commonest spinal fractures seen in clinical practice and they demand detailed consideration.

Mechanism of injury

Fractures of the thoracic or lumbar vertebral bodies are nearly always caused by a vertical force acting through the long axis of the spinal column. This force may act from above, as when a coal miner is buried by a fall of roof, or from below, as by a heavy fall on the feet or buttocks. Since the natural curve of the spine is predominantly

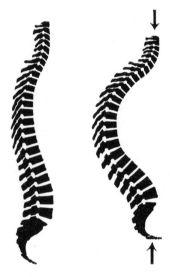

Fig. 100
Since the main natural curve of the spine is a flexion curve a force acting vertically from above or below will tend to increase the flexion. Nearly all fractures of the vertebral bodies in the thoracic and thoraco-lumbar regions are caused by hyperflexion or by combined flexion and rotation.

one of flexion, the effect of such a force is to increase the flexion (Fig. 100). Accordingly it is found that most vertebral fractures in the thoracic or thoraco-lumbar region are hyperflexion injuries and that fractures from hyperextension are uncommon. If the affected part of the spinal column is straight at the moment of impact the compression force, acting directly along the line of the vertebral bodies, may cause a 'burst' fracture like that already described in the cervical region (p. 87).

In the usual flexion injury one or more of the vertebral bodies collapses anteriorly and becomes wedge-shaped, giving rise to a localised kyphosis (Figs. 101 and 103). This is the common wedge compression fracture of a vertebral body.

When the causative violence is very severe—and especially if the flexion force is accompanied by rotation—fracture of a vertebral body may be complicated by dislocation of the intervertebral joint, with forward displacement of the upper vertebra upon the lower (Figs. 102 and 104). This is the dangerous condition of fracture-dislocation of the spine, which is so often complicated by damage to the spinal cord or cauda equina and consequent paralysis.

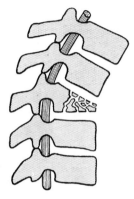

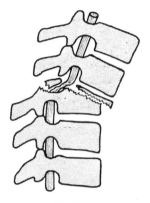

Fig. 101

Uncomplicated wedge compression fracture of a vertebral body. The spinal cord is undamaged. The injury is caused by a flexion force. The posterior ligaments are intact; so the spine is stable.

Fig. 102

Vertebral fracture-dislocation with transection of the spinal cord. Note the characteristic slice fracture of the vertebral body. The injury is caused by combined flexion and rotation.

Stable and unstable injuries

As in the case of cervical injuries (p. 86), it is important to distinguish between fractures and fracture-dislocations in which intact posterior ligaments make the spine stable against further displacement, and those unstable injuries in which rupture of the posterior ligaments might permit further displacement, with peril to the spinal cord or cauda equina. The distinction is fundamental from the point of view of treatment, because a spine that is stable does not necessarily require protection whereas an unstable spine must be protected either by external support or by internal fixation.

WEDGE COMPRESSION FRACTURE OF VERTEBRAL BODY

Diagnosis. In severe fractures there will be obvious symptoms and signs pointing to an injury of the spinal column. It should be remembered, however, that the symptoms and signs of a simple

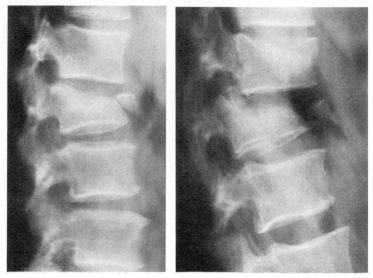

Fig. 103   Fig. 104

Typical vertebral injuries. Figure 103 shows an uncomplicated compression fracture with a corner of the vertebral body dislodged. Figure 104 shows a fracture-dislocation in which the lower end of the spinal cord was crushed.

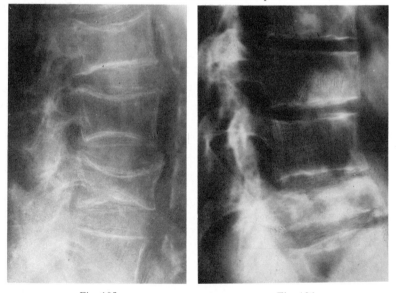

Fig. 105   Fig. 106

The spinal column is a common site for pathological fractures. The two commonest causes are senile osteoporosis (Fig. 105) and metastatic carcinomatous deposits (Fig. 106).

compression fracture are often surprisingly slight; they may be over-looked by patient and doctor alike, especially if more painful injuries to other parts of the body are also present. Careful enquiry and examination should therefore be made to determine the presence or absence of the following suggestive features: local pain; a prominent spinous process on palpation; tenderness on percussion; and painful limitation of spinal movement. In some cases a spinal fracture simulates an intra-abdominal lesion, and the abdomen may be opened in a fruitless search for a ruptured viscus if the real cause of the symptoms is overlooked. The possibility of a vertebral fracture should always be borne in mind in cases of violent injury, and it is worth remembering that a considerable proportion of cases of crush fracture of the calcaneus (an injury that is usually caused by a fall from a height on to the heels) are associated with compression fracture of the spine. If there is any doubt about the possibility of a spinal fracture radio-graphs must always be obtained, for if a fracture is overlooked and left untreated there is a possibility of persistent back pain later.

It should be remembered that the spinal column is a common site for pathological fractures (Figs. 105 and 106).

Treatment. It was formerly taught that in compression fractures of the vertebral bodies reduction should always be attempted by hyperextension, the trunk thereafter being encased in a plaster jacket (Böhler 1935; Watson-Jones 1943). It has since been found, however, that reduction is unnecessary (Nicoll 1948, 1949; Holdsworth 1970). Moreover, because the position is stable by virtue of intact posterior ligaments, there is nothing to be gained by immobilising the spine rigidly in a plaster.

Standard method. The standard method of treatment now is to nurse the patient free in bed in the early stages and to concentrate entirely on restoring function. To this end active muscle exercises—mainly for the erector spinae muscles—are begun immediately and are intensified progressively as the pain subsides. The patient is allowed up as soon as pain permits (usually one to three weeks after injury), and thereafter rehabilitation is continued under the supervision of a skilled physiotherapist by exercises designed both to strengthen the spinal muscles and to restore mobility (Fig. 107).

Alternative methods for special cases. If in the early stages pain is unusually severe it may occasionally be advisable to support the spine for three or four weeks in a plaster jacket. The plaster should be applied with the spine in the neutral position, and no attempt should be made to reduce vertebral wedging by extending the spine. The plaster may be put on while the patient stands, with or without the

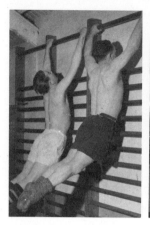
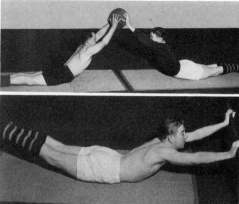

Fig. 107

Patients with vertebral compression fractures practising spinal exercises in the gymnasium. The emphasis should be on restoring the power of the posterior spinal muscles, and later on restoring full mobility.

assistance of head or shoulder harness suspended from the ceiling; or, if the patient is unable to stand, it may be applied while he lies supine upon an orthopaedic table. Vigorous muscle exercises should be encouraged while the spine is protected in the plaster and they should be intensified when the plaster is removed.

In certain special cases—especially in elderly patients and in some with pathological fractures from rarefying bone disease—semi-permanent protection by a steel-reinforced surgical corset may be required.

BURST FRACTURE OF VERTEBRAL BODY

This is a less common variant of the wedge compression fracture in which the spine is straight at the moment of injury: the compression force thus acts vertically in the line of the vertebral bodies. The intervertebral disc is forced into the affected vertebral body, causing a comminuted bursting fracture in which fragments are driven outwards in all directions. The posterior fragments may be driven into the spinal cord or cauda equina; so this injury must be regarded as more dangerous than the simple wedge compression fracture. Nevertheless the ligaments are intact and the spine is therefore stable: that is, displacement greater than that sustained at the time of the injury is not likely to occur.

Treatment. In the absence of neurological complications treatment is the same as for wedge compression fracture. A surgical corset may be worn during the first few weeks for relief of pain.

DISLOCATION AND FRACTURE-DISLOCATION

These injuries are uncommon compared with simple wedge compression fractures of the vertebral bodies.

The commonest displaced injury of the thoracic or lumbar spine is a fracture-dislocation in which one of the vertebrae is forced forwards upon the vertebra next below it (Figs. 102 and 104). This can occur only if the articular processes are fractured or if the facet joints are dislocated and the articular processes overridden. At the same time the lower of the two affected vertebral bodies is fractured near its upper surface: typically the fracture line is almost horizontal, giving the appearance in the radiograph that the vertebra has been sliced (Fig. 102). The posterior ligaments are always torn; so the spine is very unstable and further displacement may easily occur. Most of these fracture-dislocations occur in the mid-thoracic region or at the thoraco-lumbar junction, and it has been shown that the causative violence is nearly always a combined flexion and rotation force (Holdsworth, 1970).

Fracture-dislocation in the thoracic region or at the thoraco-lumbar junction is nearly always complicated by injury to the spinal cord, and the cord injury is usually a complete transection. Fracture-dislocation in the lumbar region is often complicated by injury to the cauda equina, which may be complete or incomplete.

Treatment. In most of these injuries paraplegia from injury to the spinal cord overshadows the skeletal injury. The management of such cases is considered separately in the chapter on paraplegia (Chapter 9, p. 106).

In the occasional case in which a fracture-dislocation or a dislocation is not complicated by paraplegia the patient must be handled with great care lest further vertebral displacement should injure the spinal cord. The treatment required depends upon the precise nature of the injury as revealed in the radiographs, and particularly upon the state of the articular processes.

If the articular processes are shown to be fractured it will usually be possible to reduce the vertebral displacement by gently extending the spine through a moderate range while the patient lies prone. If radiographs confirm that reduction has been achieved the spine is immobilised for three months in a closely fitting plaster jacket applied while the patient lies prone with the spine slightly extended.

If the articular processes are shown to be overridden but not fractured reduction by extending the spine should not be attempted. In such circumstances closed reduction is unlikely to be achieved, and forced extension is dangerous because it may increase the displacement and damage the spinal cord or cauda equina. Operation should therefore be advised. The vertebrae are exposed from behind and reduction is obtained under direct vision, with great care to preserve the cord or cauda equina from injury. When practicable, internal fixation is effected by a plate or wire fixed to the spinous processes, and the spine is thereafter immobilised in a plaster jacket for three months.

MINOR FRACTURES OF THE SPINAL COLUMN
Minor fractures of the vertebrae are mainly those of the transverse processes, and of the sacrum and coccyx. These injuries are referred to as minor fractures because they are not likely to be complicated

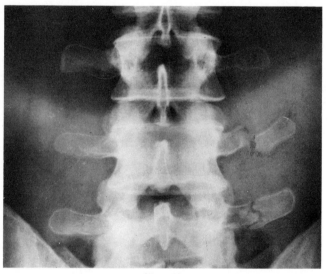

Fig. 108
Fractures of the fourth and fifth left lumbar transverse processes.

by catastrophes such as spinal cord injury, and because, if treated efficiently, they do not lead to permanent disability. On the other hand they can be very painful injuries, and they demand careful nursing and energetic physical treatment like the more serious fractures.

FRACTURES OF TRANSVERSE PROCESSES
These injuries are almost confined to the lumbar region. They are caused by direct violence such as a heavy blow or a fall against a

hard object. The injury may involve a single transverse process, but often two or more processes are fractured on the same side (Fig. 108). Occasionally there may be associated damage to the corresponding kidney.

Treatment. Treatment consists in rest in bed until the acute pain subsides. At an early stage active exercises for the spinal muscles are begun, and are intensified as the pain becomes less. After a few days or a week, according to progress, the patient begins to get up, but he should continue an active programme of rehabilitation until full function has been regained.

FRACTURE OF THE SACRUM

This uncommon injury is caused by a fall or direct blow on the sacral region. The fracture is usually no more than a crack without displacement. It may be suspected clinically from the presence of marked local tenderness, and later from the appearance of an ecchymosis. In the absence of complications no special treatment is required.

In the rare instances in which the fragments are markedly displaced there is a serious risk of injury of the cauda equina or of component nerves of the sacral plexus.

FRACTURE OF THE COCCYX

A fracture of the coccyx may be caused by a fall on the 'tail'. It is an uncommon injury. Nearly always the pain will subside gradually without special treatment, but in the exceptional case in which pain from an ununited fracture persists for many months the coccyx may be excised.

FRACTURES OF THE THORACIC CAGE

FRACTURES OF THE RIBS

Most fractures of the ribs are caused by direct injury, as by a fall against a hard object. Occasionally a rib may be fractured by laughing or coughing.

The fracture usually occurs near the angle of the rib. There is seldom severe displacement, because the fragments are held well together by the attached muscles. In the event of marked displacement a fragment may pierce the pleura or lung, with consequent haemothorax or haemo-pneumothorax.

Clinical features. There is severe pain made worse by deep breathing, with marked local tenderness on palpation over the site of fracture. Antero-posterior compression of the thorax by springing the ribs also causes pain at the site of fracture.

Treatment. Fractures of the ribs unite spontaneously, and treatment is required only to increase the patient's comfort and to

combat possible complications. The time-honoured method of applying adhesive strapping round the affected side of the chest wall is
now seldom used. It may afford some relief, but the strapping may
hinder full respiratory excursion. It is better that breathing exercises
be encouraged to ensure that the lung is fully expanded. In severe
cases pain may often be relieved by injecting a solution of long-
acting local anaesthetic about the site of fracture.

Complications. The main importance of fractures of the ribs is that
they may give rise to pulmonary complications that may sometimes
be serious or even fatal in the absence of prompt and efficient treatment. The complications include haemothorax, pneumothorax,
surgical emphysema, and pneumonia. As one might expect, they are
most common after violent direct injuries, and they are liable to be
especially serious in elderly patients with multiple rib fractures.
Treatment is outlined below.

FRACTURES OF THE STERNUM

A fracture of the sternum may be caused in two ways: 1) by direct
injury; or 2) by vertical compression of the thoracic cage, with
simultaneous fracture of the thoracic spine.

Fractures from direct injury are uncommon but serious. The sternum is
driven in from the front, reducing the antero-posterior diameter of the
thorax and impairing the vital capacity. If displacement is marked it should
be corrected by pulling the sternum forwards with a hook.

Most fractures of the sternum are of the second type, and occur in
association with a fracture of the thoracic spine. The spinal injury is caused
in the usual way by hyperflexion, and the force is transmitted to the
sternum through the ribs. The sternum is angled backwards at the fracture,
which occurs near the junction of the manubrium and the body of the
sternum, but displacement is seldom severe. Treatment is required mainly
for the associated fracture of the spine. No special treatment is needed for
the sternal fracture.

Principles of treatment of major chest injuries

In cases of severe injury to the thoracic cage, and especially when
multiple rib fractures on both sides create a flail anterior segment of
chest wall ('stove-in chest'), prompt treatment may be required to
save life.

The danger arises from the patient's inability to take proper
breaths on account of obstruction of the airway, filling of the pleural
cavity by blood or air, loss of rigidity of the thoracic cage with
consequent paradoxical respiration, severe pain, or a combination of
several or all of these hindrances. Clearly, treatment must be

designed to correct or to counteract any condition that is preventing adequate respiration. In the worst emergencies, with the patient badly cyanosed and showing paradoxical respiration, he should be anaesthetised forthwith to allow respiration to be controlled mechanically while the necessary action is taken.

Airway. It may be necessary repeatedly to remove bronchial secretions by suction. This is facilitated by tracheostomy. Tracheostomy also aids oxygenation by reducing the dead-space air, and it permits long-term mechanical control of respiration when this is required. On the other hand it is unpleasant for the patient and should not be performed needlessly.

Pleural space. Respiratory embarrassment by blood or air in the pleural cavity is corrected by drainage through a tube inserted through an upper intercostal space and led to a suction bottle. Pleural drainage is vitally necessary in cases of tension pneumothorax.

Flail anterior segment of chest wall. If the necessary equipment and staff are available paradoxical respiration from multiple rib fractures with flail anterior segment is best controlled by intermittent positive pressure respiration with a mechanical respirator. Otherwise, steps may have to be taken to fix fractures of the sternum and ribs by stiff intramedullary wires, in order to restore rigidity to the thoracic cage.

Pain. In cases of moderate severity pain may be controlled adequately by appropriate drugs and by injection of a long-acting local anaesthetic solution about the fractures. In the worst cases there is a place for long-term anaesthesia by gas and oxygen inhalation or by continuous epidural block.

References and bibliography, page 291.

CHAPTER 9

Paraplegia from spinal injuries

Damage to the spinal cord or cauda equina complicates only a small proportion of all spinal injuries. In most cases the skeletal lesion is in the thoracic region or at the thoraco-lumbar junction; less often in the cervical or lumbar region.

THE SKELETAL INJURY

In the *cervical spine* the injury that is most commonly complicated by damage to the spinal cord is a fracture-dislocation from a flexion-rotation force (Fig. 87). This usually occurs in the lower half of the cervical column—often between the fourth and fifth vertebrae or between the fifth and sixth. Dislocaton of the atlanto-axial joint is occasionally responsible. In some cases of spinal cord injury in the neck there is no radiographic evidence of any bone injury or displacement: in such cases the nerve lesion may be caused by a protruded intervertebral disc, by an infolded ligamentum flavum (p. 94), or possibly by a momentary subluxation that has become reduced spontaneously (Barnes 1951).

In the *thoracic and lumbar regions* the skeletal injury responsible for damage to the spinal cord or cauda equina is nearly always a fracture-dislocation caused by a violent flexion or rotation force (Figs. 102 and 104) (Holdsworth 1970).

THE NERVE INJURY

The character of the nerve lesion depends upon the site of the skeletal injury. In the *cervical region* the cord injury may be either complete or incomplete. Surprisingly, the extent of the nerve injury does not bear a constant relationship to the severity of the skeletal injury: severe cord damage may be found in the absence of any demonstrable bone injury; and, conversely, there may be little or no neurological disturbance despite severe vertebral displacement.

In the *thoracic region* a fracture-dislocation usually causes complete transection of the spinal cord. The force necessary to displace the

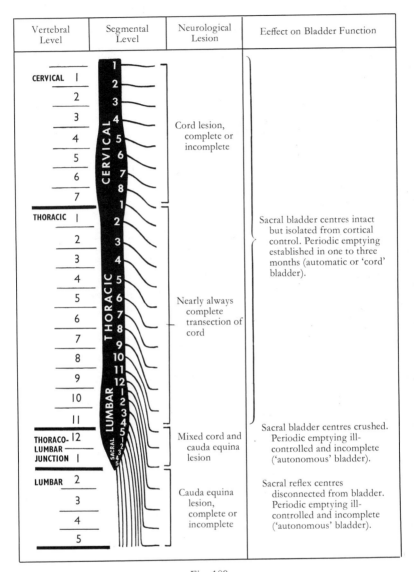

Vertebral Level	Segmental Level	Neurological Lesion	Eeffect on Bladder Function

Fig. 109

Composite diagram showing the relationship between vertebral and segmental levels, the nature of the neurological lesion and the state of the bladder after vertebral injuries involving the spinal cord or cauda equina at various sites.

vertebrae at this level is great, and the spinal cord, which is soft and friable—it may be compared in its consistence with the soft roe of a herring—is quite unable to withstand the shearing action of the displaced vertebra.

At the *thoraco-lumbar junction* (thoracic 12 to lumbar 1) the lowest segments of the spinal cord and the proximal roots of the cauda equina lie side by side in the spinal canal; so the nerve lesion caused by a fracture-dislocation may be a mixed one, due partly to cord injury and partly to nerve-root injury (Fig. 109). If the lesion is incomplete it is nearly always the nerve roots rather than the cord whose function is preserved ('lumbar root escape').

In the *lumbar region* (below the first lumbar vertebra) the spinal cord has given place to the cauda equina, which is more resistant to injury than the spinal cord itself. In fracture-dislocations at this level the neural injury may therefore be incomplete.

Characteristics of complete transection of the cord. The immediate consequence of division of the cord is total suppression of function in the segments below the lesion (spinal shock). The initial paralysis is flaccid, there is complete sensory loss, and the visceral reflexes are suppressed. This stage of spinal shock lasts usually for a few days, or sometimes weeks. As it gradually passes off the paralysis becomes spastic instead of flaccid, and there is a return of exaggerated tendon and visceral reflexes unmodified by higher control. The return of reflex activity, without recovery of sensibility or of voluntary motor power below the lesion, is diagnostic of complete transection of the spinal cord. Because of the temporary phenomena contributed by spinal shock, it is seldom possible to make an unequivocal diagnosis of complete transection of the cord until forty-eight hours or more after the injury, and accordingly repeated neurological examination is required in these first few days.

Characteristics of incomplete transection of the cord. The only certain sign of continuity of axons in the spinal cord is the preservation or early return of voluntary motor power and sensibility below the level of the lesion.

Characteristics of severe injury to the cauda equina. The paralysis remains flaccid throughout. The tendon and visceral reflexes are abolished below the lesion and do not return unless the nerve fibres recover their function.

THE BLADDER

In the normal state emptying of the bladder is governed by reflex centres in the second and third sacral segments of the spinal cord, with overriding control from the cerebral cortex. After transection of the cord above the sacral segments the overriding cerebral control is cut off, but the sacral reflex centres are left intact. In the early weeks after the injury there is retention of urine, with overflow if the retention is not relieved. But after an interval that varies from one to three months the reflex centres in the cord take over and control automatic emptying of the bladder when it is filled to a certain capacity. This reflex state has been termed automatic bladder or 'cord bladder'.

If the injury involves the sacral segments of the cord or the nerve roots that emerge from it in the cauda equina the nerve pathways for reflex control of the bladder are severed. True reflex emptying does not occur. Instead, periodic emptying of the bladder is dependent upon a local reflex in the bladder wall itself. In this state of 'autonomous bladder' the emptying action of the detrusor muscle may have to be induced by manual compression of the abdominal wall or by abdominal straining, and the emptying is less complete than it is with an automatic or cord bladder.

SPECIAL DANGERS IN CASES OF SPINAL PARAPLEGIA
The main dangers in the early months arise from pressure sores and from infection of the urinary tract. Many patients still die from these causes, but with improved methods of treatment the mortality has been greatly reduced.

PROGNOSIS
The spinal cord has no power of recovery after complete transection. On the other hand after incomplete cord lesions a remarkable degree of recovery may occur despite severe initial paralysis. Recovery may continue for many months, but the earlier and the more rapidly it begins the better the prognosis. These incomplete lesions are more common in the cervical region than in the thoracic region, where complete transection is almost the rule.

The roots of the cauda equina behave like other peripheral nerves in their capacity for recovery: that is, they are able to recover or regenerate provided their sheaths remain patent and in continuity (see p. 63). Thus if the injury is a *neurapraxia* recovery may occur early. After *axonotmesis* the nerve fibres may regenerate, but the re-establishment of function depends upon their reaching healthy end-plates. *Neurotmesis* in this region is irrecoverable because surgical repair is hardly practicable.

It will be clear from what has been said that injuries of the cauda equina have a more favourable prognosis than cord injuries in three important respects: 1) the extent of the paralysis is less; 2) the lesion is less likely to be a complete transection; and 3) the chances of recovery are much greater.

TREATMENT

It is greatly to the patient's advantage if he can be admitted immediately to a special hospital for paraplegics, where the necessary facilities and staff for the management of these difficult cases are available.

Management of the fracture. In the case of *cervical injuries,* if bony displacement is present reduction should be attempted by traction through skull calipers, as described on page 90. If there is no bony displacement but severe paralysis myelographic studies should be made. If these suggest that spinal cord compression is caused by a protruded intervertebral disc operative excision of the disc should be advised.

In fracture-dislocation of the *thoracic spine* with total distal paralysis it is to be feared that the spinal cord is completely divided. Nevertheless the surgeon cannot be certain that this is the case in the hours immediately after the injury; so there is an argument for operative correction of the displacement and fixation of the fragments by a plate. This school of thought is perhaps gaining ground over the opposing school, which prefers to disregard the fracture and to concentrate attention on skilful nursing, care of the bladder, and rehabilitation.

In fractures lower down—that is, at the *thoraco-lumbar junction* or in the *lumbar region*—the neurological injury is more likely to be incomplete, at least some of the nerve roots being spared. Operation should be undertaken immediately. Its objects are: 1) to reduce any gross displacement under direct vision to ensure that the roots of the cauda equina are free from pressure or constriction; and 2) to provide internal fixation of the fragments to prevent redisplacement and to facilitate nursing without a plaster. Internal fixation is usually effected by a metal plate bolted to the spinous processes, or occasionally by strong stainless-steel wire.

Nursing. A specialised nursing routine is essential if pressure sores are to be avoided. The old method of nursing the patient in a plaster bed has been discarded because it was found impossible to prevent the development of pressure sores in the insensitive skin. Indeed it can be stated emphatically that a plaster bed should never be used for the nursing of a patient paralysed from a spinal injury.

The accepted method now is to nurse the patient flat upon soft pillows. Every two hours throughout the day and night he is turned to a new position, so that he lies for equal periods upon his back and upon either side.

Gentle passive joint movements should be carried out regularly from an early stage to preserve mobility in the paralysed limbs. It is important, however, to avoid the use of force, which by damaging a joint may increase stiffness rather than overcome it (see p. 67).

Care and training of the bladder. The former method whereby drainage was effected by suprapubic cystostomy has been abandoned because it does not prevent infection and because it leads to shrinkage of the bladder. The most satisfactory method is probably by intermittent catheterisation, but many surgeons prefer to use an indwelling catheter with or without tidal drainage. No matter which method is used, great emphasis must be laid on the necessity for a strict aseptic technique when the catheter is changed. Some degree of infection is almost inevitable, and antibiotics may be administered as necessary to control it.

Periodic emptying of the bladder should be encouraged from an early stage by allowing the bladder to fill almost to capacity between catheterisations and by draining it at regular intervals—usually four times a day.

In most cases of transection of the cord satisfactory automatic emptying is established within one to three months of the injury. After irrecoverable damage to the sacral segments of the cord or to the cauda equina periodic spontaneous emptying is more difficult to establish and, since it is no longer governed by the reflex centres, the mechanism is less reliable. Micturition will have to be started or aided by abdominal straining or by manual compression, and a urinal may have to be worn permanently.

Rehabilitation. Despite severe permanent paralysis a proportion of patients with complete transection of the cord can be made reasonably independent and enabled to lead a useful life within the limits of their tragic disability. Though some can walk short distances with calipers and crutches, for the most part they must get about permanently in wheel chairs.

After cauda equina injuries the possibilities of rehabilitation are much greater, especially when the nerve lesion is incomplete. Even when there is considerable irrecoverable damage the patient can usually get about well with elbow crutches or sticks, perhaps with the aid of a caliper or a toe-raising spring.

Morale. An important part of the management of patients with traumatic paraplegia is the re-establishment of morale. It is natural that a person so tragically afflicted may become seriously depressed and perhaps even feel that life can no longer be worth living. In such circumstances much depends upon the personality of the doctor with charge of the case, and upon the attitude of nursing and ancillary staff. If the patient is fortunate enough to be in a centre established specially for the care of paraplegic patients, the fact of seeing other patients similarly afflicted, and especially of seeing those who are in the later stages of rehabilitation and who are already beginning to some extent to resume an active life, is always a considerable help to those freshly injured. Later, the promotion of a competitive spirit among patients, with provision of facilities for games, has also proved to be a source of encouragement. It is even more important to the patient, of course, if he can see even distantly the likelihood that he will be able to get back to some form of remunerative employment, and strenuous efforts must be directed towards this end on his behalf.

References and bibliography, page 291.

CHAPTER 10

Shoulder, upper arm and elbow

The commonest injuries in this region are fracture of the clavicle, dislocation of the shoulder, fracture of the neck of the humerus and, in children, supracondylar fracture of the humerus.

Classification
The injuries to be described may be classified as follows.

Fractures of the shoulder girdle
Fractures of the clavicle
Fractures of the scapula

Injuries of the shoulder and related joints
Dislocation of the sterno-clavicular joint
Strain of the sterno-clavicular joint
Subluxation and dislocation of the acromio-clavicular joint
Strain of the acromio-clavicular joint
Dislocation of the shoulder
Rupture of the tendinous cuff of the shoulder

Fractures of the humerus
Fracture of the neck of the humerus
Fracture of the greater tuberosity
Fracture of the shaft
Supracondylar fracture
Fractures of the condyles
Fractures of the epicondyles

Injuries of the elbow
Dislocation of the elbow
Dislocation of the head of the radius
Subluxation of the head of the radius
Contusion of the elbow

FRACTURES OF THE SHOULDER GIRDLE

The shoulder girdle comprises the clavicles and the scapulae. Fractures of the clavicle are common; they are caused by indirect violence. Fractures of the scapula are uncommon, and are usually caused by direct violence. The fractures to be described are classified in Figure 110.

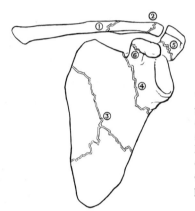

Fig. 110
Visual classification of fractures of the shoulder girdle. 1. Fracture of clavicle at junction of middle and outermost thirds. 2. Fracture of lateral end of clavicle. 3. Fracture of body of scapula. 4. Fracture of neck of scapula. 5. Fracture of acromion process. 6. Fracture of coracoid process.

FRACTURES OF THE CLAVICLE

Most fractures of the clavicle are caused by a fall on the outstretched hand. The commonest site is at the junction of the middle and outermost thirds (Fig. 111). Less often a fracture occurs near the outer end of the clavicle. If displacement occurs—as it usually does—the lateral fragment is displaced downwards and medially.

Treatment. Displacement is reduced so far as possible by the simple method of holding the shoulders braced back in a figure-of-eight bandage (Fig. 112). This should be applied snugly, but it is important to ensure that it is not wrapped too tightly: otherwise the venous return from the upper limb may be obstructed or one or more of the nerve trunks in the axilla may be injured. It is seldom possible to restore perfect position of the fragments, but moderate displacement does not hinder union and should be accepted. At first the arm is rested in a sling, but active shoulder exercises are begun as soon as the pain begins to subside—usually about a week after the injury. The figure-of-eight bandage is discarded after two weeks.

Fractures of the clavicle unite readily, and the only common residual disability is a palpable or visible irregularity of the bone at the site of fracture. In children, remodelling quickly restores a normal contour. In adults some thickening may remain permanently, but it is

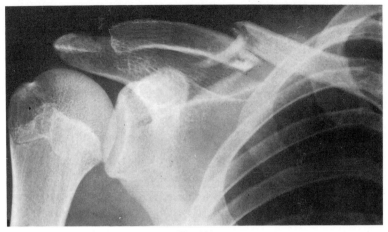

Fig. 111
Fracture of the clavicle at the usual site, with typical displacement.

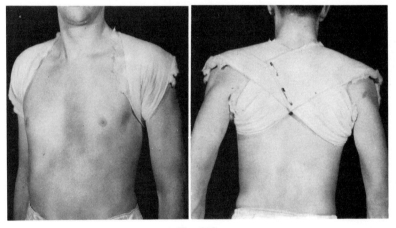

Fig. 112
Figure-of-eight bandage used to brace the shoulders back in a case of fractured clavicle.

seldom prominent. If the patient is seriously concerned about the cosmetic blemish operative smoothing of bony prominences is justified. In old persons there is a risk of stiffness of the shoulder if exercises are not practised from an early stage.

FRACTURES OF THE SCAPULA
The scapula is fractured usually by direct injury. Such fractures are uncommon, and in most cases unimportant because the patients do

well without special treatment. Nevertheless there is often severe pain, and there may be extensive extravasation of blood into the tissues, with widespread ecchymosis.

Four fractures will be considered (Fig. 110): 1) fracture of the body of the scapula; 2) fracture of the neck of the scapula; 3) fracture of the acromion process; and 4) fracture of the coracoid process.

FRACTURE OF THE BODY OF THE SCAPULA

Although the fracture may be comminuted there is no important displacement because the fragments are held in position by their extensive muscle attachments.

Treatment. Attention should be directed mainly to the restoration of shoulder function. A sling is worn at first, but as soon as the pain begins to subside active shoulder exercises are begun, and continued until a full range of movement is regained.

FRACTURE OF THE NECK OF THE SCAPULA

The fracture extends from the scapular notch to the axillary border of the scapula, so that the part bearing the articular surface is detached in one piece from the body of the bone. The glenoid fragment may be displaced downwards, but the displacement is seldom severe.

Treatment. Again the main necessity is not to provide rigid splintage but to restore shoulder function by early active exercises as soon as pain allows. Indeed immobilisation, except to the extent provided by a sling, is unnecessary.

FRACTURE OF THE ACROMION PROCESS

The fracture occurs at a variable distance from the tip of the acromion. There may be no more than a crack without displacement, or the acromion may be comminuted and displaced downwards.

Treatment. If the fracture is simply a crack without displacement it is sufficient to arrange active shoulder exercises as soon as the pain begins to subside; meanwhile a sling is worn.

If the acromion is comminuted or markedly depressed operation is advised. The acromion is excised back to the acromio-clavicular joint, and the deltoid muscle is sutured to the periosteum covering the stump of the bone. The shoulder is held abducted on a frame or in plaster for three weeks, after which intensive mobilising exercises are begun.

FRACTURE OF THE CORACOID PROCESS

The injury may be no more than a crack, or there may be a complete fracture with separation and downward displacement of the coracoid process.

Treatment. The fracture should be disregarded and attention concentrated on restoring shoulder function by early active exercises.

INJURIES OF THE SHOULDER AND RELATED JOINTS

DISLOCATION OF THE STERNO-CLAVICULAR JOINT

When the sterno-clavicular joint is dislocated the medial end of the clavicle is usually displaced forwards. The injury is uncommon. Rarely the clavicle is displaced backwards (retrosternal dislocation) and may press dangerously upon the trachea or great vessels (Tyer, Sturrock and Callow 1963).

Treatment. Anterior displacement is easily reduced by direct pressure over the medial end of the clavicle while the shoulders are arched forwards. A pad should be applied over the front of the joint and held in place by firm adhesive strapping. A sling is worn for two weeks, and thereafter active shoulder exercises are encouraged. The rare posterior dislocation may demand operative reduction.

RECURRENT DISLOCATION

In a rather high proportion of cases dislocation of the sterno-clavicular joint becomes recurrent or permanent despite early reduction of the first dislocation. In recurrent dislocation the clavicle springs forwards when the shoulders are braced back and clicks back into place when the shoulders are arched forward.

Treatment. In most cases the disability is slight or negligible, and treatment is not required. In the occasional case in which the repeated displacement is troublesome operation is advised. The joint may be stabilised by constructing a new retaining ligament from the tendon of the subclavius muscle (Burrows 1951; Lunseth, Chapman and Frankel 1975) or from a strip of fascia (Bankart 1938).

STRAIN OF THE STERNO-CLAVICULAR JOINT

Strain of the sterno-clavicular joint is followed by local pain and swelling. The area of the joint is tender on palpation, but the clavicle is not displaced. Spontaneous recovery may be expected and no special treatment is required.

SUBLUXATION AND DISLOCATION OF THE ACROMIO-CLAVICULAR JOINT

Injuries of the acromio-clavicular joint are much more common than injuries of the sterno-clavicular joint. They are caused by falls on the outer prominence of the shoulder, tending to force the acromion downwards. Such injuries are especially common among rugby football players.

Pathology. SUBLUXATION. In cases of subluxation the capsule of the joint is torn and the acromion is displaced slightly downwards from the lateral end of the clavicle (Fig. 113); but severe displacement is

References and bibliography, page 291.

prevented by the intact conoid and trapezoid ligaments, which anchor the clavicle to the coracoid process.

DISLOCATION. When the joint is dislocated the mechanism is the same but the violence is more severe: the conoid and trapezoid

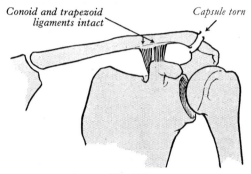

Conoid and trapezoid
ligaments intact

Capsule torn

Fig. 113

Subluxation of acromio-clavicular joint. The joint capsule is torn and the tip of the clavicle is slightly elevated, but severe displacement is prevented by the intact conoid and trapezoid ligaments, which hold the clavicle to the coracoid process.

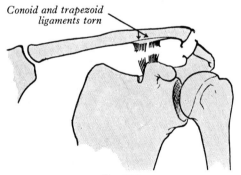

Conoid and trapezoid
ligaments torn

Fig. 114

Dislocation of acromio-clavicular joint. Not only the joint capsule but also the conoid and trapezoid ligaments are torn; so there is nothing to prevent severe displacement.

ligaments are torn and the acromion is displaced markedly downwards (or the clavicle upwards) (Fig. 114).

Treatment. The time-honoured method in which encircling strapping is applied from the mid-part of the clavicle round the under side of the flexed elbow is not recommended: it is ineffective and unnecessary in cases of subluxation, and it is seldom adequate for a complete dislocation.

SUBLUXATION. Slight displacement of the acromio-clavicular joint is harmless and may be accepted. The only treatment advised if pain is severe is to support the limb with a sling for two weeks or so, and to encourage active shoulder exercises from an early stage.

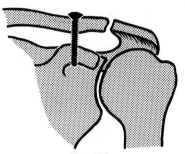

Fig. 115

Stabilisation of the acromio-clavicular joint after dislocation. A screw is passed through a drill hole in the clavicle to engage the coracoid process.

DISLOCATION. Since it is difficult to control a complete dislocation of this joint adequately by external splintage, operation should usually be advised. A simple method is to hold the clavicle in place by means of a screw passed through a drill hole in the clavicle to engage a pilot hole in the coracoid process (Fig. 115). Alternatively, reduction may be maintained by a stiff wire passed horizontally from the tip of the acromion, across the acromio-clavicular joint, into the clavicle. The screw or wire should be removed after six or eight weeks, when it may be assumed that the torn ligaments will have healed. For old persistent displacement a new ligament may be constructed from fascia, to hold the clavicle to the coracoid process; or the outer end of the clavicle may be excised.

STRAIN OF THE ACROMIO-CLAVICULAR JOINT

When the violence is insufficient to subluxate or dislocate the joint, a fall on the point of the shoulder may cause a strain of the joint capsule. There is pain localised accurately to the region of the joint, with marked tenderness on palpation. Pain is aggravated by attempted full abduction of the arm, which entails movement of the acromio-clavicular joint to the limit of its range.

Treatment. Recovery occurs spontaneously with time and use. A sling may be worn if pain is severe, but active shoulder exercises should be encouraged from the beginning.

DISLOCATION OF THE SHOULDER

The shoulder is dislocated commonly in adults but seldom in children.

Pathology. For practical purposes dislocations of the shoulder may be grouped into two main types—anterior and posterior. Anterior dislocation is very much the more common. The cause is nearly always a fall on the outstretched hand or on the region of the shoulder itself. In most cases the humeral head is displaced through a rent in the capsule and comes to lie in the infraclavicular fossa just below the coracoid process; hence the term subcoracoid dislocation often used to describe this injury.

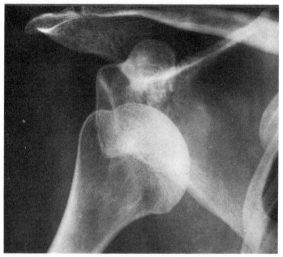

Fig. 116
Typical radiographic appearance in anterior
dislocation of the shoulder.

When the dislocation is posterior there may be a history of a direct blow to the front of the shoulder, driving the humeral head backwards. More often, however, posterior dislocation is the consequence of an electric shock or an epileptiform convulsion, which perhaps acts by causing violent medial rotation.

Clinical features. ANTERIOR DISLOCATION. Pain is severe, and the patient is unwilling to attempt movements of the shoulder. On examination, the contour of the shoulder below the tip of the acromion—normally made strongly convex by the prominence of the humeral head—is flattened, so that the tip of the acromion is now the most lateral point of the shoulder region. A noticeable prominence, caused by the displaced humeral head, is seen and felt in the infra-clavicular fossa. Radiographs show that the outline of the humeral articular surface is not congruous with the articular surface of the glenoid fossa (Fig. 116).

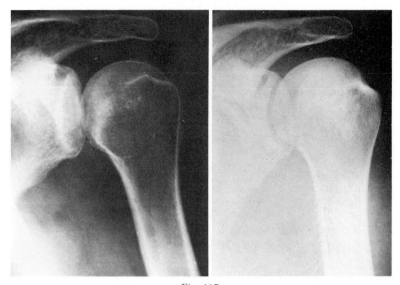

Fig. 117

Left—Antero-posterior radiograph in a case of posterior dislocation of the shoulder. Displacement is not obvious and might be overlooked. *Right*—The same shoulder after reduction of the dislocation, showing normal congruity of the joint surfaces.

POSTERIOR DISLOCATION. The features of a posterior dislocation of the shoulder are not very striking, and for that reason the injury is often overlooked. The most obvious sign is fixed medial rotation of the arm, which cannot be rotated outwards even as far as the neutral position. There is also flattening anteriorly below the front of the acromion, where the head of the humerus normally forms a rounded bulge. *Radiography* may be misleading if only the ordinary antero-posterior film is available, because the dislocation may not be apparent—or at least not obvious—in this projection (Fig. 117). It is therefore important, in doubtful injuries of the shoulder, to insist on a more detailed radiological study. A lateral projection, obtained by directing the rays upwards from the axilla, with the arm abducted to a right angle, is the most valuable (Fig. 118), but if it is impossible to get the arm abducted widely enough for this examination a through-the-chest lateral radiograph may suffice.

Treatment. The dislocation should be reduced as soon as possible. An anaesthetic is usually necessary.

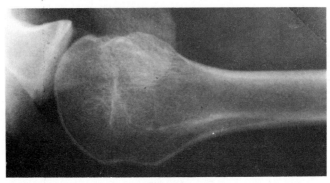

Fig. 118

True lateral radiograph of normal gleno-humeral joint obtained by axillary projection with the arm abducted 90 degrees. This view is especially valuable in the diagnosis of posterior dislocation of the shoulder.

ANTERIOR DISLOCATION. The well known Kocher manoeuvre is nearly always effective. The steps are as follows: 1) With the elbow flexed to a right angle steady traction is applied in the line of the humerus; 2) the arm is rotated laterally; 3) the arm is adducted by carrying the elbow across the body towards the midline; 4) the arm is rotated medially so that the hand falls across the opposite side of the chest.

An alternative method of reducing an anterior dislocation of the shoulder is to pull firmly and steadily upon the semi-abducted arm against counter-traction in the axilla, which may be provided either by an assistant or by the surgeon's stockinged foot; at the same time direct backward pressure may be applied over the humeral head. This method is useful if the more convenient Kocher's manoeuvre fails.

Reduction should be confirmed both by clinical tests and by radiographic examination. Thereafter the limb should be rested in a sling for a few days, but as soon as the pain has subsided active movements may be encouraged.

POSTERIOR DISLOCATION. Reduction is effected by rotating the arm laterally while direct forward pressure is applied over the displaced humeral head. The after-treatment is the same as for anterior dislocation.

Complications. Injury to axillary nerve. The axillary [circumflex] nerve is often damaged in anterior dislocations of the shoulder. There is consequent paralysis of the deltoid muscle, with a small area of anaesthesia at the lateral aspect of the upper arm. *Treatment* is expectant, as for other nerve injuries complicating closed injuries of the limbs (p. 63). Recovery in a few weeks or months is the rule, but if the nerve has been severely damaged by traction the changes may be irreversible and the paralysis permanent.

Other nerve injuries. Occasionally other branches of the brachial plexus are damaged—especially the posterior cord.

Vascular injury. In anterior dislocation the displaced humeral head may occasionally damage the axillary artery, especially if the vessel is atheromatous; or the artery may be damaged during attempted late reduction of a dislocation that has been overlooked (Johnston and Lowry 1962; Curr 1970).

Associated fracture. Dislocation of the shoulder is often accompanied by fracture of the greater tuberosity of the humerus. Treatment is not difficult, because once the dislocation has been reduced the fracture may be treated along the usual lines.

A more serious association is that between dislocation of the shoulder and fracture of the neck of the humerus. Again the plan of treatment should be first to reduce the dislocation (if necessary by operation) and then to deal with the fracture.

RECURRENT ANTERIOR DISLOCATION OF THE SHOULDER

In some instances the damage sustained by a shoulder in a violent dislocation is permanent, and of such a nature that it predisposes to further dislocations. These tend to occur with increasing frequency and with decreasing violence.

Pathology. Whereas in ordinary or non-recurrent dislocation of the shoulder there is probably a tear of the capsule which heals spontaneously when the dislocation has been reduced, in recurrent dislocation the pathology is different, and is such that spontaneous healing does not occur (Bankart 1923) (Figs. 119–122). The changes are two-fold: 1) the capsule is stripped from the anterior margin of the glenoid rim; and 2) the articular surface of the humeral head is dented postero-laterally (probably from violent impingement against the sharp anterior margin of the glenoid fossa) (Figs. 120–122).

Recurrent dislocation occurs most easily when the arm is abducted, extended and rotated laterally.

Treatment. If the disability is troublesome operation is advised. A reliable operation, and the one commonly employed, is the Putti-

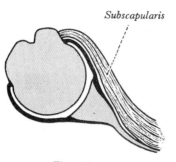

Subscapularis

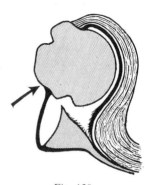

Fig. 119   Fig. 120

Horizontal section of left shoulder showing the pathology of recurrent dislocation. Figure 119 shows the normal condition. In Figure 120 the humeral head is shown dislocated forwards. It has stripped the capsule from the margin of the glenoid, creating a pocket in front of the neck of the scapula into which the humeral head is displaced. Note that the humeral head has been dented by the sharp glenoid margin. The defect thus caused in the articular surface is a typical feature.

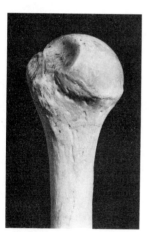

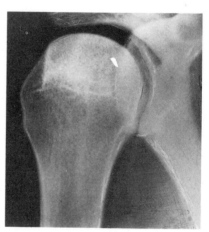

Fig. 121   Fig. 122

Figure 121—Typical defect of articular surface of humeral head, found in most cases of recurrent dislocation of the shoulder. Figure 122—Radiographic appearance. The defect is seen at the upper and outer quadrant of the humeral head. It is shown best when the arm is in medial rotation, as in this radiograph.

Platt procedure, in which the subscapularis muscle is shortened by overlapping or 'reefing' in order to limit lateral rotation (Adams 1948; Osmond-Clarke 1948). In an alternative operation, that of Bankart (1938), the detached capsule and glenoid labrum are re-attached to the front of the glenoid rim.

RUPTURE OF THE TENDINOUS CUFF OF THE SHOULDER
(Torn supraspinatus)

As age advances the tendinous cuff[1] of the shoulder, of which the supraspinatus tendon forms the central part, degenerates and is liable to rupture if subjected to sudden stress, as from a fall on the shoulder or even from an everyday action such as pushing a swing door.

A clear distinction must be made between major tears of the tendinous cuff and minor tears or strains.

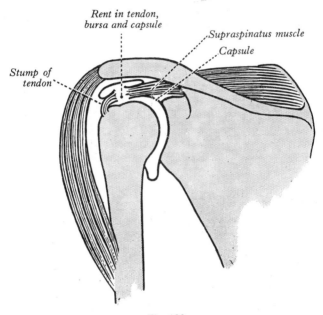

Fig. 123

Tear of supraspinatus shown diagrammatically. Note that the subacromial bursa communicates with the shoulder joint through the rent.

MAJOR TEARS. After a major tear of the cuff the action of the supraspinatus is lost. The clinical features are characteristic. The patient is unable to initiate abduction of the shoulder because the early phase of abduction demands the combined action of the supraspinatus (which stabilises the humeral head in the glenoid fossa)

---

[1] The *tendinous cuff* includes the supraspinatus tendon and the adjoining flat tendons that are blended with it—namely, the infraspinatus behind and the subscapularis in front. They form a cuff over the shoulder that has also been termed, inaccurately, the *rotator cuff*. Distally, the tendons forming the cuff blend with the capsule of the shoulder.

and the deltoid (which lifts the arm). But when the arm is raised passively to the right angle the patient can sustain abduction by deltoid action alone (Figs. 123–125). *Treatment:* When the patient is old operation should usually be avoided, because the degenerate nature of the tendon makes satisfactory repair impracticable. Even though untreated, some patients eventually regain the ability to abduct the arm by deltoid action alone. In younger patients operative repair is advised. It entails exposure of the tendon from above by

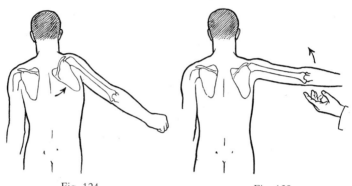

Fig. 124   Fig. 125

Complete tear of tendinous cuff (torn supraspinatus). Figure 124—Active abduction from the resting position is possible only by rotation of the scapula; there is no active abduction at the gleno-humeral joint, because the deltoid is unable to initiate abduction without the help of the supraspinatus. Figure 125—When the limb is raised passively beyond the horizontal abduction can be sustained actively by the deltoid.

splitting the acromion in the coronal plane, and re-attachment of the tendon by sutures through drill holes in the tuberosity of the humerus (Debeyre, Patte and Elmelik 1965). Thereafter a long course of supervised exercises may be required before a full range of active movement is restored.

MINOR TEARS. If the tendon is only strained the action of the supraspinatus is not lost. There is a full range of active shoulder movement, but there is pain during the mid-part of the range of abduction, caused by impingement of the damaged part of the tendon beneath the acromion or coraco-acromial ligament. A minor tear of the supraspinatus is thus one cause of the well known 'painful arc' syndrome (supraspinatus syndrome), for a full description of which the reader is referred to textbooks on orthopaedics. *Treatment* is conservative, by rest, short-wave diathermy, and graduated exercises.

FRACTURES OF THE HUMERUS

Classification
Fractures of the humerus may be classified into six groups (Fig. 126):
1) fracture of the neck of the humerus; 2) fracture of the greater
tuberosity; 3) fracture of the shaft; 4) supracondylar fracture; 5)
fractures of the condyles; and 6) fractures of the epicondyles.

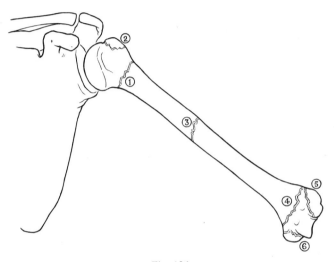

Fig. 126
Visual classification of fractures of the humerus. 1. Fracture of
neck of humerus. 2. Fracture of greater tuberosity. 3. Fracture of
shaft of humerus. 4. Supracondylar fracture of humerus. 5. Fracture
of condyle (usually lateral). 6. Fracture of epicondyle (usually
medial).

FRACTURE OF THE NECK OF THE HUMERUS
Fracture of the neck of the humerus occurs most often in elderly
women, in whom it is a common injury. In a high proportion of
such persons there is some degree of rarefaction of the skeleton, so
that the bones are relatively weak (Solomon 1977). The fracture is
usually caused by a fall on the limb. Displacement is variable: there
may be none; or there may be moderate or severe tilting of the head
fragment so that the shaft appears either abducted or adducted in
relation to it (Fig. 127). A notable feature is that in well over half the
cases the fragments are firmly impacted together so that the bone
moves as one piece. Impaction is important because it has a bearing on
treatment.

Diagnosis. The fracture may be easily overlooked if it is impacted, because the patient may be able to use the arm to some extent without severe pain. The possibility of a fracture should be suspected from the nature of the injury—especially when the patient is an elderly woman—and after a day or two from the appearance of extensive bruising in the upper and middle parts of the upper arm (Fig. 128). (The visible bruise tends to gravitate down the arm, and may extend almost to the elbow after a few days.)

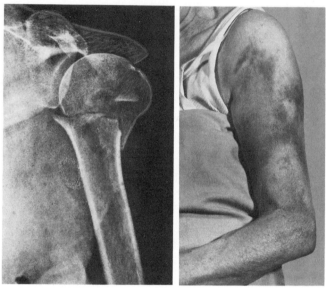

Fig. 127   Fig. 128

Figure 127—Fracture of neck of humerus with moderate displacement. Radiographs do not indicate with certainty whether such a fracture is impacted or not, but the matter is easily decided by clinical examination (see text). Figure 128—Photograph showing extensive bruising gravitating down the arm, a feature typical of these fractures.

Radiographs do not indicate with certainty whether or not the fracture is impacted. This can best be determined by clinical examination: if the limb can be handled and moved passively through a reasonable range without causing severe pain the fracture is impacted; if the slightest attempt to move the limb causes severe pain the fracture is not impacted.

Treatment. In a discussion on the best method of treatment of this injury three points should be borne constantly in mind: first, that even severe displacement is compatible with the restoration of excellent function; secondly, that it is often impossible to hold the fragments in normal relationship except by an extensive plaster or by operation; and thirdly, that the shoulder is prone to become stiff if it is immobilised for a long time, especially in old persons. In most cases, therefore, the most satisfactory method of treatment is that which permits early mobilisation of the shoulder, even if this means that an imperfect position of the fragments must be accepted.

Standard method. In the usually elderly victim of this injury displacement should be ignored and attention concentrated on the restoration of function. Whether or not immobilisation is necessary will depend upon the state of the fracture. *Impacted fractures:* If the fracture is impacted immobilisation is unnecessary. Active and assisted shoulder movements should be begun immediately and continued daily, the arm being carried in a sling in the intervals between treatment. *Unimpacted fractures:* If the fracture is not impacted, immediate shoulder exercises are impracticable because of the pain that movement causes. The arm should be supported in a sling, supplemented if necessary by a bandage to hold the arm to the chest wall. Elbow, wrist, and finger exercises should be practised from the beginning, but shoulder movements are deferred for three weeks. By that time the fragments are generally glued together sufficiently by granulation tissue to allow assisted shoulder exercises with little or no pain, and without fear of retarding union.

Alternative methods for special cases. Although a result adequate for an elderly patient can be achieved when even considerable displacement is left unreduced, in younger patients there is a place for deliberate reduction if the fragments are in poor position. Reduction can often be achieved by manipulation under anaesthesia, the distal (shaft) fragment being brought into line with the head fragment. To maintain reduction it is sometimes necessary to immobilise the limb in abduction in a plaster shoulder spica or on an abduction frame for four weeks.

Operative reduction is occasionally justified when it is impossible to secure a satisfactory reduction by manipulation. If operation is resorted to, internal fixation should be used to secure the fragments. The choice lies between a metal plate fixed with screws, or an intra-medullary nail driven up the bone from the olecranon fossa. In either case it may be difficult to secure rigid fixation because of the small size of the proximal fragment.

Complications. JOINT STIFFNESS. In old persons the shoulder is prone to become stiff after injuries in the vicinity of the joint, especially if it is immobilised for a long time. Hence it is important to get the shoulder moving by active or assisted exercises as soon as the condition of the fracture will allow. The sooner movements can be begun the less is the risk of serious stiffness.

NERVE INJURY. Occasionally a fracture of the neck of the humerus is complicated by injury to the axillary nerve, evidenced by the patient's inability to contract the deltoid muscle during attempted abduction of the shoulder, and by numbness or anaesthesia over a small area at the outer side of the upper arm. *Treatment* is expectant (p. 63).

DISLOCATION OF THE SHOULDER. Rarely the fracture is associated with dislocation of the shoulder. *Treatment:* The dislocation should be reduced first (if necessary by operation) and the fracture should then be treated along the usual lines.

JUXTA-EPIPHYSIAL FRACTURE-SEPARATION

In children the injury that corresponds to a fracture of the neck of the humerus is separation of the capital epiphysis at the epiphysial line, usually with detachment of a marginal fragment from the shaft (juxta-epiphysial fracture-separation). If there is severe displacement an attempt at reduction should be made, but if a perfect position cannot be restored the surgeon should be content with the best position that can be obtained. With the vigorous capacity for remodelling that accompanies bone growth in childhood, even severe displacement is effaced and the bone becomes almost indistinguishable from normal within a year or so (Aitken 1936).

FRACTURE OF THE GREATER TUBEROSITY OF THE HUMERUS

Fracture of the greater tuberosity is usually caused by a fall on the shoulder. It occurs in adults of any age, but particularly in old persons. Usually there is no marked displacement (Fig. 129), but the tuberosity may be comminuted. In a few cases a fragment of bone is lifted away from the tuberosity by the action of the attached muscles and is separated widely from its bed.

Treatment. The treatment depends on whether or not the tuberosity fragment is severely displaced. If it is not—as is usually the case—splintage is unnecessary and all that is needed is to arrange shoulder exercises to restore movement and function.

If a fragment of bone is avulsed and separated widely from its bed in the tuberosity the problem of treatment is more difficult. The displacement must be reduced and immobilisation must be provided. Adequate reduction can sometimes be effected by abducting the arm to a right angle and applying pressure over the displaced fragment. If this fails, operative replacement may be required. After manipulative or operative reduction, the limb may have to be immobilised in the abducted position in a plaster shoulder spica or on an abduction frame for three weeks. Thereafter shoulder exercises should be practised until satisfactory movement is restored.

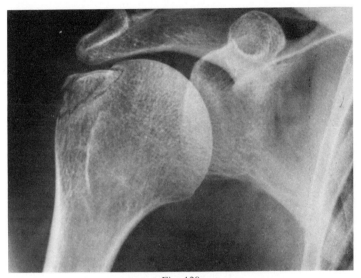

Fig. 129

Fracture of greater tuberosity of humerus. In this case there was no displacement of the fragment. Sometimes the fragment is avulsed from its bed and pulled upwards by the muscles attached to it.

Complications. PAINFUL ARC SYNDROME (supraspinatus syndrome). Thickening or irregularity of the greater tuberosity may interfere with free abduction at the gleno-humeral joint, because the thickened area may impinge against the acromion process or coraco-acromial ligament, with consequent pain. Impingement occurs mainly during the middle phase of abduction.

Treatment. In most cases the symptoms gradually subside under prolonged treatment by exercises, perhaps supplemented by short-wave diathermy. Exceptionally, if severe symptoms persist for many months, there is a place for excision of the acromion.

FRACTURE OF THE SHAFT OF THE HUMERUS

The shaft of the humerus is usually fractured in its middle third, either from an indirect twisting force (which causes a spiral fracture) or from direct violence (which causes a transverse, short oblique, or comminuted fracture). The fracture occurs in adults of any age, but seldom in children. Displacement is variable: there may be no loss of position, or there may be marked angulation or overlapping of the fragments (Fig. 130).

The proximal half of the humerus is a common site for pathological fracture from carcinomatous metastases (Fig. 131).

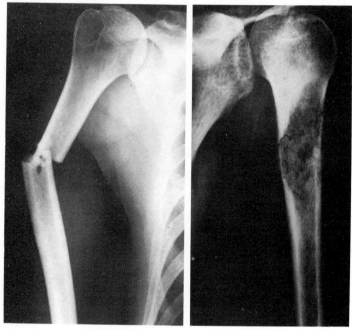

Fig. 130   Fig. 131

Figure 130—A typical fracture of the shaft of the humerus, of transverse type. Long oblique or spiral fractures are equally common. Figure 131—Pathological fracture of the humerus from a carcinomatous metastasis. This is a common site for metastatic deposits in the upper limb.

Treatment. Provided the alignment of the fragments is good it is unnecessary to secure perfect end-to-end apposition. Contact over a quarter or a third of the area of the fracture is sufficient. Nor is it usually necessary to enforce strict immobilisation, because most of these fractures unite readily with a minimum of external splintage.

Standard method. If displacement is greater than can be accepted reduction is carried out by manipulation under anaesthesia. A plaster is applied to maintain alignment of the fragments, but as a rule it need not give absolute immobility. Most surgeons rely upon a plaster cylinder encircling only the upper arm from the axilla to the elbow (Fig. 132). Some prefer to extend the plaster downwards to include the forearm, with the elbow flexed to a right angle (Fig. 133). In

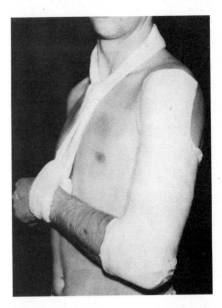

Fig. 132
Upper arm plaster, as commonly used for fractures of the shaft of the humerus—an alternative to that shown in Figure 133. The plaster grips the elbow but the forearm, supported by a sling, is free to rotate.

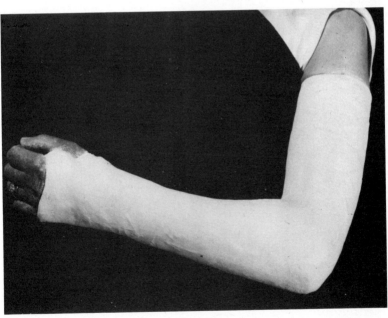

Fig. 133
Full length arm plaster with elbow flexed 90 degrees. This plaster is sometimes used for fractures of the shaft of the humerus. It is also the standard type of plaster for many injuries of the elbow and forearm.

either case further support is provided by a sling. Assisted shoulder exercises and active finger exercises should be practised under the supervision of a physiotherapist.

Alternative methods for special cases. When the fragments are very unstable a more positive method of fixation is required. If adequate closed reduction is possible one solution is to control the fragments by a plaster shoulder spica. This encloses the trunk and the whole upper limb with the exception of the fingers, the shoulder being held semi-abducted and the elbow flexed to a right angle. The alternative is to resort to internal fixation, and because of the rather severe discomfort that a cumbersome shoulder spica imposes on the patient this is often to be preferred so long as there is no special reason to avoid operation. Internal fixation may be effected by a plate and screws or, often better when the fracture is near the middle of the shaft, by a long intramedullary nail. The nail is preferably inserted from below, entering just above the olecranon fossa: insertion from above, through the greater tuberosity, may impair shoulder movement. Whenever possible nailing should be done 'closed'—that is, without exposing the fracture itself.

Complications. NERVE INJURY. Fracture of the shaft of the humerus may be complicated by injury to the radial nerve, which winds round the bone in close contact with it. The nerve injury is usually no more than a contusion, seldom a complete division. The effects of paralysis of the radial nerve in the upper arm are chiefly motor: there is paralysis of the extensor muscles of the wrist, fingers, and thumb ('wrist-drop'), and of the brachioradialis and the supinator. The only sensory change is a small area of anaesthesia or blunting of sensibility on the radial side of the back of the hand. *Treatment:* The principles of treatment of nerve injuries complicating fractures were considered in Chapter 4 (p. 63). In closed fractures it is assumed that the nerve is in continuity and spontaneous recovery is awaited. If re-innervation of the most proximal muscle has not occurred in the expected time, as calculated from the distance from the site of injury to the neuromuscular junction, the nerve should be explored. In most cases of injury to the radial nerve the prognosis is good. In neglected cases, or when efficient suture of a divided nerve is impracticable, function can be improved greatly by suitable tendon transfers. A satisfactory plan is as follows: the pronator teres is transferred to the extensor carpi radialis brevis; flexor carpi ulnaris or flexor carpi radialis is transferred to the extensor digitorum and extensor pollicis longus; and palmaris longus is transferred to the abductor pollicis longus.

NON-UNION. Although most fractures of the shaft of the humerus unite readily despite imperfect immobilisation, there are a few that are extremely obstinate and defy the ordinary methods of conservative treatment, no matter for how long they are continued. Indeed the mid-shaft of the humerus is recognised as a site of some of the most

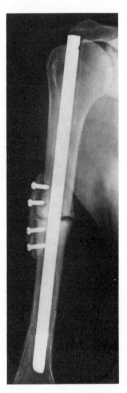

Fig. 134

Non-union of a fracture of the humerus for which operative treatment by intra-medullary nail and onlay bone graft was unsuccessful. Although most fractures of the humeral shaft unite readily a small proportion are extremely obstinate and may defy many attempts by operation to induce union.

resistant cases of non-union (Fig. 134). *Treatment:* If it is clear that union is not occurring with conservative treatment a bone-grafting operation should be advised. The fracture may be bridged by a slab graft of cortical bone from the tibia, fixed with four screws; or cancellous grafts of iliac bone may be combined with fixation by a long intramedullary nail.

SUPRACONDYLAR FRACTURE OF THE HUMERUS

Supracondylar fracture of the humerus is one of the commonest and most important fractures of childhood. It is seldom seen in adults. It should always be regarded as potentially dangerous because of the risk of injury to the brachial artery.

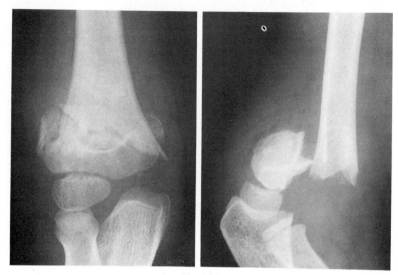

Fig. 135
Supracondylar fracture of the humerus in a child,
showing the typical displacement.

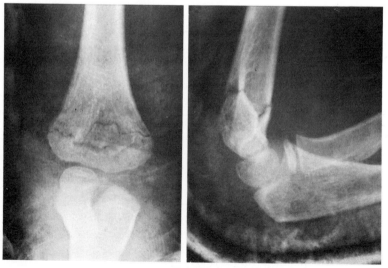

Fig. 136
The same elbow as shown in Figure 135, after
manipulative reduction of the displacement.

The injury occurs through a fall on the outstretched arm. Displacement, when it occurs, is characteristic: the lower fragment is displaced backwards and tilted backwards (Fig. 135).

Treatment. Undisplaced fractures in children require no more than three weeks' protection in plaster (Fig. 133). When the fragments are displaced manipulative reduction under anaesthesia should be undertaken (Fig. 136). The lower fragment is brought back into position by longitudinal traction on the limb and direct pressure behind the olecranon with the elbow flexed 90 degrees or more. Perfect anatomical reposition is not essential provided any lateral tilting of the lower fragment is corrected, for remodelling can gradually efface a moderate displacement as the bone grows (Attenborough 1953; Holdsworth 1954). After reduction the limb is immobilised in plaster with the elbow flexed a little more acutely than the right angle.

Precautions. A careful watch should be kept on the condition of the circulation in the forearm and hand. The plaster should be cut away at the radial side of the wrist to allow the surgeon to feel for the radial pulse.

Complications. The main importance of this fracture lies in the risk of damage to the brachial artery, a possibility that must always be borne in mind. Other complications include injury to the median nerve, and mal-union with consequent deformity.

ARTERIAL OCCLUSION. Injury to the brachial artery by the sharp upper fragment may lead to impairment of the circulation to the forearm and hand (Fig. 137). The artery may be severed or simply contused. If it is contused, its lumen may be occluded by thrombosis or by spasm of the vessel wall.

The effects of arterial occlusion at the elbow vary from case to case. In a small proportion the circulation is impaired so severely that gangrene of the digits ensues. More often, enough blood gets through the collateral vessels to keep the hand alive, but the flexor muscles of the forearm, and sometimes the peripheral nerve trunks, may suffer ischaemic changes. The affected muscles are replaced by fibrous tissue, which contracts and draws the wrist and fingers into flexion (Volkmann's ischaemic contracture) (Fig. 138). If the peripheral nerve trunks are also damaged by ischaemia there will be sensory and motor paralysis in the forearm and hand, which may be temporary or permanent according to the severity of the ischaemic damage.

Diagnosis. In the incipient stage vascular occlusion is suggested by signs of impaired circulation in the hand and fingers (see p. 23), and by the patient's inability to extend the fingers fully, with marked pain in the forearm if passive extension is attempted. In the established stage the diagnosis is clear from the history and the characteristic flexion contracture of wrist and fingers.

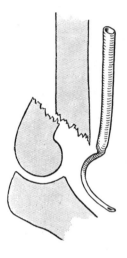

Fig. 137
To show how a supracondylar fracture of the humerus may damage the brachial artery, with risk of consequent ischaemia in the forearm and hand. Ischaemia may also be caused by over-tight plaster or dressings.

Treatment. In the **incipient stage** the problem is that of dealing with a sudden occlusion of the brachial artery. The case must be handled as an emergency, because the effects of the occlusion become irreversible after a few hours. The following action must be taken. *First step:* Any external splint or bandage that might be causing constriction is removed. Displacement of the fragments, if not already reduced, is corrected so far as possible by gentle manipulation. Heat cradles or hot bottles are applied over the other three limbs and trunk to promote general vasodilation. If these measures fail to bring about a return of adequate circulation within half an hour, the next step is taken. *Second step:* At operation the brachial artery is explored. If the occlusion is due to kinking or spasm of the artery an attempt is made to relieve it by freeing the vessel and applying papaverine. If this fails, the artery may be distended by the injection of saline between clamps. In the last resort, the artery may have to be opened and damaged intima removed, repair being effected thereafter with a vein patch.

In the **established stage** restoration to normal is impossible: reconstructive surgery at best can only improve what function remains. The choice of treatment depends upon the circumstances of each case. In mild cases acceptable function may be restored by intensive exercises guided by a physiotherapist. In more severe cases the muscle shortening has been counteracted by shortening of the forearm bones or by detachment and distal displacement of the flexor muscle origin (muscle slide operation). In selected cases with severe muscle infarction, however, the best results are probably obtained by

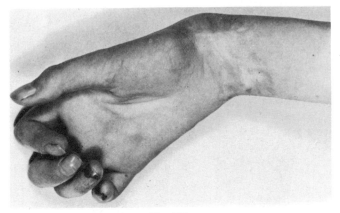

Fig. 138
Typical appearance of the hand in established
Volkmann's ischaemic contracture.

excision of the dead muscles and subsequent transfer of a healthy muscle (for example, a wrist flexor or a wrist extensor) to the tendons of flexor digitorum profundus and of flexor pollicis longus to restore active flexion of the digits (Seddon 1956). These muscle transfers may be combined, in appropriate cases, with arthrodesis of the wrist. When the median nerve is irreparably damaged by ischaemia nerve grafting is sometimes successful in restoring its function (Seddon 1976).

INJURY TO MEDIAN NERVE. The median nerve is occasionally injured by the protruding lower end of the proximal fragment. *Treatment* should be expectant at first, on the assumption that the lesion is no more than a neurapraxia (p. 63).

DEFORMITY FROM MAL-UNION. It has been mentioned already that in children it is not essential to restore perfect anatomical apposition of the fragments, because remodelling will gradually efface a moderate backward or lateral shift of the lower fragment. But an alteration of alignment cannot be corrected spontaneously: so if a fracture has been allowed to unite with appreciable tilting of the distal fragment there will be permanent deformity. The commonest deformity to be seen clinically is outward bowing at the site of fracture, causing cubitus varus (Fig. 139). *Treatment:* When the deformity is slight it can usually be accepted; but if the angulation is marked it may be corrected by osteotomy in the supracondylar region of the humerus (Fig. 140).

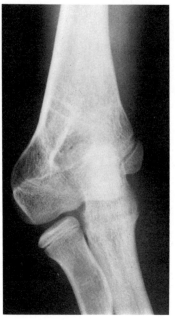 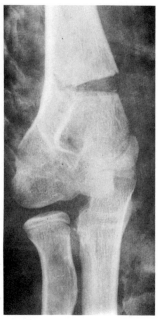

Fig. 139   Fig. 140

Figure 139—Cubitus varus after a supracondylar fracture of the humerus in which medial tilting of the lower fragment was left uncorrected. Figure 140—Radiograph after corrective osteotomy.

FRACTURES OF THE CONDYLES OF THE HUMERUS

Condylar fractures are relatively uncommon, but often troublesome. Like supracondylar fractures, they occur mainly in children. The usual cause is a fall. The lateral condyle is fractured much more commonly than the medial, and the description that follows relates mainly to injuries of the lateral condyle.

The usual lateral condylar fracture (fractured capitulum) extends obliquely upwards and laterally from the capitular surface. In young children the greater part of the detached fragment may be cartilaginous, so that the fragment appears much smaller as seen radiographically than it is in fact (Fig. 141). Displacement is seldom severe, but even moderate displacement is important because the fracture involves the joint surface.

Treatment. A simple crack fracture without displacement requires no more than a few weeks' protection in plaster, followed by a course of mobilising exercises for the elbow.

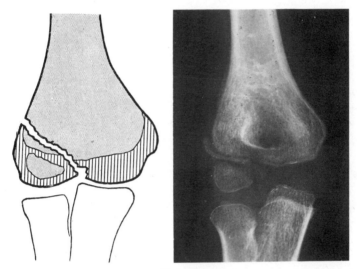

Fig. 141

Fracture of lateral condyle of humerus. In children (the usual victims of this injury) the lower end of the humerus is largely cartilaginous and therefore invisible in radiographs. What might appear from the radiographs to be a minor flake fracture in fact represents the injury shown in the diagram, with separation of a large fragment including the whole of the articular surface of the capitulum. Accurate reduction is essential.

Displaced fractures must be regarded seriously because they are potentially a cause of permanent disability. An attempt should be made first to reduce the displacement by manipulation under anaesthesia. If this is successful a plaster is applied with the elbow at 90 degrees and retained until union occurs. If manipulation fails to give perfect reduction operation is advised. The fracture is exposed and reduced under direct vision, and the condylar fragment is fixed in position, usually by a small screw introduced through the diaphysial part of the detached fragment.

Complications. Condylar fractures are prone to non-union, and may lead to deformity of the elbow and to osteoarthritis.

NON-UNION. The fracture line remains clearly visible and the condylar fragment—usually consisting of a large part of the capitulum—is displaced slightly upwards (Fig. 142). *Treatment:* If non-union is recognised before the elbow has become seriously disorganised by persistent displacement of the condylar fragment operation is advised. The fracture surfaces are freshened and brought accurately into position, and the condylar fragment is secured with autogenous bone pegs or a screw. In neglected cases with long-

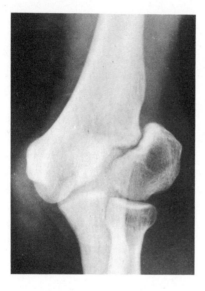

Fig. 142

Fracture of lateral condyle of humerus with persistent non-union eight years after the injury. The separated condyle (capitulum) is displaced slightly upwards.

established non-union the disability may have to be accepted. The elbow is already considerably disorganised and function is unlikely to be improved by late operation.

DEFORMITY. Deformity at the elbow may be caused by persistent upward displacement of the fractured condyle, or by retardation of epiphysial growth on the affected side from damage to the growing epiphysial cartilage. If the lateral condyle is affected the deformity will be that of cubitus valgus, whereas involvement of the medial condyle causes cubitus varus. In cases of cubitus valgus there is a risk of ulnar paralysis from friction neuritis where the nerve is angled behind the medial epicondyle. *Treatment:* If the deformity is slight it may be accepted; but if angulation is marked it should be corrected by supracondylar osteotomy of the humerus (Fig. 140). If symptoms of ulnar neuritis develop the nerve should be transposed from its post-epicondylar groove to a new bed in front of the elbow.

OSTEOARTHRITIS. Osteoarthritis is liable to occur when a condylar fracture leaves permanent deformity or irregularity of the articular surface. As a rule it does not become troublesome until several years after the original injury, and if the elbow is not subjected to heavy stress the arthritis may never cause serious disablement.

FRACTURES OF THE EPICONDYLES

Whereas most condylar fractures affect the lateral side, epicondylar fractures usually affect the medial (Fig. 143). The injury occurs rather more often in children than in adults. It may be caused by direct violence, but it is often an avulsion injury, the epicondyle being pulled off by the attached flexor muscles during a fall; this latter type is usually associated with dislocation or momentary subluxation of the elbow.

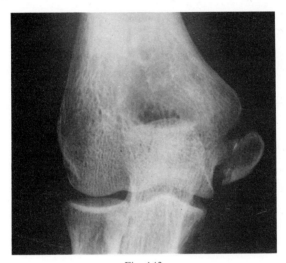

Fig. 143
Fracture of medial epicondyle of humerus. There was transient damage to the ulnar nerve.

Treatment. In an uncomplicated case only symptomatic treatment is required. Displacement is seldom severe and it need not be corrected. The elbow should be immobilised in plaster for three weeks to relieve pain, and thereafter joint movement should be restored by active exercises.

Complications. The important complications are: 1) inclusion of the medial epicondylar fragment in the joint; and 2) injury to the ulnar nerve.

INCLUSION OF EPICONDYLAR FRAGMENT IN THE JOINT. This complication occurs in children. The separated fragment of the medial epicondyle is 'sucked' into the joint cavity and may become jammed between the joint surfaces (Fig. 144). The fragment is not completely loose, however, for it retains its attachment to the forearm flexor muscles. *Treatment:* It is

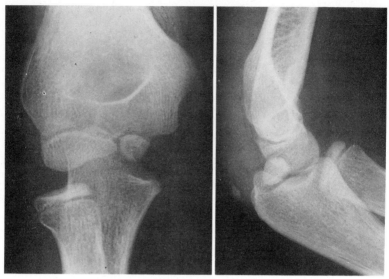

Fig. 144
Avulsion of medial epicondyle with inclusion of the fragment in the joint.
Operation was required to release the fragment.

imperative that the fragment be removed from the joint. Sometimes, with the patient anaesthetised, it may be extracted by extending fully the wrist and fingers to put the flexor muscles on the stretch, while the joint is widened at the medial side by abduction of the forearm and the negative pressure within the joint is released by the insertion of a hypodermic needle. If this manoeuvre fails operation is required. After the fragment has been extracted by operation it should be secured in the normal position by sutures through the overlying soft tissues.

INJURY TO THE ULNAR NERVE. The ulnar nerve is clearly in danger of immediate direct injury in displaced fractures of the medial epicondyle. It may also suffer gradual damage later from friction upon a roughened groove. *Treatment:* Whenever there is interference with the ulnar nerve at the elbow it should be transposed from its groove behind the medial epicondyle to a new bed in the soft tissues at the front of the elbow.

INJURIES OF THE ELBOW

DISLOCATION OF THE ELBOW

Dislocation of the elbow is usually caused by a heavy fall on the outstretched hand. It is a fairly common injury both in children and in adults.

Pathology. The dislocation is nearly always posterior or postero-lateral (Fig. 145). That is to say, the ulna and the radius are displaced backwards, or backwards and laterally, relative to the humerus. There may be an associated fracture of the coronoid process, or of the radial head, the capitulum or the medial epicondyle, but in most such cases the fracture is of a minor nature.

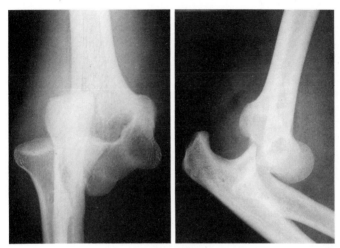

Fig. 145
Postero-lateral dislocation of the elbow in an adult.

Treatment. The dislocation should be reduced under anaesthesia as soon as possible. Reduction is usually easy: all that is necessary is to pull steadily upon the forearm with the elbow semi-flexed, while direct pressure is applied behind the olecranon. Reduction should be confirmed by radiographic examination as well as by clinical tests. Thereafter it is recommended that the elbow be rested in a plaster in 90 degrees of flexion for three weeks before mobilising exercises are begun. A plaster affords the best conditions for healing of the injury to the soft tissues, which is often extensive; furthermore, it allows greater freedom of movement at the shoulder and hand than does the collar-and-cuff sling that is so often prescribed for this injury.

Complications. VASCULAR OR NERVE INJURY. Occasionally the brachial artery or one of the major nerve trunks is damaged in a dislocation of the elbow. But when the severity of the displacement is considered it is remarkable how uncommon these complications are. *Treatment:* The treatment of injuries to the brachial artery was considered on page 138, and the treatment of closed nerve injuries on page 64.

JOINT STIFFNESS. The elbow is prone to troublesome stiffness after injury, and especially after dislocation. The stiffness is usually caused by intra-articular and peri-articular adhesions (p. 65), and it will gradually yield to active exercises, provided they are persevered with for long enough. Manipulation and passive stretching should be avoided.

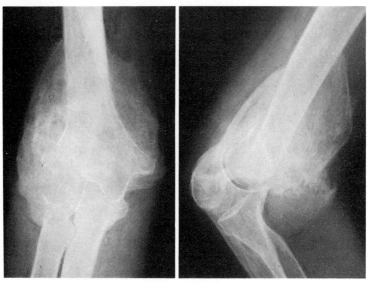

Fig. 146
Ossified haematoma (so-called myositis ossificans)
about the elbow after a fracture-dislocation.

A less common but more serious cause of stiffness is post-traumatic ossification (wrongly termed myositis ossificans), a condition in which new bone forms in the haematoma beneath the stripped-up periosteum and joint capsule (Fig. 146). The treatment of this complication was considered on page 68.

DISLOCATION OF THE HEAD OF THE RADIUS
Very occasionally the head of the radius may be dislocated forwards without any disturbance of the humero-ulnar relationship and without a fracture. The injury is probably caused by forced pronation (Evans 1949). Reduction should be attempted by supinating the forearm while direct pressure is applied over the displaced radial head.

Caution. It should be noted that dislocation of the head of the radius as an isolated injury is rare, and that it is more often associated with a fracture of the shaft of the ulna (Monteggia fracture, p. 154). Radiographic examination should always include the whole length of the ulna lest a fracture be overlooked.

The head of the radius is sometimes congenitally dislocated, in which case it tends to be somewhat globular and lacks the normal concavity of its upper articular surface. Care must be taken to avoid confusing this congenital deformity with a traumatic dislocation.

SUBLUXATION OF THE HEAD OF THE RADIUS
(*Pulled elbow*)

If a young child is lifted by the wrist the head of the radius may be pulled partly out of the annular ligament. This injury is sometimes termed 'pulled elbow'. There is local pain, and movements of the elbow are restricted. The displacement is easily reduced by pushing the forearm upwards and rotating it alternately into supination and pronation.

CONTUSION OR STRAIN OF THE ELBOW

In children an injury of the elbow may cause severe pain and limitation of movement even in the absence of bone injury or displacement. The lesion is probably a strain of the capsule or a contusion of the periosteum. The only treatment required is two weeks' rest in a plaster or sling, followed by active exercises. As in all elbow injuries, manipulation and passive stretching should be avoided.

References and bibliography, page 291.

CHAPTER 11

Forearm, wrist and hand

Injuries of the forearm, wrist and hand are without doubt those most commonly encountered in an accident unit. The hand in particular is so vital to man's ability to earn his living that tremendous resources have been expended in studying its intricate mechanism and function—an essential background to restorative surgery. Indeed, hand surgery is fast becoming a distinct speciality, demanding experience both of orthopaedic and of plastic surgery. In the United States of America there are already many surgeons who have dedicated their whole careers to the surgery of the hand, and a similar trend is becoming evident in Britain. Nevertheless, the management of fractures in the hand does not usually present undue difficulty so long as general orthopaedic principles are applied.

Classification
The injuries to be described may be classified as follows.

Fractures of the forearm bones
Fracture of the olecranon process
Fracture of the coronoid process
Fracture of the head of the radius
Fracture of the upper end of the ulna with dislocation of the head of the radius
Fractures of the shafts of the forearm bones
Fracture of the shaft of the radius with dislocation of the inferior radio-ulnar joint
Fracture of the lower end of the radius
Fracture of lower end of radius with anterior displacement
Fracture-separation of lower radial epiphysis

Injuries of the carpus
Dislocations of the carpal bones
Fracture of the scaphoid bone
Fractures of other carpal bones

Injuries of the metacarpal bones and phalanges
Fracture of the base of the first metacarpal
Other fractures of the metacarpal bones
Fractures of the phalanges
Dislocation of the metacarpo-phalangeal and interphalangeal joints
Strains of the interphalangeal joints

FRACTURES OF THE FOREARM BONES

Classification
The injuries to be considered in this section are classified visually in Figure 147.

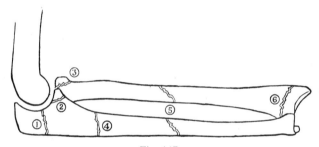

Fig. 147

Visual classification of fractures of the forearm bones. 1. Fracture of olecranon process. 2. Fracture of coronoid process. 3. Fracture of head of radius. 4. Fracture of uppermost third of ulna with dislocation of head of radius. 5. Fractures of radius and ulna (separately or together). 6. Fracture of lower end of radius.

FRACTURE OF THE OLECRANON PROCESS
The olecranon is fractured by a fall on the point of the elbow, usually in an adult. The fracture may take three forms (Fig. 148): it may be a crack without displacement; it may be a clean break with separation of the two fragments; or it may be a comminuted fracture. The fracture line nearly always enters the joint near the middle of the trochlear notch.

Treatment. The treatment depends upon the type of fracture, and will be considered in relation to the three types mentioned above.

CRACK FRACTURE. The only treatment necessary is to protect the elbow by a plaster for two or three weeks. It is unnecessary to apply the plaster with the elbow fully extended; the joint may safely be flexed to a right angle without fear of distracting the fragments, which are held together by the surrounding aponeurosis. The right-angled position is more comfortable for the patient and it allows functional activity of the hand and fingers.

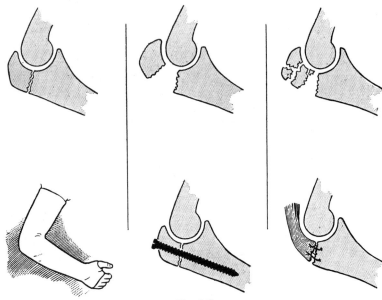

Fig. 148

Fractures of the olecranon and their treatment. The diagrams in the upper row show the three types of fracture, and those below depict the treatment for each type. 1. Crack without displacement. *Treatment:* Rest in plaster. 2. Clean break with separation. *Treatment:* Open reduction and fixation by screw. 3. Comminuted fracture. *Treatment:* Excision of fragments and re-attachment of triceps.

CLEAN FRACTURE WITH SEPARATION. It is impracticable to gain and hold perfect reduction by closed methods; so operation should be advised. The fragments are exposed and fitted together accurately under direct vision, with care to ensure that the articular surface is perfectly smooth. Rigid fixation is attained by a long coarse-threaded screw passed down the bone from the upper surface of the olecranon (Fig. 148). After operation the elbow should be protected in plaster for three weeks before mobilising exercises are begun.

COMMINUTED FRACTURE. Perfect replacement and fixation of the fragments are impracticable. The correct treatment for this type is to excise the olecranon fragments by dissecting them out from the aponeurosis that forms the insertion of the triceps, and to secure the triceps to the stump of the ulna by strong sutures passed through small drill holes in the bone. After operation the elbow is protected in plaster for three weeks and thereafter mobilised by active exercises.

Complications. These are: 1) non-union; and 2) osteoarthritis.

NON-UNION. Olecranon fractures usually fail to unite by bone if a gap is allowed to remain between the fragments. The gap is bridged by fibrous tissue, so the continuity of the triceps is restored. Nevertheless the power of extension is weakened. *Treatment:* In old patients the disability can usually be accepted. In younger persons it may be advisable to excise the scar tissue, freshen the fracture surfaces, and secure the fragments in close apposition by a long screw.

OSTEOARTHRITIS. Osteoarthritis may develop some years after the injury if the articular surface of the olecranon is left roughened or 'stepped'. It is unlikely to become severe unless the arm is used for heavy work.

FRACTURE OF THE CORONOID PROCESS

The coronoid process is seldom fractured except in association with posterior dislocation of the elbow. Marked displacement is prevented by the strong aponeurotic fibres that invest the bone. No special treatment is needed other than that for the associated dislocation.

FRACTURE OF THE HEAD OF THE RADIUS

Fracture of the head of the radius is one of the commonest fractures of the upper limb in young adults. It is caused by a fall on the outstretched hand, the force being transmitted axially along the shaft of the radius. In more than half the cases the fracture is no more than a crack without displacement (Fig. 149): in most of the remainder a segment of the disc-shaped radial head is broken away and depressed below the plane of the articular surface (Fig. 150). Sometimes the whole of the head is extensively comminuted. The cartilage covering the articular surface is often badly bruised, as is also the articular cartilage of the capitulum—a feature that is not evident from the radiographs.

Diagnosis. A fracture of the head of the radius is easily overlooked because it is sometimes not immediately obvious in the radiographs. Features that should suggest the true nature of the injury are a history of a fall on the outstretched arm, with marked local tenderness on palpation over the head of the radius, impaired movement at the elbow, and sharp pain at the lateral side of the joint at the extremes of rotation. If in the presence of these symptoms and signs a fracture is not seen in the initial radiographs further films should be obtained to show the radial head in different positions of rotation.

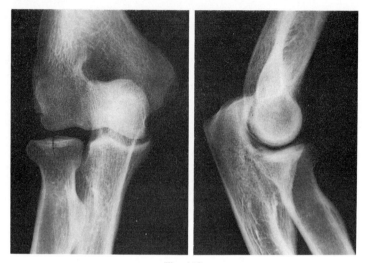

Fig. 149

Fracture of head of radius without displacement. Note the vertical crack extending downwards from the articular surface. Rest in plaster is the only treatment required. In these minor injuries the fracture line is often ill-defined and it may easily be overlooked.

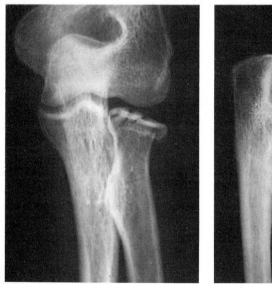

Fig. 150   Fig. 151

Figure 150—Fracture of head of radius with comminution. Figure 151— After excision of head of radius. In severe injuries of this type excision of the radial head gives more reliable results than conservative treatment.

Treatment. The treatment required depends upon the severity of the damage to the radial head.

Slight damage. If radiographs suggest that the radial head has been only slightly damaged, and that after union has occurred the articular surface will be reasonably smooth, conservative treatment is recommended (Fig. 149). A plaster is applied with the elbow at a right angle and with the forearm midway between pronation and supination (Fig. 133). The plaster is worn for three weeks, after which active mobilising exercises are arranged. A plaster is to be preferred to the more usual collar-and-cuff sling, because it is more effective in relieving pain and allows freer use of the shoulder and hand.

Severe damage. If the radial head is severely comminuted, with inevitable permanent distortion of the articular surface, operation should be advised (Figs. 150 and 151). The entire head of the radius should be excised. After operation the elbow is rested in plaster for two weeks before active mobilising exercises are begun.

In children the fracture is usually through the neck of the radius, with tilting of the radial head. Reduction is achieved by manipulation or if necessary by operation. Excision of the head should never be advised in children, because as growth occurs the radius is liable to ride up towards the humerus, with consequent disturbance of its relationship to the ulna.

Complications. Complications are infrequent: usually the function of the elbow is restored to normal or almost so. Occasional complications are: 1) joint stiffness; and 2) osteoarthritis.

JOINT STIFFNESS. The range of flexion-extension and of rotation movement at the elbow may be impaired for a long time after a badly comminuted fracture even when it has been treated promptly by excision of the radial head. In most cases the stiffness yields slowly but surely to active exercises if they are carried out with sufficient perseverance. It should be remembered that the elbow is a joint that does not tolerate manipulation or forced passive movements. Indeed recovery may be retarded rather than hastened by the injudicious use of force in an attempt to increase the range, especially in children.

OSTEOARTHRITIS. If the articular surface of the radial head is left roughened and irregular, wear and tear of the joint will be accelerated and osteoarthritis may supervene. It is partly to forestall this complication that excision of the radial head is recommended in cases of severely comminuted fracture. *Treatment:* In the early stage, when arthritis is incipient rather than established, timely excision of the radial head may delay its progress. When osteoarthritis is established excision of the radial head cannot be expected to bring full relief.

FRACTURE OF THE UPPER END OF THE ULNA WITH DISLOCATION OF THE HEAD OF THE RADIUS

This injury is often termed a Monteggia[1] fracture-dislocation. It is usually caused by a fall associated with forced pronation of the forearm; but a similar injury may be caused by a direct blow on the back of the upper forearm. The usual displacement is characteristic: the ulna is angled forwards and the head of the radius is dislocated forwards (Fig. 152). Much more rarely, the reverse deformity occurs.

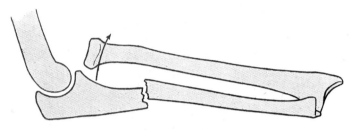

Fig. 152

The Monteggia fracture-dislocation, a combination of fracture of the upper half of the ulna with dislocation of the head of the radius. The displacement is usually forwards, as shown here, but the reverse deformity may occur.

Treatment. In this fracture accurate reduction is essential. It is seldom possible to reduce both the dislocation and the fracture by closed methods, but an attempt should be made to do so by manipulation with full supination of the forearm. If this succeeds a plaster should be applied with the elbow at a right angle and the forearm supinated. The plaster is retained until union occurs—usually a matter of about twelve weeks.

More often closed reduction is imperfect, or redisplacement occurs in the plaster: operation is then required. The head of the radius is first replaced within the annular ligament; or in late neglected cases it may be excised. At the same operation, but through a separate incision, the ulnar fracture is reduced and fixed internally either by a plate with screws or by a long intramedullary nail introduced through the olecranon. After operation the limb is protected in a plaster until union occurs.

FRACTURES OF THE SHAFTS OF THE FOREARM BONES

A fracture may involve either the radius alone or the ulna alone, or both bones may be fractured. These injuries will be considered together because similar principles of treatment apply to them all.

[1] Monteggia, an Italian surgeon, described the injury in 1814.

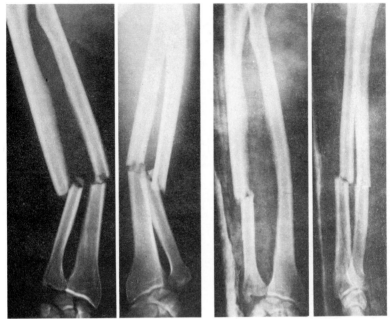

Fig. 153   Fig. 154

Figure 153—A typical fracture of both bones of the forearm, with marked displacement. Figure 154—After manipulative reduction and immobilisation in plaster. Though successful in this case, manipulation often fails to restore an acceptable position, and operative reduction will then be required.

The cause may be either an indirect force such as a fall on the hand, or a direct blow upon the forearm. Displacement may be absent or slight, but these fractures are notoriously prone to severe displacement which is often very difficult to correct without open operation (Fig. 153). In general, displacement is more frequent and more severe in adults than in children, who often sustain no more than a greenstick fracture with minor angulation.

Treatment. In fractures of the forearm bones accurate reduction is important because even slight displacement may disturb the relationship between radius and ulna, with consequent impairment of rotation, and with subluxation of the inferior radio-ulnar joint.

Conservative treatment. It is worth while first to attempt manipulative reduction under anaesthesia, and if this is successful a full-length arm plaster is applied with the elbow at a right angle and the forearm in a position midway between pronation and supination (Figs. 133 and 154). Check radiographs should be taken weekly for the first three weeks to ensure that redisplacement within the plaster does not go undetected. The plaster is retained until union occurs—usually a matter of ten or twelve weeks in an adult.

Operative treatment. In a high proportion of cases, especially in adults, it is impossible to obtain satisfactory reduction by manipulation, or to maintain reduction by splintage in plaster. Failure is almost inevitable when the plane of the fractures is oblique or spiral. In these cases operative reduction and internal fixation are required.

The fracture is exposed and the fragments are fitted together accurately under direct vision. If both the radius and the ulna are injured they should be approached through separate incisions. Internal fixation is effected usually by a metal plate held by four screws, two in each fragment. An alternative method is to use a long intramedullary nail. The ulna lends itself well to this method because the olecranon process offers a convenient place for the introduction of the nail. After the operation the limb should usually be protected by a full-length plaster with the elbow at a right angle until union occurs, to prevent rotatory strains. Thereafter a course of active mobilising exercises is arranged.

From time to time attempts have been made to fix the fragments so rigidly by strong plates or by intramedullary nails that external protection by plaster may be dispensed with (Hicks 1961). But this is not always practicable, and the surgeon must judge each case on its merits in deciding whether or not a plaster is necessary. As a general rule the author prefers to have the safeguard of a plaster, especially for the first few weeks.

Complications. As with any bone that lies superficially beneath the skin there is a risk of infection from contamination of an open fracture. Another possibility that must always be borne in mind is arterial occlusion from soft-tissue swelling within a rigid plaster (p. 61). Complications that are seen more often are delayed union, non-union, and mal-union.

DELAYED UNION AND NON-UNION. Fractures of the shafts of the forearm bones are prone to delayed union or non-union, and this applies particularly to the ulna near the junction of its middle and lowest thirds (Fig. 155). In most cases the cause is believed to be either impairment of the blood supply to one of the fragments, or imperfect immobilisation with consequent rotatory shearing movement between the fragments. *Treatment:* Most cases of delayed union or non-union of the forearm bones lend themselves well to bone-grafting operations. If the fragments remain in good position and

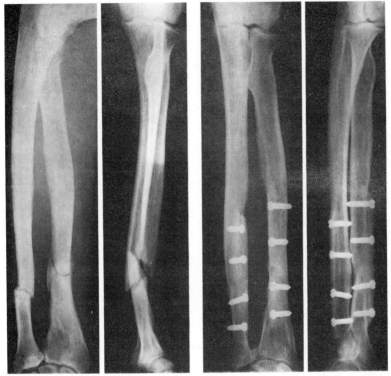

Fig. 155   Fig. 156

Delayed union of fractures of radius and ulna. Figure 155—Both fractures ununited five months after injury. Figure 156—Sound consolidation of the fractures four months after onlay bone grafting.

alignment it may be sufficient to lay slivers of cancellous bone from the ilium under the periosteum without disturbing the fracture itself (Phemister graft; see p. 57). But if the position of the fragments is imperfect the fracture surfaces should be cleared of fibrous tissue, full reduction should be obtained under direct vision, and the fracture should be bridged by a cortical slab graft (usually obtained from the tibia) held rigidly by four screws (Fig. 156). Alternatively—and especially in the ulna—fixation by a long intramedullary nail may be combined with grafting by cancellous bone slivers. When both bones are ununited they should each be grafted at the same operation through separate incisions. After operation a full-length plaster should be worn until union occurs.

When non-union occurs in a fracture of the ulna within five centimetres of its lower end bone grafting is unnecessary, because good results can be secured simply by excising the short distal fragment of the ulna. (If the radius is also ununited the excised piece of ulna may sometimes be used as a graft for the radius.)

MAL-UNION. It has been emphasised already that without operation it is often difficult or impossible to secure accurate coaptation of the fragments in fractures of the forearm bones. If an imperfect position is accepted there is a risk of impaired function of the forearm and wrist; and the more severe the mal-position the more likely it is to cause trouble.

Impairment of function may arise in three ways: it may be caused by angulation of the fragments, by relative shortening of one of the bones, or occasionally by cross union between the radius and ulna. Angulation of the radius or ulna, or of both bones, can produce a mechanical block to rotation beyond a certain limited range. Cross union between the two bones, of course, prevents rotation altogether. Shortening of one of the two bones, or unequal shortening of both bones, leads to subluxation at the inferior radio-ulnar joint, with consequent pain and restriction of movement.

Treatment. In many cases slight or moderate disability from mal-union can be accepted. Only occasionally is it justifiable to reproduce the fracture at operation in order to restore correct apposition and alignment. Pain and stiffness from subluxation of the inferior radio-ulnar joint may be relieved by excising the lower end of the ulna (Figs. 168–169).

FRACTURE OF SHAFT OF RADIUS WITH DISLOCATION OF INFERIOR RADIO-ULNAR JOINT

In this injury, often referred to as the Galeazzi[1] fracture-dislocation, the shaft of the radius is fractured near the junction of its middle and lowest thirds, the ligaments of the inferior radio-ulnar joint are ruptured and the head of the ulna is displaced from the ulnar notch of the radius. The fragments of the radius are usually tilted medially towards the ulna (Fig. 157). The head of the ulna may be shifted medially, anteriorly or posteriorly. The injury is analogous to the Monteggia fracture-dislocation in the upper part of the forearm (p. 154): it is said to be more common than the Monteggia injury. The cause is usually a fall on to the hand.

Treatment. Perfect reduction is essential for restoration of full function. Only occasionally—and then usually in children—can adequate reduction be gained and maintained by conservative methods. In adults redisplacement is common after reduction by manual traction and supination; so resort must usually be had to operative reduction and internal fixation of

---

[1] Riccardo Galeazzi of Milan published a full description of this injury in 1935. The injury had been recognised long before that but had been referred to only briefly in published work.

the radial fracture, preferably by a metal plate with screws. Once the radius has been secured in anatomical position, stable reduction of the inferior radio-ulnar dislocation is usually achieved without difficulty. The position

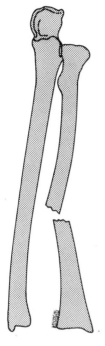

Fig. 157
The Galeazzi fracture-dislocation, a combination of fracture of the shaft of the radius with dislocation of the inferior radio-ulnar joint.

is held by a full length arm plaster with the elbow flexed to the right angle and the forearm supinated: the plaster is retained until union occurs.

FRACTURE OF THE LOWER END OF THE RADIUS
(Colles's fracture)

The Colles's[1] fracture is seen more often than any other injury in fracture clinics in civilian practice. It is not the commonest fracture at all ages—indeed it occurs rather infrequently in young adults—but it is certainly the commonest fracture in persons over forty years of age, and especially in women. It is nearly always caused by a fall on the outstretched hand.

The typical deformity. In a few cases there is simply a crack without displacement, but in the great majority the fracture and the

---

[1] Abraham Colles, a Dublin surgeon, published a report *On Fracture of the Carpal Extremity of the Radius* in 1814. It should be remembered that at that time x-rays were not available, and it is probable that the injury, though often seen, had previously been confused with dislocation of the wrist.

displacement are characteristic. The fracture occurs transversely about two centimetres above the lower articular surface of the radius. The lower fragment is displaced slightly backwards and laterally and is tilted backwards so that the articular surface, instead of pointing downwards and slightly forwards as in the normal wrist, is directed

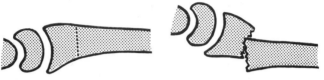

Fig. 158

The typical displacement in Colles's fracture. The distal fragment of the radius is tilted backwards so that the articular surface is directed downwards and backwards instead of downwards and slightly forwards as in the normal state. The distal fragment is often also shifted backwards, as depicted here. The normal state is shown for comparison.

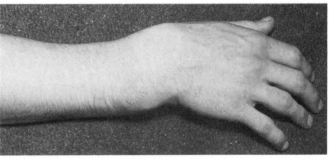

Fig. 159

Typical deformity from displaced fracture of the lower end of the radius (Colles's fracture).

downwards and backwards (Figs. 158–160). The lower fragment is also driven upwards and impacted into the upper fragment. Sometimes a vertical extension from the main transverse fracture enters the wrist joint. The styloid process of the ulna is commonly detached, but not always.

This typical displacement is reflected in a characteristic clinical appearance that has been termed the 'dinner-fork' deformity (Fig. 159). There is a dorsal hollow or depression in the lowest third of the forearm (proximal to the fracture), but immediately below this there

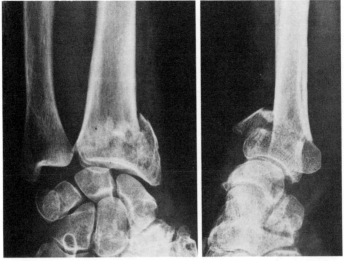

Fig. 160
A typical fracture of lower end of radius. Note the backward displacement and backward tilt of the lower fragment, whose articular surface now points downwards and backwards.

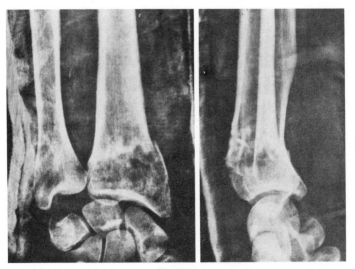

Fig. 161
The fracture seen through plaster after manipulative reduction. Normal alignment restored. Note in the lateral radiograph that the articular surface of the radius is directed downwards and slightly forwards.

is a marked prominence caused by the lower fragment's being displaced backwards, carrying with it the whole of the carpus and hand. Anteriorly there is a fullness where the soft tissues are stretched over the forward-projecting upper fragment.

Reversed deformity. In a small proportion of fractures of the lower end of the radius the deformity is the reverse of that just described. That is, the lower fragment is displaced forwards and rotated forwards so that the articular surface is directed too far anteriorly. This variation is described separately on page 169.

Treatment. In displaced fractures the standard method of treatment is to undertake manipulative reduction under anaesthesia and to immobilise the forearm and wrist in a below-elbow plaster. In effecting the reduction the fragments must first be disimpacted and the bone drawn out to full length; the distal fragment can then be repositioned accurately by firm pressure over its dorsal surface (Fig. 161).

Technique of reduction. The muscles of the forearm should be relaxed, either by general anaesthesia (supplemented if necessary by a relaxant) or by regional anaesthesia. The first step is to disimpact the fragments, which have often been driven together firmly in the position of deformity. Disimpaction is achieved by firm longitudinal traction upon the hand and thumb, against the counter-traction of an assistant who grips the arm above the flexed elbow (Fig. 162). When the fragments have been disimpacted, their mobility can be demonstrated by grasping the distal fragment between the finger and thumb of one hand and the proximal fragment likewise with the other hand. Reposition of the distal fragment may then be achieved by firm forward pressure (best applied by the thenar eminence) over the distal fragment, with counter-pressure (directed backwards) against the proximal fragment just above the fracture. This key manoeuvre is illustrated in Figure 163. After reduction a plaster is applied with the wrist in the neutral position, and while it is setting the 'thenar grip' manoeuvre is repeated to mould the plaster snugly to the bones as a safeguard against redisplacement.

Immobilisation. The type of plaster depends upon individual preference. Two variations are in common use: the complete encircling plaster and the dorsal plaster slab. The complete encircling plaster is shown in Figure 164. The dorsal plaster slab covers only three-quarters of the circumference of the limb—namely, the dorsum and the medial and lateral sides (Fig. 165): the front of the limb is left uncovered by plaster. The slab is held in position by cotton bandages. Theoretical advantages of the incomplete dorsal slab are that it may be more easily loosened if serious swelling should occur, and that it can be tightened down repeatedly by re-applying the cotton bandage as the swelling subsides. In practice, however, there is probably little to choose between the two methods.

In the management of a Colles's fracture it is important that the position of the fragments be checked by radiography a week after the

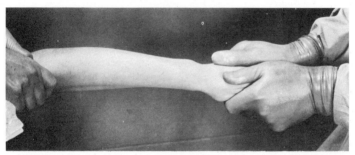

Fig. 162

First step in the reduction of a fracture of the lower end of the radius with backward tilting of the distal fragment: traction is being applied to disimpact the fragments

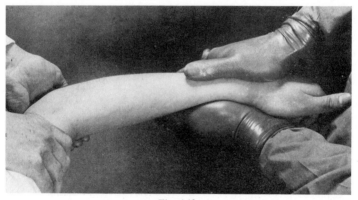

Fig. 163

The 'thenar grip' recommended for correcting the backward displacement and tilting of the distal fragment of the radius. Note the position of the surgeon's hands: the thenar eminence of one hand is placed over the distal fragment to press it forwards against the counter-pressure of the other thenar eminence upon the shaft of the radius just above the fracture. It will be found easiest to use the right hand to control the distal fragment when the fracture involves the left radius (as shown here), and the left hand in a fracture of the right radius.

initial reduction and again after a further week, because there is a risk of redisplacement in the early days despite immobilisation in plaster. If the check radiographs show that redisplacement has occurred, further manipulative reduction under anaesthesia should be advised. Usually it is impossible to correct a redisplacement by manipulation if it has been allowed to persist for more than two weeks; so it is important to ensure that any redisplacement is detected early.

While the limb is in plaster the patient should be encouraged to use the hand freely for everyday activities, and deliberate exercises should be carried out for the fingers, elbow, and shoulder.

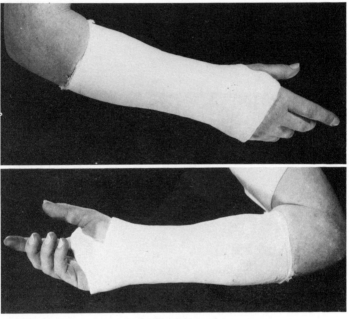

Fig. 164

Plaster used for fractures of lower end of radius. The wrist is in a neutral position. The plaster is moulded closely to grip the lower fragment. The palm is left free beyond the proximal transverse skin crease, to allow full flexion at the metacarpo-phalangeal joints.

The plaster should be retained usually for six weeks, though it may be discarded earlier in undisplaced crack fractures. Although union is far from consolidated at six weeks, it is firm enough to ensure that no further displacement will occur, because the leverage acting through the short lower fragment is slight. After the plaster has been removed a course of mobilising and muscle-strengthening exercises for the wrist and fingers should be arranged.

Complications. Most patients progress rapidly towards full recovery of function, and complications are infrequent considering the large number of these fractures that are treated every day. Nevertheless the incidence of mal-union is disconcertingly high. Other complications that are seen occasionally are subluxation of the inferior radio-ulnar joint, stiffness of the fingers or shoulder from neglected use, rupture of the tendon of extensor pollicis longus, and Sudeck's atrophy of the bones of the wrist and hand.

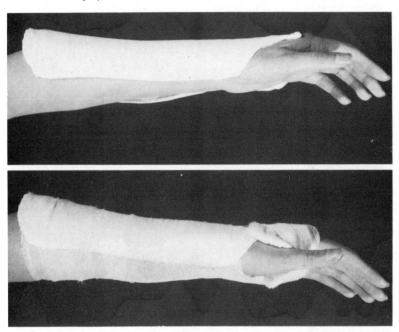

Fig. 165

Dorsal plaster slab, an alternative method of immobilisation for fracture of the lower end of the radius. The slab covers the dorsum and sides of the forearm and wrist. It is secured firmly in position with cotton bandages. The fingers and thumb must be left free so that the hand may be used.

MAL-UNION. It has been mentioned already that redisplacement of the fragments is liable to occur despite immobilisation in plaster, especially in the first week after reduction. If redisplacement is not detected the fragments will unite in the deformed position—that is, with backward displacement and backward tilting of the distal fragment (Fig. 166). This is associated with a rather ugly clinical deformity, and function of the wrist is impaired. *Treatment:* Each case must be considered on its merits. Often the disability is slight and can be accepted. But if the deformity is severe and function considerably impaired operation should usually be advised, unless the

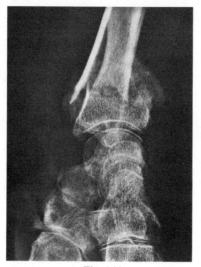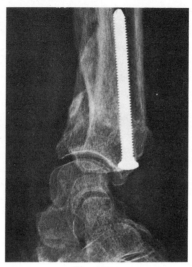

Fig. 166   Fig. 167

Mal-union of a fracture of the lower end of the radius corrected by operation. Figure 166—Five weeks after injury: marked backward displacement and backward tilt of lower fragment. Figure 167—Three months after operative reduction and fixation by a screw.

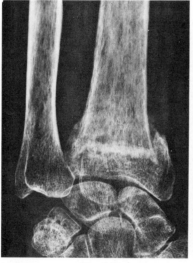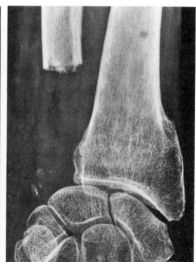

Fig. 168   Fig. 169

Figure 168—Subluxation of inferior radio-ulnar joint after fracture of lower end of radius. There was pain over the joint, the head of the ulna was prominent, and rotation of the forearm was impaired. Figure 169—After excision of lower end of ulna.

patient is very old. The fracture site is exposed through a dorsal incision and the bone is divided with an osteotome. The lower fragment is realigned in normal position and fixed with a screw, a staple, or a small bone graft (Fig. 167). Thereafter the wrist is immobilised in plaster until union occurs.

SUBLUXATION OF THE INFERIOR RADIO-ULNAR JOINT. This complication is caused by persistent upward displacement of the distal fragment of the radius, which is thus slightly shortened while the ulna remains of normal length. Clinically, there is pain in the region of the radio-ulnar joint, especially during active use of the wrist. The head of the ulna is unduly prominent at the back of the wrist, and it lies on a level with, or even below, the tip of the radial styloid process, whereas normally it lies above the level of the radial styloid (Fig. 168). Wrist movements are impaired, especially adduction (ulnar deviation) and rotation. *Treatment:* A minor degree of subluxation may be accepted without treatment, especially in an old person. But if the disability is troublesome operation should be advised. A simple and reliable method is to excise the lower end of the ulna, including its head and about three centimetres of the shaft (Fig. 169).

SUDECK'S POST-TRAUMATIC OSTEODYSTROPHY. Sudeck's osteodystrophy (Sudeck's atrophy) was described on page 68. It is an ill-understood condition in which the hand and fingers become markedly swollen, so that the overlying skin is stretched and glossy, and the joints become stiff. It seems to be distinct from the ordinary stiffness that may arise from disuse. A Colles's fracture is one of the commonest causes of Sudeck's atrophy in the upper limb, but the incidence of the complication is nevertheless small. Most patients eventually do well with conservative treatment by elevation and intensive active exercises, provided these are carried out with sufficient perseverance, though full recovery may take several months.

STIFFNESS OF FINGERS OR SHOULDER. If while the wrist is in plaster the patient is encouraged to use the hand and is supervised in appropriate exercises for the fingers and shoulder, stiffness from disuse will be avoided; but if the hand and shoulder are not exercised there is a serious risk of stiffness, especially in an old person.

RUPTURE OF EXTENSOR POLLICIS LONGUS. The tendon of the extensor pollicis longus sometimes ruptures spontaneously without a preceding injury to the wrist; but the accident is much more frequent after a fracture of the lower end of the radius. The tendon is more liable to give way than its neighbours because it takes a sharp bend laterally as it leaves its groove on the back of the lower end of the radius: it therefore bears heavily against the bone as it glides to and fro with movements of the thumb. Rupture is preceded by fraying of the tendon over a length of one or two centimetres. The fracture of the lower end of the radius is not necessarily severe: indeed the tendon seems to rupture more often after a minor crack fracture than after a major fracture with marked displacement.

Clinical features. The usual interval between fracture of the radius and rupture of the tendon is four to eight weeks. Thus the symptons may develop either while the wrist is still immobilised in plaster or soon after the plaster has been removed. In some cases the patient feels something give way at the back of the wrist, and notices immediately that she is unable to extend the thumb. In other cases the onset is less dramatic, the first thing to call attention to the rupture being difficulty in using the thumb. On

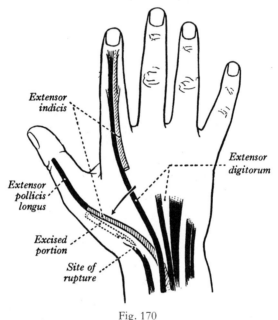

Fig. 170

Transfer of extensor indicis to replace a ruptured extensor pollicis longus. This transfer is to be preferred to direct suture when the ends of the ruptured tendon are frayed.

examination there is a full range of passive movement at the thumb joints, but active extension at the interphalangeal joint is impossible and active extension at the metacarpo-phalangeal joint is greatly impaired. If the plaster has been removed there may be slight local discomfort or tenderness on palpation over the course of the tendon over the lower end of the radius.

Treatment. Operation should be advised. Because of the extensive fraying of the tendon it is unsatisfactory to attempt end-to-end suture of the torn ends. The most reliable method is to transfer the tendon of extensor indicis to activate the distal stump of the extensor pollicis longus. The tendon of extensor indicis is divided opposite the neck of the index metacarpal, re-routed in the direction of the extensor pollicis longus, and sutured to the distal stump of the extensor pollicis longus at about the level of the base of the first metacarpal (Fig. 170). The loss of the extensor indicis does not noticeably impair extension of the index finger.

FRACTURE OF LOWER END OF RADIUS WITH ANTERIOR DISPLACEMENT
(Smith's fracture; Barton's fracture)

As already mentioned (p. 162), in a small proportion of cases fracture of the lower end of the radius is associated not with the typical posterior displacement and posterior tilting of the distal fragment that characterise the Colles's fracture, but with the reverse deformity: the distal fragment is displaced forwards and tilted forwards (Fig. 171). This injury is often termed Smith's[1] or Barton's fracture or, loosely, reversed Colles's fracture. It is usually caused by a fall on to the back of the hand, which at the time of impact is flexed at the wrist.

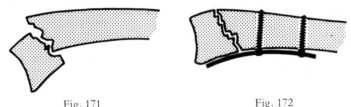

Fig. 171   Fig. 172

Figure 171—Smith's fracture. Diagram showing typical anterior displacement and anterior tilting of the distal fragment of the radius. Figure 172—Stabilisation of the fracture by a buttress plate screwed to the front of the proximal fragment. The flared lower half of the plate prevents the small distal fragment from slipping forward.

Treatment. Reduction by closed manipulation should be attempted, and if it is successful the wrist should be supported in a well moulded forearm plaster for at least six weeks, with weekly check radiographs in the first three weeks to ensure that redisplacement within the plaster does not go undetected. The fracture is a difficult one to manage by conservative methods: reduction is often imperfect and tends to be unstable, so that redisplacement often occurs in the first two weeks. If an acceptable position cannot be secured and maintained by manipulation and plaster operation is advised. The lower fragment is restored to its proper position and held against redisplacement by a special buttressing plate screwed to the front of the upper fragment (Ellis 1965). The splayed lower end of the plate lies snugly against the mobile lower fragment of the radius and prevents it from slipping forward (Fig. 172).

[1] R. W. Smith published his original description of this fracture from Dublin in 1847.

FRACTURE-SEPARATION OF LOWER RADIAL EPIPHYSIS

In young children fractures of the lower end of the radius are usually of the greenstick type, without much displacement. Less often an injury occurs which is the counterpart of the severely displaced Colles's fracture in adults—namely, fracture-separation of the lower radial epiphysis (with or without the lower ulnar epiphysis). As the name implies, the epiphysis is separated through the epiphysial line, but a small fragment from the metaphysis is usually carried with it (Fig. 173). As in the typical Colles's fracture in adults, the lower fragment is usually displaced backwards. Often the displacement is severe—so much so that there may be no remaining point of contact between the separated surfaces.

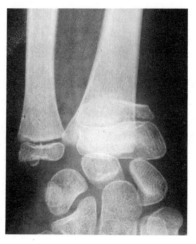 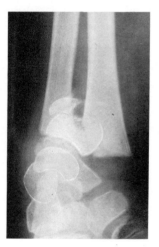

Fig. 173

Fracture-separation of lower radial epiphysis in a child. The distal fragment is displaced backwards and laterally. It has carried with it a triangular fragment of the metaphysis of the radius.

Treatment. Displacement should be corrected by manipulation under anaesthesia and a plaster applied, as for fractures of the lower end of the radius in adults. Since bone healing is rapid in children the plaster need be retained for only three or four weeks.

In some cases perfect reduction is not secured by manipulation. In that event there is no need to resort to operative reduction. Although one should always strive for accurate reduction, a somewhat imperfect position can be accepted in these young children because the deformity is rapidly effaced by the remodelling that occurs with growth.

Complications. ARREST OF EPIPHYSIAL GROWTH. In crushing injuries of the epiphysial cartilage there is a risk of arrest of epiphysial growth. This is uncommon after the ordinary fracture-separation.

INJURIES OF THE CARPUS

DISLOCATIONS OF THE CARPAL BONES

Complete dislocation of the wrist—that is, dislocation of the carpus as a whole from the radius—is very uncommon and need not be described here. Various types of incomplete carpal dislocation are recognised, in which one or more of the carpal bones are displaced, and the dislocation may be associated with a fracture. The injuries seen most frequently are dislocation of the lunate bone and perilunar dislocation of the carpus.

DISLOCATION OF THE LUNATE BONE

It is surprising that a bone that nestles so snugly between its neighbours, and which has strong ligamentous attachments, should be liable to dislocation through a fall on the hand. But the lunate bone is somewhat wedge-shaped with its base anteriorly, and with the hand extended in a fall the bone may be squeezed out from between the capitate bone and the radius. The displacement is characteristic: the lunate bone lies at the front of the wrist and it is rotated through 90 degrees or more on a horizontal axis so that its concave lower articular surface faces forwards (Fig. 174). For the lunate bone to reach this position it is clear that its posterior ligamentous attachments must be torn, so that it hinges on its anterior ligaments.

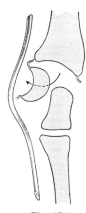

Figure 174—Dislocation of the lunate bone. Note the position of the median nerve, which may suffer injury.

Figure 175—Perilunar dislocation of the carpus. This is basically the same injury as dislocation of the lunate bone, in that the remainder of the carpus is separated from the lunate bone. The two may thus be regarded as variations of the same injury.

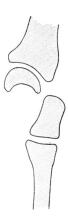

Fig. 174   Fig. 175

Treatment. Manipulative reduction should be attempted under anaesthesia. Strong traction is first applied to the hand to open up the space for the lunate bone. Direct pressure is then applied over the displaced bone and it may pop back into position. If so, a plaster is applied and retained for four weeks before active mobilising exercises are begun.

In cases seen early closed reduction will often be achieved. But in many cases—and especially if there has been delay—manipulation is unsuccessful. In that event the bone should usually be replaced by operation; but in neglected cases in which the dislocation has been present for a long time it is better to excise the bone than to attempt to replace it. In such a case considerable permanent impairment of wrist function is inevitable.

Complications. The blood supply of the displaced lunate bone is precarious because many of its soft-tissue attachments are torn; so there is a risk of avascular necrosis and later of osteoarthritis. There is also a risk of injury to the median nerve.

AVASCULAR NECROSIS. After a dislocated lunate bone has been replaced—whether by manipulation or by operation—its condition should be observed by radiography at monthly intervals. If its blood supply is inadequate, signs of avascular necrosis may appear within one to four months. These signs are: 1) relative density of the bone compared with the adjacent bones which become osteoporotic from disuse while in plaster; and 2) collapse or 'squashing' of the bone. *Treatment:* If clear evidence of avascular necrosis is seen the lunate bone should be excised without further delay. Excision of the lunate bone—like excision of the scaphoid—leaves a wrist that is far from normal, but the results are better than those of leaving a 'dead' bone in the wrist. The results are probably better if the excised lunate bone is replaced by a silicone rubber ('Silastic') prosthesis, though the outcome of this operation in the long term is not yet known with certainty.

OSTEOARTHRITIS. Osteoarthritis will occur inevitably if the lunate bone is avascular and if it is not excised. When osteoarthritis is already established it is too late to hope for improvement from excision of the bone. *Treatment* should be conservative at first—for instance, by a leather or plastic wrist support (Fig. 181)—but if the disability becomes severe the only satisfactory treatment is by arthrodesis of the wrist.

INJURY TO MEDIAN NERVE. The median nerve is liable to be trapped between the displaced lunate bone and the flexor retinaculum. If the nerve is injured there will be signs of sensory and motor impairment in the median distribution in the hand. *Treatment:* The nerve must be decompressed as soon as possible by reduction of the lunate dislocation or, in long-standing cases, by excision of the lunate bone.

DISLOCATION OF LUNATE AND HALF SCAPHOID
This is exactly the same injury as that just described except that the displaced lunate bone carries with it the proximal half of the scaphoid bone, which is fractured into two roughly equal halves through its waist. The principles of treatment are the same.

PERILUNAR DISLOCATION OF THE CARPUS
In this injury the whole carpus is dislocated backwards except for the lunate bone, which remains in normal relationship with the radius (Fig. 175).

So far as the relationship between the lunate bone and the rest of the carpus is concerned there is no difference between this injury and a dislocation of the lunate bone (Fig. 174). Indeed a perilunar dislocation of the carpus is sometimes converted into a dislocation of the lunate bone during attempted reduction.

Treatment. Manipulative reduction should be attempted, but if it is unsuccessful operative reduction should be resorted to.

TRANS-SCAPHO-PERILUNAR DISLOCATION OF CARPUS

This is exactly the same injury as perilunar dislocation of the carpus except that the scaphoid bone is fractured and its proximal half remains attached to the lunate bone, in normal relationship with the radius.

FRACTURE OF THE SCAPHOID BONE

Fracture of the scaphoid bone is common in young adults. It is not common in children or in patients beyond middle age. The usual cause is a fall on the outstretched hand, or comparable violence such as a kick-back from the starting handle of a motor.

The fracture nearly always occurs transversely through the middle, or waist, of the scaphoid; so the proximal and distal fragments are of about equal size (Fig. 176). There is seldom any appreciable displacement of the fragments.

Diagnosis. Fractures of the scaphoid bone are often overlooked, either through failure to get the wrist radiographed or through failure to detect the fracture in the radiographs. In many cases the pain from the injury is slight and the patient can continue to use the hand. Thus he may regard the injury as a strain and may not even consult his doctor. In other cases the doctor may be at fault because, finding little in the nature of clinical signs, he neglects to send the patient for radiography. In yet other instances radiographs may be obtained but the fracture is overlooked because it is not shown clearly in the films.

The only safeguard against overlooking this fracture is to insist upon thorough radiographic examination in every case of wrist injury in which clinical examination shows tenderness in the scaphoid region (especially in the 'anatomical snuff-box') or impairment of wrist movements.

In radiographing a wrist for suspected fracture of the scaphoid bone the surgeon should request two oblique projections in addition to the antero-posterior and lateral projections. Often a fracture is visible only in an oblique radiograph and gives no indication of its presence in the other films.

When the clinical features suggest fracture of the scaphoid bone but the initial radiographs give no confirmation of it the radiographic examination should be repeated after an interval of two weeks. A fracture may sometimes become obvious after an interval even though

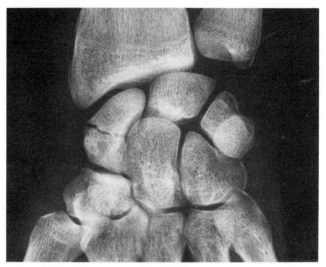

Fig. 176
A typical fracture through the waist of the scaphoid bone.

it was not apparent in the initial films. In the interval it is advisable to immobilise the injured wrist in a plaster. As well as affording rest, the plaster serves the purpose of ensuring that the patient will return for re-examination.

Treatment. The standard method of treatment in uncomplicated cases is to immobilise the wrist firmly in a plaster until the fracture is shown radiologically to be united, usually in two to three months. Since there is usually no displacement reduction is not required.

The plaster generally used for a scaphoid fracture is slightly more extensive than that used for a fracture of the lower end of the radius. It should extend down the thumb to the level of the interphalangeal joint, and it must be moulded firmly round the first metacarpal bone (Fig. 177). The palm is left free beyond the proximal skin crease to allow a full range of movement at the metacarpo-phalangeal joints of the fingers; and the thumb should be free to move at the inter-phalangeal joint.

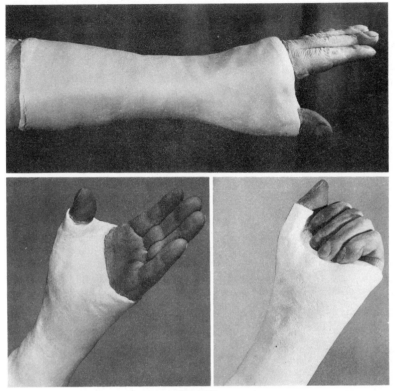

Fig. 177

Plaster used for fractures of the scaphoid bone. The plaster grips the first metacarpal and the proximal segment of the thumb, but the interphalangeal joint is left free. The palm is left free beyond the proximal transverse skin crease, to allow a full range of finger movements.

Complications. Fractures of the scaphoid bone are potentially troublesome and the incidence of complications is high. The most important complications are: 1) delayed union; 2) non-union; 3) avascular necrosis; and 4) osteoarthritis.

DELAYED UNION. The general subject of delayed union was discussed on page 54, where it was emphasised that there can be no hard-and-fast time limit beyond which union is said to be delayed. In a rather high proportion of cases fractures of the scaphoid bone unite slowly, and despite fixation in plaster a fracture may be still ununited four, five, or even six months after the injury. It is uncertain whether delay in union is caused by imperfect immobilisation or by impaired blood supply to one of the fragments. *Treatment:* If union has not occurred by the end of six months despite continuous rest in plaster, a decision must be made whether to continue with further immobilisation, whether to accept the situation and allow active mobilisation of the wrist, or whether to advise a bone-grafting operation. Most surgeons now agree that immobilisation for longer than six months is hardly justified by the likely gain, and some put the outside limit as three or four months. On the other hand, opinion is divided on the relative merits of encouraging active movement and use of the wrist in disregard of the fracture, as against a bone-grafting operation. A good case can be made for bone grafting (by impacting an autogenous graft into a deep slot cut in both fragments, across the fracture), and it should probably be advised if significant symptoms persist for two months after removal of the plaster—especially in a young person. On the other hand the results of bone grafting are not uniformly satisfactory, and among some surgeons there is a trend towards deliberate neglect of the fracture and the encouragement of exercises and active use in preference to bone grafting. Many such fractures will be found to unite eventually, and even if permanent non-union ensues, the disability is often slight provided the blood supply to the fragments has not been impaired (see under 'non-union' below).

NON-UNION. Although most fractures of the scaphoid bone unite readily (albeit sometimes slowly), there is a somewhat greater liability to non-union than in most other bones (with the notable exception of the neck of the femur). In some cases non-union may be ascribed to imperfect immobilisation, or possibly, since the fracture is intra-articular, to the action of synovial fluid in hindering the formation of a fibrinous bridge between the fragments. In other cases non-union can be ascribed to impairment of the blood supply to one of the fragments, and it is a common, if not inevitable, accompaniment of avascular necrosis of the proximal fragment.

When non-union has been present for a long time the fracture surfaces become rounded and sharply defined, as if a joint were forming between them (Fig. 178). There may also be cystic changes in one or both fragments. Later still, the radiographs may show the beginnings of osteoarthritis.

Treatment. The treatment of non-union of a fracture of the scaphoid bone is unsatisfactory: permanent disability is often unavoidable.

If there is no radiographic evidence of avascular necrosis it must be assumed, for lack of more accurate knowledge, that the failure of union has been due to imperfect immobilisation, or to dissolution of the fracture haematoma by synovial fluid. In such a case it has been found that by the time non-union (as distinct from delayed union) is clearly established early osteoarthritic changes are usually already present in the radio-carpal joint, and that attempts to cause the fracture to unite (as by a bone-grafting operation) may do more harm than good by aggravating the arthritis. On the other hand the disability from an ununited fracture of the scaphoid bone is often slight or insignificant, especially if heavy strains to the wrist can be avoided. Indeed the disability depends almost entirely upon the

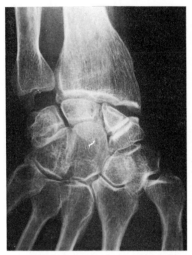

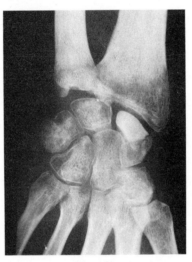

Fig. 178

Established non-union of a fracture of the scaphoid bone. Note the well defined fracture line and the sclerotic bone margins, suggesting a false joint between the fragments.

Fig. 179

Avascular necrosis of proximal half of fractured scaphoid bone. The dead fragment has not shared in the disuse osteoporosis that has affected the other bones.

secondary osteoarthritis rather than upon the ununited fracture as such, and varies proportionately to the degree of arthritis. A wise policy, therefore, is to advise the patient to accept the condition of non-union and to have no treatment so long as the disability remains within reasonable bounds, and to resort to active treatment only if disabling osteoarthritis supervenes (see p. 179).

AVASCULAR NECROSIS OF PROXIMAL FRAGMENT. The blood supply to the proximal fragment of the scaphoid bone is precarious after a fracture through the waist or proximal half of the bone, because the main nutrient vessels enter the distal half of the bone and must clearly be damaged by the fracture in their intra-osseous course. If the remaining blood supply is inadequate the proximal fragment may die and, since it does not lie in a vascular bed, there is little chance of its becoming revascularised before irreversible changes develop which lead to crumbling of the bone. Although not common, avascular necrosis is a serious complication because it is likely to cause troublesome and permanent disability (Fig. 180).

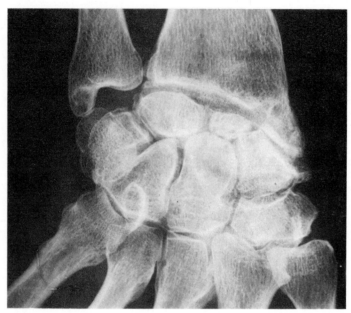

Fig. 180

Osteoarthritis of wrist complicating an ununited fracture of the scaphoid bone. The marked collapse of the proximal fragment suggests that it suffered avascular necrosis.

In many instances (though probably not in all) avascular necrosis of a scaphoid fragment may be diagnosed from the radiographic appearance, because the avascular bone does not share in the general osteoporosis of the carpal bones that occurs from disuse, and it therefore stands out in sharp contrast to the other bones by virtue of its relatively greater density (Fig. 179). This appearance is not usually manifest until about one to three months after the injury.

Treatment. There is no treatment available that can restore the wrist to normal, and some permanent disability must be accepted. If the dead fragment of bone is left in the wrist it may cause early osteoarthritis because its surface is irregular. It is therefore advised that the avascular fragment be excised. It is true that excision of the fragment leaves a wrist that is far from normal—it may be weak and lack a full range of movement—but the results are nevertheless probably better than those of non-intervention. If the operation is unsuccessful in alleviating pain and disability—as is sometimes the case—the more radical operation of arthrodesis may have to be resorted to (see under 'osteoarthritis' below). Replacement of the damaged scaphoid bone by a silicone rubber ('Silastic') or metal prosthesis is an alternative to simple excision, but long-term results must be awaited before the method can be assessed for general application.

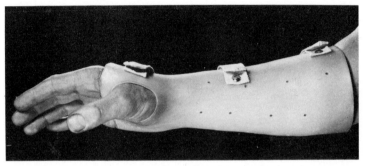

Fig. 181
Polythene wrist support. A splint such as this is sometimes used in the conservative treatment of osteoarthritis of the wrist.

OSTEOARTHRITIS. Osteoarthritis is a common sequel to fractures of the scaphoid bone with non-union, because repeated movement of the damaged articular surface upon the adjacent bones leads to increased wear of the articular cartilage. At first confined to the radial side of the carpus, the arthritis sooner or later involves the whole of the radio-carpal joint and the intercarpal joints (Fig. 180). The development and progress of the arthritis vary widely from case to case, and depend largely upon the condition of the ununited scaphoid fragments and upon the use to which the wrist is put. If the fragments retain good shape and close contact, and if the wrist is used only for light activities, arthritis may be slight, and the disability negligible; whereas if the scaphoid is grossly distorted, as it often is after un-treated avascular necrosis (Fig. 180), and if the wrist is used for heavy work, arthritis may soon become disabling. *Treatment:* In mild cases it may be sufficient to prescribe a wrist support (Fig. 181) and to advise the patient to avoid subjecting the wrist to heavy stress. In severe cases operation is required: the only reliable method is to eliminate the source of pain by arthrodesis of the wrist. The fusion should include the radio-carpal joint and all the intercarpal joints, but the radio-ulnar joint must be left undisturbed to preserve rotation.

FRACTURE OF THE TUBEROSITY OF THE SCAPHOID BONE
Fractures of the tuberosity are rare in comparison with those of the waist of the scaphoid bone, but they are relatively common in adolescent boys. They are not of great importance because they generally unite readily and cause little trouble.

Treatment. Immobilisation in plaster for about six weeks is usually sufficient to ensure union.

CONGENITAL BIPARTITE SCAPHOID BONE
In a small number of individuals the scaphoid bone is in two parts, with a joint between them. Radiographs of such a bone may be wrongly interpreted as showing a fracture. But the gap between the halves of a congenitally bipartite scaphoid is clear-cut like the other intercarpal joints, and the articulating surfaces are smooth. Moreover radiographs will usually show an identical appearance in the other wrist.

FRACTURES OF OTHER CARPAL BONES
Apart from the scaphoid bone, the carpal bones are seldom the site of serious fractures, though isolated examples are seen from time to time. In general, the principles of treatment are like those for uncomplicated fractures of the scaphoid bone.

FLAKE FRACTURE OF THE TRIQUETRAL BONE
A minor fracture that is seen fairly often is a flake or chip fracture of the triquetral bone. It is caused by a fall. There is pain at the back of the wrist, and the radiographs show a small flake of bone detached from the dorsal surface of the triquetrum, but not markedly displaced.

Treatment. Rest in plaster for three weeks is sufficient to relieve pain, and thereafter full function is quickly restored.

KIENBÖCK'S DISEASE OF THE LUNATE BONE
Injury to the lunate bone (whether it be a contusion or a minor fracture) is occasionally followed by a pathological condition in which the bone substance becomes soft, granular, and fragmented. In this state the bone tends to become squashed and flattened, and in the absence of treatment the deformity and irregularity of the articular surface quickly lead to severe osteoarthritis. The precise nature of the affection is unknown, but it is thought to be caused by interference with the blood supply of the bone. It is described fully in textbooks of orthopaedics.

INJURIES OF THE METACARPAL BONES AND PHALANGES

FRACTURE OF THE BASE OF THE FIRST METACARPAL BONE

A fracture of the base of the first metacarpal bone is usually sustained from longitudinal violence applied by a blow, as in boxing.

Pathology. There are two distinct types of this injury (Figs. 182 and 183): 1) a transverse or short oblique fracture across the base of

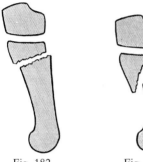

Fig. 182   Fig. 183

Two fractures of base of first metacarpal. Figure 182—Fracture not involving joint. Figure 183—Fracture entering joint, with displacement (Bennett's fracture). Whereas the first type is relatively stable the second may be difficult to control by plaster alone.

the metacarpal, but not entering the joint; and 2) an oblique fracture entering the carpo-metacarpal joint at about the middle of the articular surface (Bennett's fracture[1]). The second type is the more serious, because unless a smooth joint surface can be restored there is a risk of the development of osteoarthritis. When the fracture is oblique there is a strong tendency for the large distal fragment to be displaced backwards and upwards upon the small proximal fragment (Fig. 183).

Two methods of stabilising a fracture-subluxation of the base of the first metacarpal bone. Figure 184—Fixation by a screw. Figure 185—Stabilisation by pins driven into the trapezium. Operation is advised only when reduction cannot be held by a plaster.

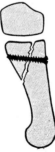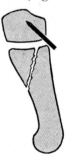

Fig. 184   Fig. 185

Treatment. Displacement can nearly always be reduced by manipulation under anaesthesia. But it is often difficult, in oblique fractures, to maintain the reduction. An attempt should be made to

[1] Edward Hallaran Bennett, an Irish surgeon, described this injury in 1880.

do this by applying a well moulded plaster, which should include the forearm and wrist and should hold the thumb metacarpal well extended at the carpo-metacarpal joint. Check radiographs should be taken twice during the first week to determine whether a good position has been maintained.

Slight loss of position matters little in the case of a fracture that does not involve the joint, but nothing short of perfect reduction should be accepted if the joint surface is involved. In such a case, therefore, if reduction cannot be maintained by plaster alone operation should be advised. At operation it may be feasible to fix the fragments together with a small screw (Fig. 184). If not, an alternative method of preventing redisplacement after operative reduction is to drive two small pins of stainless steel into the trapezium in such a position that their protruding ends abut against the base of the metacarpal and prevent its riding upwards (Fig. 185). The pins should be removed after three or four weeks, by which time the fracture will be stable. After internal fixation by either method a well fitting plaster should be retained until the fracture is united—usually about eight weeks.

Complications. OSTEOARTHRITIS. The risk of osteoarthritis has been mentioned already. It will occur only after a fracture that has damaged the joint surface and left it irregular, but it may be a cause of troublesome disability if the hand is used for heavy work. Exceptionally it may demand operation, which may take the form either of arthrodesis of the trapezio-metacarpal joint or—more often—of excision of the trapezium.

OTHER FRACTURES OF THE METACARPAL BONES

Fractures of the metacarpal bones are fairly common at all ages. The commonest causes are a fall on the hand, and a blow upon the knuckles as in boxing. There are three main patterns of fracture: 1) a fracture through the base of the metacarpal bone (Fig. 186); 2) an oblique fracture of the shaft (Fig. 187); and 3) a transverse fracture through the neck of the bone (Fig. 188). In the great majority of cases displacement is slight and unimportant. In the exceptional case there is wide separation of the fragments, marked angulation at the site of a fracture of the metacarpal neck, or unacceptable shortening from telescoping of an oblique fracture of the shaft.

Treatment. The treatment depends upon the degree of displacement. There are thus two groups to be considered—those in which the existing position is acceptable, and those in which the position cannot be accepted.

Undisplaced fractures (including those with insignificant displacement). These comprise a large proportion of the total. Treatment is simple—indeed sound union and perfect recovery of function may be expected without treatment of any kind, but simply with active use of the hand. It is nevertheless wise in most cases to provide some form of temporary support for relief of pain. The usual method is

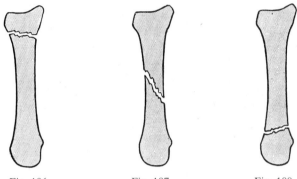

| Fig. 186 | Fig. 187 | Fig. 188 |

Fractures of metacarpal bones. The diagrams show the three sites of fracture—base, shaft, and neck. In the absence of displacement treatment is hardly necessary, but a dorsal plaster slab is usually applied for comfort's sake. It extends to the heads of the metacarpals but should not interfere with movement of the fingers.

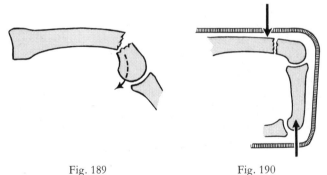

| Fig. 189 | Fig. 190 |

Figure 189—The only metacarpal fracture that commonly demands reduction—a fracture through the neck with forward tilting of the head fragment. Figure 190—Diagram showing the method of reduction by a force applied dorsalwards through the flexed proximal phalanx. The position is held by a splint made from malleable aluminium strip.

to apply a light dorsal plaster slab for three weeks. Finger movements and active use of the hand must be encouraged from the beginning.

Displaced fractures. In the exceptional case with severe displacement or angulation, reduction and splintage must be advised. The commonest of these special fractures is a fracture of the neck of the fifth metacarpal in which the distal or head fragment is tilted sharply forwards so that it may form an angle of nearly 90 degrees with the shaft fragment (Fig. 189). This fracture can usually be reduced by flexing the metacarpo-phalangeal joint to a right angle and then

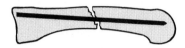

Fig. 191

A method of internal fixation (by an intramedullary wire) for the rare metacarpal fractures with severe uncontrollable displacement.

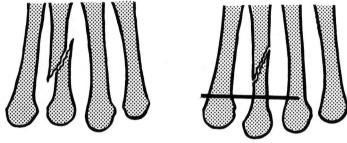

Fig. 192

A method of maintaining length after oblique fracture of the third or fourth metacarpal with recession of the knuckle.

pushing the flexed finger dorsalwards against counter-pressure over the site of fracture (Fig. 190). The finger is immobilised in this position on a malleable metal strip splint for three weeks.

If a badly displaced metacarpal fracture cannot be reduced by manipulation, operative reduction and internal fixation should be undertaken. The most satisfactory technique of fixation is to pass a stiff wire along the medullary canal and across the fracture (Fig. 191). The wire can best be introduced at the dorsal aspect of the base of the metacarpal.

Alternatively, for unacceptable shortening of an obliquely fractured metacarpal shaft of the middle or ring finger it may be practicable to draw out the fragments to full length under anaesthesia, and to maintain the position by transfixing the necks of the injured metacarpal and of the two adjacent metacarpals with a slender stiff wire (Fig. 192). The wire should be removed after three weeks.

FRACTURES OF THE PHALANGES

The various patterns of fracture that are met with in the phalanges of the fingers are shown diagrammatically in Figure 193.

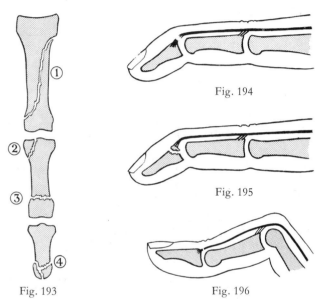

Fig. 194

Fig. 195

Fig. 193   Fig. 196

Injuries of the fingers. Figure 193—Fractures of the phalanges. 1. Long spiral fracture of shaft. 2. Oblique fracture of base. 3. Transverse fracture of shaft. 4. Comminuted fracture of distal phalanx. Figure 194—Mallet finger from rupture of extensor tendon near insertion. Figure 195—Mallet finger from avulsion fracture of base of phalanx. Figure 196—Recommended position of finger joints splinted for mallet finger.

Treatment. It should be remembered that fingers tolerate immobilisation badly. To immobilise an injured finger for a long time is to court disaster in the form of prolonged or even permanent stiffness. It should be regarded as a sound working rule that a fractured finger should never be immobilised for more than three weeks. After that time active exercises must be begun, irrespective of the condition of the fracture. Nearly all phalangeal fractures will proceed to bony union whether they are splinted or not; so the main purposes of splintage are to prevent redisplacement of fractures that have required reduction, and to relieve pain. Both these purposes will have been achieved within two or three weeks, and therefore there is no further need for splintage after that time.

Undisplaced fractures of shaft. The fragments are held together by the periosteal sheath. There is no fear of displacement. Treatment is unnecessary except to relieve pain. A simple method of affording support without immobilisation is to bind the phalanges of the injured finger to the corresponding segments of an adjacent normal finger with adhesive strapping.

Comminuted fractures of distal phalanx. The pulp or the nail bed may be torn, and the nail may often separate. The fracture should be ignored and attention directed solely to the soft-tissue injury, for which dry dressings covered by protective soft wool and a cotton bandage will usually be required.

Displaced fractures, and fractures involving joint surfaces. The displacement is corrected by manipulation under anaesthesia, and the finger is immobilised on an aluminium strip splint shaped to hold the interphalangeal joints semi-flexed (Fig. 43, p. 39). Splintage should be discarded in favour of active exercises after two weeks.

Occasionally, when serious displacement cannot be corrected by manipulation, there may be need for operative reduction and internal fixation. This is often best effected by an intramedullary wire.

MALLET FINGER
(Baseball finger)

This is caused by an injury at the insertion of the extensor tendon at the base of the distal phalanx, usually from sudden flexion violence. In most cases the tendon is torn away from the bone at its point of insertion (Fig. 194), but sometimes a fragment of bone is avulsed with the tendon (Fig. 195). In both types the patient is unable actively to extend the distal interphalangeal joint.

Treatment. The finger should be immobilised for three weeks with the proximal interphalangeal joint flexed and the distal interphalangeal joint extended—a position which ensures that the distal part of the extensor expansion is fully relaxed (Fig. 196).

If a large fragment of bone has been avulsed and is lying away from its bed operative reposition and fixation with wire sutures should be advised.

Neglected and unsuccessfully treated cases. Even without treatment, the avulsed tendon or bone fragment will unite with the phalanx by fibrous tissue, but with slight lengthening. Since the attachment of the tendon to the middle phalanx prevents the slack from being taken up by the muscle belly, the lengthening causes permanent loss of full active extension at the distal interphalangeal joint, usually by about 20 or 30 degrees. When the local pain and tenderness have subsided most patients are willing to accept the disability, which is slight. If not, an attempt may be made to correct the lengthening of the tendon by excising a piece about two millimetres long. This is best done through healthy tendon over the middle of the middle phalanx.

DISLOCATIONS OF THE METACARPO-PHALANGEAL AND INTERPHALANGEAL JOINTS

Most dislocations of the finger and thumb joints are caused by forced hyperextension. The distal segment is usually displaced backwards from the proximal (Fig. 197).

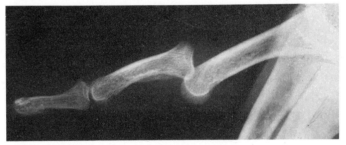

Fig. 197
A typical dislocation of a finger. The middle phalanx is displaced
backwards upon the proximal.

Treatment. The dislocation should be reduced with the least possible delay. Reduction is usually effected easily by pulling upon the digit and applying direct pressure over the base of the displaced phalanx. This can often be done without anaesthesia. Radiographs should be taken to check the reduction. Immobilisation is not required, and active movements of the joint should be encouraged from an early stage.

'Button-hole' injuries. Sometimes in metacarpo-phalangeal dislocations the head of the metacarpal bone is driven forwards through a rent in the front of the capsule at the same time as the phalanx is dislocated backwards. In this event manipulative reduction may be impossible and operation is required. The capsular slit is enlarged sufficiently to allow it to be hooked back over the metacarpal head.

STRAINS OF THE INTERPHALANGEAL JOINTS

Strains of the interphalangeal joints are notorious for their chronicity. The joint may remain swollen and painful for as long as six or nine months after a relatively minor injury. Yet there is little or no restriction of movement and full recovery occurs eventually.

The causative injury is usually an angulation force with incomplete disruption of the medial or lateral ligament and of the joint capsule. The consequent periarticular thickening causes a characteristic fusiform swelling about the joint. Radiographs may show no bone injury, but sometimes a tiny flake of bone is avulsed at the point of attachment of the capsule.

Treatment. In mild cases treatment is unnecessary. If pain is severe the finger may be supported by strapping or by a malleable metal splint for a week before active movements are begun. The tendency to slow rather than rapid recovery should be explained to the patient.

References and bibliography, page 291.

CHAPTER 12

Pelvis, thigh and knee

In this chapter much space is necessarily devoted to fractures of the upper end of the femur—that is, fractures of the neck of the femur proper and of the trochanteric region. Not only are these fractures common in elderly people; they are also important because they are so seriously disabling, often depriving a patient of independence. Because of this, such injuries account for a sizeable proportion of the admissions to orthopaedic hospital beds. In comparison with these fractures of the upper end of the femur, fractures of the pelvis and of the shaft of the femur are relatively uncommon.

At the lower end of the region to be considered in this chapter, injuries of the knee are particularly common. In most instances these are not bone injuries but rather injuries to the soft parts—mainly the menisci and the ligaments of the knee. In contrast to fractures of the upper end of the femur, knee injuries are common in young athletic individuals, and particularly in those who play football.

Classification
The injuries to be described may be classified as follows.

Fractures of the pelvis
Isolated fractures
Fractures with disruption of the pelvic ring

Dislocations and fracture-dislocations of the hip
Posterior dislocation and fracture-dislocation
Anterior dislocation
Central fracture-dislocation

Fractures of the femur
Fracture of the neck of the femur
Fracture of the trochanteric region
Fracture of the shaft
Supracondylar fracture
Fractures of the condyles

Injuries of the knee
Fracture of the patella
Other injuries of the extensor mechanism of the knee
Dislocation of the knee
Lateral dislocation of the patella
Tears of the ligaments of the knee
Strain of the medial or lateral ligament
Tears of the menisci
Traumatic effusions in the knee

FRACTURES OF THE PELVIS

Fractures of the pelvis are not serious injuries in themselves but may be so by reason of their complications. They are usually caused by direct injury, or by violence transmitted through the femur.

Classification
Two groups of fractures will be described (Figs. 198 and 199): 1) isolated fractures not destroying the integrity of the pelvic ring; and 2) fractures with disruption of the pelvic ring.

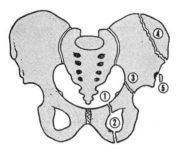 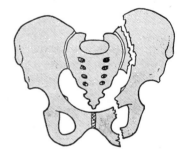

Fig. 198   Fig. 199

Two types of injury of the pelvis. Figure 198—Isolated fractures. The pelvic ring remains intact. (1. Fracture of superior ischio-pubic ramus. 2. Fracture of inferior ischio-pubic ramus. 3. Fracture entering acetabulum. 4. Fracture of wing of ilium. 5. Avulsion of anterior inferior spine.) Figure 199—Displaced fractures with disruption of the pelvic ring.

ISOLATED FRACTURES
Any part of the pelvis may be affected (Fig. 198). The commonest fractures occur through the superior or inferior ischio-pubic ramus, or through both rami. Less often there is an isolated fracture of the wing of the ilium. Rarely, in boys, the anterior inferior spine of the

ilium may be pulled off by a violent contraction of the rectus femoris muscle.

Treatment. No special treatment is needed for these injuries, except to relieve pain. Rest in bed for one to three weeks is usually sufficient. Exercises for the lower limbs should be encouraged from the beginning.

Complications. Complications are uncommon in these minor fractures of the pelvis. The bladder or urethra may be damaged by a fragment of bone, or the articular surface of the acetabulum may be injured, with a risk of consequent osteoarthritis. These complications will be described in the next section.

FRACTURES WITH DISRUPTION OF THE PELVIC RING

The pelvic ring is composed of the sacrum and the two innominate bones. Disruption of the ring can occur only if there are fractures or dislocations at *two* points approximately opposite one another. Thus a fracture in the anterior half of the ring with separation of the fragments must be associated with an injury in the posterior half of the ring (Fig. 199). In most cases of this type the anterior injury takes the form of a fracture through both ischio-pubic rami with separation, or of disruption of the symphysis pubis (Fig. 200). The posterior

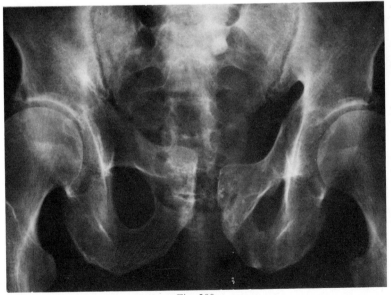

Fig. 200
Disruption of symphysis pubis. In this case the posterior injury was a subluxation of the left sacro-iliac joint.

injury is usually a subluxation of the sacro-iliac joint, or a fracture through the ilium or the lateral mass [ala] of the sacrum near the sacro-iliac joint. Displacement between the two halves of the pelvis is usually slight, but it may be severe.

Treatment. If displacement is slight all that is required is rest in bed until the two halves of the pelvis become united reasonably firmly—a matter of about four or six weeks. During the period of rest exercises for the lower limbs should be carried out daily to keep the joints mobile and the muscles active.

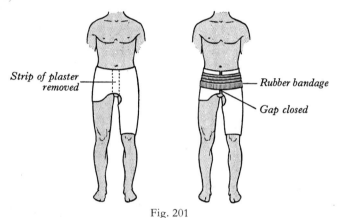

Strip of plaster removed

Rubber bandage

Gap closed

Fig. 201
A method of holding a disrupted pubic symphysis reduced.

Disruption of symphysis pubis. If the pubic bones are widely separated at the symphysis an attempt should usually be made to bring them together. A short plaster hip spica is applied over protective sponge padding, and when it is dry a vertical strip three or four centimetres wide is removed from the front (Fig. 201). The jacket is then encircled with a rubber bandage of the Esmarch type, applied with just enough tension to close the gap in the plaster. Radiographs will usually show that this has been sufficient to bring together the halves of the symphysis pubis. The plaster should be retained for four weeks.

An alternative method is to expose the pubic bones at operation and to secure them together with strong stainless-steel wire looped through drill holes, or with a small plate and screws. This operative method has been little used in the past but it may well find a wider application.

Upward displacement of the half pelvis. In disruption injuries from severe violence one half of the pelvis is occasionally displaced markedly upwards. In that event an attempt should be made to reduce the displacement by heavy weight traction applied through a tibial pin (Fig. 230).

Complications. RUPTURE OF BLADDER. The bladder may be torn open in disruptions of the symphysis pubis or it may be penetrated by a spike of bone. The rupture is usually extra-peritoneal, and urine is extravasated into the perivesical space. The patient is shocked: he complains of a desire to pass urine but is unable to do so. A catheter passes easily into the bladder but only a few drops of blood-stained fluid escape.

Treatment. Urgent operation is required, and whenever possible it should be undertaken by a urological surgeon. The principles of treatment are: 1) to suture the rent; 2) to drain the bladder; and 3) to drain the perivesical space.

RUPTURE OF URETHRA. This also is commonest in cases of wide disruption of the symphysis pubis. The rupture is usually in the membranous part. Extravasation will occur into the perineum if the patient attempts to pass urine. If a ruptured urethra is suspected the patient should be warned not to attempt to pass urine. A catheter should be introduced. Inability to pass the catheter into the bladder, and the escape of a little blood at the meatus, confirm the diagnosis.

Treatment. Urgent operation is required, and the cooperation of a urological surgeon should be sought. The principles of treatment are: 1) to identify the torn ends of the urethra through incisions in the perineum and, if necessary, in the bladder; 2) to suture the ends, if necessary over a rubber catheter passed into the bladder; 3) to drain the bladder suprapubically; and 4) to close the perineal wound with drainage.

INJURY TO RECTUM. This is a rare complication, and it need not be considered fully here.

INJURY TO MAJOR BLOOD VESSEL. Rarely the common iliac artery or one of its branches may be damaged by a spike of bone. In the case of a main vessel, with threat to the viability of the limb, the torn ends of the vessel should be sutured or, if direct suture is impracticable, continuity may be restored by a vein graft. Severance of a smaller artery with formation of a massive haematoma may necessitate ligation of the vessel itself or occasionally of its parent trunk: for instance, in haemorrhage from the superior gluteal artery near the point of its emergence from the pelvis into the buttock it may be expedient to ligate the internal iliac artery proximal to the superior gluteal branch.

INJURY TO NERVES. In a case of major disruption of the pelvic ring with marked upward displacement of the half pelvis, it is common for nerves of the lumbo-sacral plexus to be injured. In some of these cases there is a vertical fracture of the sacrum with wide displacement, and individual nerves may be damaged as they lie within the sacral foramina. In other cases the disruption occurs through the sacro-iliac joint, and then presumably the nerve trunks may be damaged by stretching. Although these nerve injuries may sometimes fall within the groups of neurapraxia or axonotmesis and show partial or full recovery, in most cases the injury is irrecoverable and the consequent weakness or paralysis—which may be of patchy distribution—is permanent.

INVOLVEMENT OF ACETABULUM WITH SUBSEQUENT OSTEOARTHRITIS. A fracture extending into the acetabulum may leave the articular surface roughened. The increased wear-and-tear may then lead gradually to the development of osteoarthritis of the hip.

DISLOCATIONS AND
FRACTURE-DISLOCATIONS OF THE HIP

Classification. Only three types of dislocation and fracture-dislocation of the hip need be considered: 1) posterior dislocation or fracture-dislocation; 2) anterior dislocation; and 3) central fracture-dislocation. All these injuries are uncommon when compared, for example, with dislocation of the shoulder. Of the three types, the posterior dislocation is the commonest.

Diagnosis. It is surprising but nevertheless true that a dislocation or fracture-dislocation of the hip has often been overlooked even by experienced surgeons. This grave mistake is liable to be made when there are other serious injuries in the same limb—particularly a fracture of the shaft of the femur (Helal and Skevis 1967). In such a case the symptoms and signs of the shaft fracture may so over-shadow those of the hip injury that neither the patient's nor the surgeon's attention is drawn to the hip. The essential safeguards against this error are, firstly, to insist always on a full clinical survey of the whole body in cases of major injury, and secondly, to make sure that the radiographs in every case of fractured femoral shaft take in the whole length of the bone and include the hip joint.

POSTERIOR DISLOCATION AND FRACTURE-DISLOCATION
The femoral head is forced out of the back of the acetabulum by violence applied along the shaft of the femur while the hip is flexed or

semiflexed (Fig. 202). The injury often occurs as a result of a motor accident in which the occupant of a car involved in a collision is thrown forwards and strikes the front of his flexed knee against a part of the body-work. Another common cause is a motor-cycle crash.

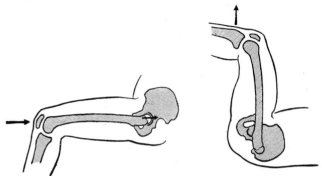

Fig. 202   Fig. 203

Figure 202—Posterior dislocation of the hip is usually caused by a force acting along the axis of the femoral shaft while the hip is semi-flexed. Figure 203—Diagram showing the method of reduction, by traction upwards in the line of the femur with the hip and knee flexed 90 degrees. As traction is applied the hip is gradually rotated laterally.

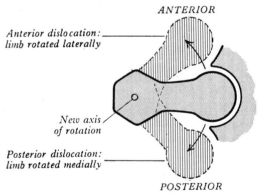

ANTERIOR

Anterior dislocation:
limb rotated laterally

New axis
of rotation

Posterior dislocation:
limb rotated medially

POSTERIOR

Fig. 204

Diagram to show the position of the limb in anterior dislocation and in posterior dislocation of the hip.

In about half the cases of posterior dislocation of the hip the head of the femur carries with it a small or large fragment of bone from the rim of the acetabulum (fracture-dislocation). It should be noted that the sciatic nerve is almost directly in the path of displacement and may easily be damaged.

Clinical features. To remember the clinical deformity it is easiest to think of the greater trochanter as being held more or less in its normal position by the attached muscles, and forming the centre of a new vertical axis about which the femoral head may swing forwards or backwards (Fig. 204). Thus in a posterior dislocation the femur—

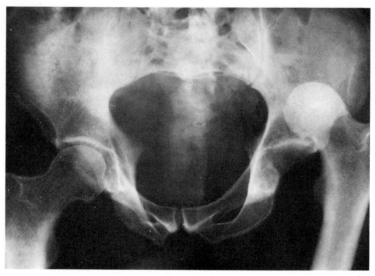

Fig. 205
Posterior dislocation of left hip sustained in a motor-cycle crash.

and with it the whole lower limb—is rotated medially (Fig. 204). There will also be true shortening of the limb, perhaps by two or three centimetres. Radiographs will confirm the dislocation (Fig. 205) and show whether or not there is an associated fracture. Careful examination should always be made for signs of injury to the sciatic nerve.

Treatment. The dislocation should be reduced under general anaesthesia as soon as possible. Reduction is usually effected without difficulty by pulling longitudinally upon the femur while the hip is flexed to a right angle and rotated laterally. *Technique:* The patient is placed supine, and an assistant grasps the pelvis firmly through the iliac crests. The surgeon flexes the hip and knee to a right angle so that the line of the femur points vertically upwards. He then pulls the thigh steadily upwards, at the same time gradually rotating the femur laterally (Fig. 203).

After the dislocation has been reduced the limb is supported from a beam, with light traction, for three to six weeks (Fig. 226). Meanwhile mobilising exercises for the hip and knee are begun after a few days and are gradually intensified.

Persistent displacement of acetabular fragment. A small marginal fragment from the acetabulum will usually fall back into place when the dislocation is reduced. If a large acetabular fragment remains unreduced operation is required. The fragment is exposed through a posterior incision, reduced under direct vision, and fixed in place by a screw.

Complications. These are: 1) injury to the sciatic nerve; 2) post-traumatic ossification; 3) avascular necrosis of the femoral head; and 4) osteoarthritis.

INJURY TO SCIATIC NERVE. The nerve is vulnerable to injury where it lies behind the posterior wall of the acetabulum. It may be damaged in a dislocation without fracture of the acetabulum, but it is particularly liable to severe injury when a large fragment of the acetabular wall is driven backwards with the head of the femur. The nerve lesion is usually a neurapraxia or an axonotmesis (p. 63).

Treatment. Pressure upon the nerve must be relieved at the earliest moment by reduction of the dislocation and replacement of displaced bone fragments, if necessary by operation. Thereafter treatment is usually expectant at first, as for other closed nerve injuries (p. 64); but if operation has to be undertaken to replace a large acetabular fragment the opportunity should be taken to examine the nerve at the same time. *Prognosis:* The outlook for recovery is good after a minor nerve lesion of the type classed as neurapraxia. But after severe injuries of the sciatic nerve at this high level the prognosis for recovery of good muscle power is poor because of the length to be regenerated and the likelihood that the distal muscles will have suffered irreversible changes before they are re-innervated. The prognosis for sensory recovery is also doubtful.

In cases of permanent paralysis function can be improved by appliances or by stabilising operations upon the ankle and foot. When the sole of the foot is insensitive there is a risk of persistent 'trophic' ulceration, but if fixed deformity of the foot is prevented or corrected ulceration is seldom troublesome, and nowadays it should be rare for amputation to become necessary on that account.

POST-TRAUMATIC OSSIFICATION. Occasionally a mass of new bone forms about the hip, from ossification in the haematoma that collects beneath the stripped-up periosteum and capsule (so-called myositis ossificans—see p. 67).

AVASCULAR NECROSIS OF FEMORAL HEAD. The general subject of avascular necrosis was discussed on page 57. There is a rather high incidence of avascular necrosis of the femoral head after dislocation of the hip—in the order of 15 to 20 per cent according to Stewart and Milford (1954), though the higher rate probably obtains only when there has been delay in reduction. The complication is presumably

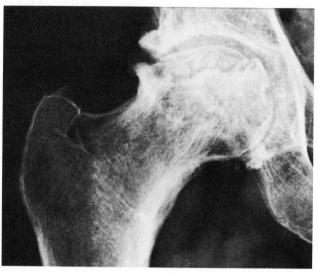

Fig. 206
Marked irregularity and partial collapse of the femoral head a year and a half after posterior dislocation of the hip. The changes suggest that part of the femoral head suffered avascular necrosis from damage to its blood supply at the time of the injury.

caused by damage to blood vessels in the ligament of the femoral head [ligamentum teres] and in the capsule, which may be extensively torn. In the course of several months the avascular head gradually collapses, wholly or in part, and osteoarthritis of the hip is the inevitable sequel (Fig. 206).

OSTEOARTHRITIS. After a dislocation of the hip osteoarthritis may arise from two distinct causes—avascular necrosis of the femoral head (see above), and roughening of the acetabulum from a fracture involving its articular surface.

When avascular necrosis is responsible, the features of osteo-arthritis usually begin to be evident within a few months of the dislocation, though often there is a latent period of up to a year or more before arthritis becomes incapacitating.

When osteoarthritis follows roughening of the acetabulum consequent upon a fracture, it tends to develop more slowly, and if the damage has been slight many years may elapse before the arthritis becomes troublesome.

Treatment. If osteoarthritis becomes disabling the only effective treatment is by operation. The choice usually lies between arthrodesis and replacement arthroplasty. Arthrodesis has the advantage of permanence, and provided the hip is fixed in the optimal position (15 to 20 degrees of flexion; no abduction or adduction; no rotation), and provided the adjacent joints are healthy, function is good. Arthrodesis is therefore often preferred for a relatively young patient (say, under 50) because of the serious drawback of replacement arthroplasty that it may fail—usually from loosening—after a number of years. In older patients total replacement arthroplasty is the natural choice.

ANTERIOR DISLOCATION

Anterior dislocation of the hip is much less common than posterior dislocation. Indeed it is a very uncommon injury. It is caused by forced abduction and lateral rotation of the limb, usually in a violent injury such as a motor accident or aircraft crash. There is not usually an associated fracture of the acetabular margin. *Clinically*, the limb rests in marked lateral rotation (Fig. 204).

Treatment. Reduction under anaesthesia is effected by traction upon the flexed limb combined with medial rotation. Thereafter treatment is the same as for posterior dislocation.

Complications. There is not the same risk of damage to the sciatic nerve as there is in posterior dislocations, but the risk of osteoarthritis from avascular necrosis is the same.

CENTRAL FRACTURE-DISLOCATION

In central fracture-dislocation of the hip the femoral head is driven through the medial wall, or 'floor', of the acetabulum towards the pelvic cavity. It differs from anterior and posterior dislocations in that the capsule remains intact; but there is inevitably a fracture of the acetabulum, usually with much comminution.

This injury is caused by a heavy lateral blow upon the femur, as in a fall from a height on to the side; or it may be caused by a longitudinal force acting upon the femur (as from a blow upon the flexed knee) while the hip is abducted. The degree of displacement varies with the severity of the violence. Thus in the minor varieties of the injury the femoral head and the medial wall of the acetabulum may be displaced inwards by only a few millimetres (Fig. 207), whereas in the most severe type the head may be driven right through the acetabulum into the pelvis (Fig. 208).

Treatment. Treatment tends to be rather unsatisfactory in so far as it often fails to prevent the later development of osteoarthritis, from roughening of the articular surface of the acetabulum. Treatment depends largely upon the degree of comminution and displacement of the acetabular fragments and upon whether or not it is possible to restore the articular surface to its normal shape. In practice the cases thus fall into two groups: those in which the main part of the weight-bearing surface of the acetabulum can be restored to its normal position, congruous with the femoral head; and those in which this is impossible on account of severe comminution of the weight-bearing surface.

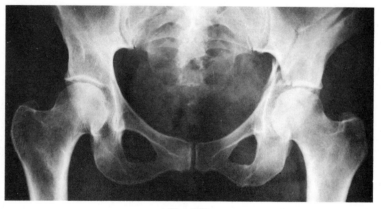

Fig. 207

Fracture of the acetabulum with slight medial displacement of the femoral head and acetabular floor. The main part of the weight-bearing surface of the acetabulum is intact. With traction, or failing that by operation, a reasonably smooth acetabular surface may be restored, but there is nevertheless a serious risk that osteoarthritis will develop later.

Cases in which restoration of articular surface is possible. These are mainly the cases in which the major part of the weight-bearing area of the acetabulum remains in one piece (Fig. 207). In this event it is worth pursuing energetic measures to restore this key fragment to its anatomical position. The fragment is usually displaced upwards and medially with the femoral head, and an attempt should first be made to pull it back into place by heavy traction upon the femur through a Steinmann pin passed antero-posteriorly through the greater trochanter. The direction of pull should be downwards and outwards. In a favourable case the acetabular fragment will follow the femoral head, and satisfactory reduction may be achieved by traction alone.

If not, resort may be had to operation: it may be possible to push the main fragment out from within the pelvis and to secure it in position with screws or transfixion wires. After reduction, whether it be by traction or by operation, moderate weight traction should be maintained for four to six weeks to allow the position to become stable. Meanwhile exercises for the hip are encouraged.

Cases in which severe comminution precludes accurate reduction. This is unfortunately by far the commoner type of case. The medial and superior walls of the acetabulum are shattered into small fragments and the femoral head is often driven far medially, part way into the pelvis (Fig. 208).

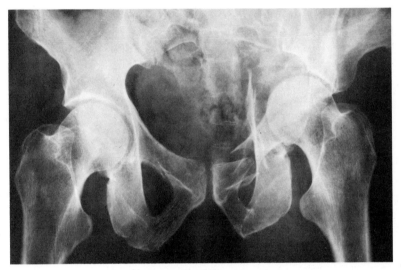

Fig. 208

Severe central fracture-dislocation of the hip. There is no possibility of restoring a smooth acetabular surface.

Restoration of a smooth articular surface is clearly impossible, and there seems little point in attempting it. It may be better to leave the femoral head in the displaced position, for it has been found that a centrally dislocated hip is stable and often painless (Charnley 1952): moreover a useful though restricted range of movement may sometimes be restored by intensive exercises. The suggested plan of treatment for this second category of case, therefore, is that light traction on the limb, applied through adhesive strapping on the lower leg, should be maintained for three weeks simply for the sake of comfort, and that thereafter the patient should be encouraged to walk with crutches, gradually taking an increasing proportion of the body weight on the injured limb. Hip exercises should be practised from the beginning, in an attempt to mould the healing granulations into a congruous surface.

Complications. If the articular surface of the acetabulum is left rough and irregular, as is usually the case, there is a serious risk that osteoarthritis will develop gradually in the ensuing months or years. If the disability from arthritis becomes severe the only effective treatment is by operation. The choice usually lies between arthrodesis and total replacement arthroplasty. Arthrodesis may be appropriate for a patient below the age of 50, but in older patients replacement arthroplasty (by a prosthetic femoral head articulating with a plastic socket) is to be preferred.

FRACTURES OF THE FEMUR

Classification

The behaviour and treatment of fractures of the femur differ markedly according to the site of the injury. On this basis femoral fractures

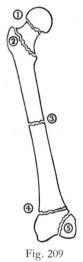

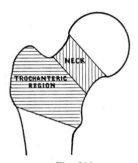

Fig. 210

Figure 209—Visual classification of fractures of the femur. 1. Fracture of femoral neck. 2. Trochanteric fracture. 3. Fracture of femoral shaft. 4. Supracondylar fracture. 5. Condylar fracture. Figure 210 shows the upper end of the femur with the zones of femoral neck fractures and trochanteric fractures demarcated.

Fig. 209

may be classified in five groups (Figs. 209 and 210): 1) fracture of the neck of the femur; 2) fracture of the trochanteric region[1]; 3) fracture of the shaft of the femur; 4) supracondylar fracture; 5) condylar fractures.

---

[1] It must be made clear that some surgeons use the term 'fracture of the neck of the femur' loosely to include trochanteric fractures as well as fractures of the femoral neck proper. Thus they recognise two types of femoral neck fracture: 1) intracapsular or transcervical fracture (=fracture of femoral neck proper); and 2) extracapsular or trochanteric fracture. Less confusion will arise if the classification suggested above is adopted.

FRACTURE OF THE NECK OF THE FEMUR

Fracture of the neck of the femur is common in persons over the age of 60, in whom there is a tendency for the bone to become increasingly fragile in consequence of generalised osteoporosis (Solomon 1973; 1977). The causative injury is often slight—usually a fall or stumble. In most cases the fracture is probably caused by a rotational force. In about nineteen cases out of twenty there is marked displacement, the shaft fragment being rotated laterally and displaced upwards (Fig. 211). In the remaining small minority the two fragments are firmly impacted together, with slight abduction of the distal fragment upon the proximal (impacted abduction fracture, Fig. 214).

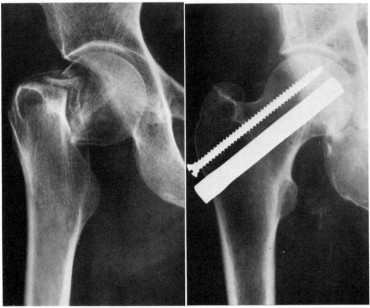

Fig. 211   Fig. 212

A typical fracture of the neck of the femur before and after reduction and internal fixation with a three-flanged nail and a screw.

Clinical features. In a case of displaced fracture a typical history is that the patient—usually an elderly woman—tripped and fell, and was unable to get up again unaided. She was subsequently unable to take weight on the injured limb. *On examination* the most striking feature is the marked lateral rotation of the limb. This is often as much as 90 degrees, so that the patella and the foot point laterally. The limb is shortened by about two or three centimetres. Any movement of the hip causes severe pain.

Impacted abduction fracture (Fig. 214). In the exceptional case in which the fracture is impacted the history and signs are different. The patient may have been able to pick herself up after falling, and she may even have walked a short distance afterwards. Indeed some patients have carried on and have not sought medical advice for several days. *On examination* there is no detectable shortening and no rotational deformity. The patient can move the hip through a moderate range without severe pain.

Radiographic examination. In the ordinary case with displacement of the fragments the fracture is obvious and cannot be mistaken (Fig. 211); but in some cases of impacted abduction fracture the radiographic changes are slight and the fracture may be overlooked (Fig. 214). Lateral radiographs should always be obtained as well as antero-posterior films.

Treatment. Displaced fractures and impacted abduction fractures must be considered separately.

DISPLACED FRACTURES. Unimpacted fracture of the neck of the femur is one of the few fractures that needs rigid immobilisation if it is to have any chance of uniting.

Standard method. Except in children (in whom this fracture is rare), immobilisation in plaster is unreliable as well as cumbersome; so the accepted treatment is to fix the fragments internally by a suitable metal device. Hitherto the device most commonly used has been the three-flanged Smith-Petersen nail or one of its modifications (Fig. 213); but most surgeons now believe that a nail alone can seldom provide adequate fixation, and accordingly they prefer to use either a three-flanged nail in conjunction with a screw (Fig. 212), or a combined nail and femoral plate, some models of which embody a telescopically sliding nail to allow for the absorption and consequent slight shortening of the femoral neck that are sometimes unavoidable. The author's own preference is for a three-flanged nail in conjunction with a Venable hip screw, the screw being placed parallel to, and just above, the nail, as described below.

Technique of internal fixation for femoral neck fracture. With the patient upon an orthopaedic table the fracture is reduced by flexion and medial rotation of the thigh combined with traction in the line of the femur. After this manipulation the position of the fragments is maintained pending insertion of the screw and nail by binding the foot to the soleplate of the orthopaedic table in a position of slight medial rotation, and the reduction is confirmed by antero-posterior and lateral radiographs or by viewing with the television-monitored image intensifier. Through a lateral incision in the upper thigh a guide wire is passed along the neck of the femur from a point on the shaft a little below the greater trochanter, and its position is checked by radiographs in two planes. When this first wire has been placed centrally in the neck—or preferably just below the central axis—a second wire is inserted 1·25 centimetres above the first wire and

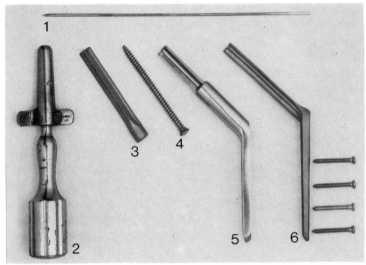

Fig. 213

Instruments and internal appliances for operative treatment of fractures of neck and trochanteric region of femur. 1. Guide wire. 2. Guide wire introducer. 3. Three-flanged nail for fractures of neck of femur. 4. Venable hip screw. 5. Telescopically sliding nail and plate (Tulloch Brown pattern) for fracture of neck of femur. 6. Nail-plate (Jewett pattern) and screws for fracture of the trochanteric region.

parallel to it. After its position has been checked this second wire is removed and its track is enlarged to 4 millimetres in diameter by a special drill, to allow the insertion of a Venable hip screw of appropriate length. Finally the selected three-flanged nail, which has a central cannula, is threaded over the lower guide wire and driven home with hammer and punch (Fig. 212). If a nail-plate is to be used instead of a nail and a screw, a single guide wire only is required. The nail-plate is threaded over the guide wire and hammered home, and finally the plate part is fixed to the femoral shaft with screws.

After operation the patient is nursed free in bed and active hip movements are encouraged. Ideally, perhaps, weight-bearing on the injured limb should be avoided for three months to afford the greatest chance of union. But in old patients the advantages to the general health of being up and about outweigh the theoretical advantages to the fracture of rest; so most surgeons allow a limited amount of walking with the aid of sticks or elbow crutches from an early stage—often within the first week or two after operation.

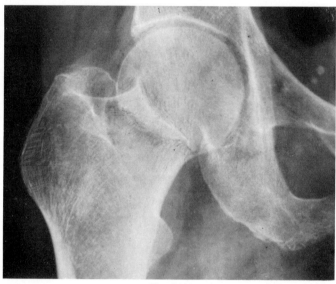

Fig. 214

Impacted abduction fracture of neck of femur. Note that the shaft fragment is slightly abducted in relation to the femoral head, so that the upper corner of the fracture surface is driven into the cancellous bone of the femoral head. This is the only type of femoral neck fracture in adults that can be treated successfully without operation.

Alternative methods for special cases. Because of the uncertain results of nailing these fractures, especially in the aged, many surgeons have advocated immediate excision of the femoral head and its replacement by a metal prosthesis (replacement arthroplasty, Fig. 217). Some go even farther and advise the fitting of a plastic socket as well as a prosthetic femoral head (total replacement arthroplasty) (Fig. 218) if the bones are very soft. These operations are a little more severe than that of introducing a nail, but the results are sufficiently encouraging to suggest that they may have a place in primary treatment, especially in old persons who are unlikely to place heavy demands upon the hip. It is accordingly common practice now at many centres to recommend primary prosthetic replacement as a routine method in preference to fixation by a nail or nail-plate in patients over 70.

Treatment in children. In children, manipulative reduction followed by immobilisation in plaster is often effective. Nevertheless most surgeons advise operative fixation, usually by two or three threaded pins.

IMPACTED ABDUCTION FRACTURES. An impacted abduction fracture (Fig. 214) will usually unite readily without operation, and conservative treatment should therefore be advised. The patient should rest in bed for three weeks but should be encouraged to practise hip and knee flexion exercises under the supervision of a physiotherapist. Check radiographs are obtained weekly at first to make sure that the original impacted position has been maintained. After three weeks the patient is usually able to sit out of bed and to begin walking with crutches. After a further three weeks elbow crutches are substituted. Full weight bearing is avoided until about the eighth week.

It should be mentioned that some surgeons distrust this conservative approach to impacted abduction fractures, fearing that the fragments may become separated and displaced (Bentley 1968). Accordingly they advocate nailing as a routine practice, as for unimpacted fractures. The decision is arbitrary, but there seems to be full justification for avoiding operation because the incidence of late displacement is very small, provided always that the clinical and radiographic criteria of impaction are interpreted strictly.

Complications. Fractures of the neck of the femur are more prone to complications than any other fracture. The important complications are avascular necrosis, non-union, and late osteoarthritis. All these complications affect fractures with displacement rather than impacted abduction fractures.

AVASCULAR NECROSIS. After fracture of the femoral neck the blood supply to the head of the femur is very precarious. Normally, blood is supplied to the femoral head by three routes (Fig. 215): through the vessels in the ligament of the head of the femur (ligamentum teres), through the capsular vessels reflected onto the femoral neck, and through branches of the nutrient vessels within the substance of the bone. When the neck of the femur is fractured the nutrient vessels within the bone are necessarily severed. Some at least of the capsular vessels are likely to be interrupted, and the higher the fracture the more complete is the interruption of these channels likely to be. Thus the viability of the femoral head may depend almost entirely upon the blood supplied through the ligament of the head of the femur (ligamentum teres). This is a variable quantity, and it is often insufficient to keep the head alive. In that event the bone cells die (avascular necrosis) and the fracture may fail to unite; or if it does unite it may not do so quickly enough to allow revascularisation of the head fragment before irreversible changes in bone or cartilage have occurred. Avascular changes may be total, affecting the whole of the head, or they may be partial, affecting only a segment of the head.

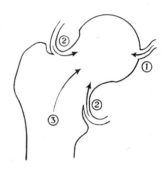

Fig. 215
Normal blood supply of the femoral head. The three groups of vessels are: 1. vessels in ligament of femoral head; 2. capsular vessels; 3. nutrient vessels from the femoral shaft. A fracture through the femoral neck may leave only the vessels in the ligament of the femoral head intact, but some of the capsular vessels may also escape.

Consequences of avascular necrosis. The main consequence of avascular necrosis of the head of the femur is collapse of the bone structure, leading to fragmentation. This does not occur immediately but is delayed for a matter of months or even for as long as two or three years. Necrosis and collapse involving the fracture surface may lead to failure of union of the fracture, whereas collapse at the articular surface leads to degenerative arthritis (osteoarthritis). If necrosis is total the whole femoral head may collapse, with complete disorganisation of the hip. The complication of avascular necrosis is thus closely related to both of the other two complications to be described—non-union and osteoarthritis.

Treatment. Treatment is mainly that of the secondary effects and will be described in the succeeding sections on non-union and osteoarthritis.

NON-UNION. Non-union occurs in about a third of all cases of fracture of the neck of the femur despite competent primary treatment. Three causes of non-union have to be considered: 1) inadequate blood supply to the femoral head with consequent avascular necrosis; 2) incomplete immobilisation; and 3) flushing of the fracture haematoma by synovial fluid.

Avascular necrosis was described above and it must be accepted as a potent source of non-union—perhaps the most important factor of all.

Incomplete immobilisation is probably also an important cause of non-union in that it prevents the formation of a satisfactory bridge of bone-forming tissue. Movement between the fragments occurs particularly when the fracture has been insecurely fixed by a badly placed nail, or when the bone is soft and allows the nail to cut through. Unlike avascular necrosis, this factor is to a large extent under the control of the surgeon.

Flushing of the fracture haematoma by synovial fluid is a possible factor that needs further investigation. In so far as a flow of synovial fluid between the fracture surfaces may prevent the formation of a haematoma and of

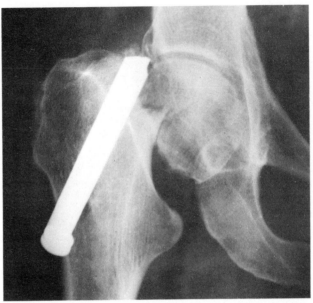

Fig. 216
Ununited fracture of the neck of the femur with extrusion of the nail and redisplacement of the fragments. Much of the femoral neck has been absorbed.

bone-forming tissue it is certainly reasonable to suggest that it may prevent union, or that it may help to perpetuate a state of non-union initiated by some other cause. This factor may prove to be more important than has hitherto been realised.

Pathology and clinical features. When the fracture fails to unite the neck of the femur undergoes progressive absorption, so that the femoral head sinks down towards the trochanters. At the same time the nail or other fixation device loosens and is partly extruded along the path through which it was driven in. Finally the point of the nail breaks away from the femoral head and the fragments become redisplaced (Fig. 216). As noted already, if the bone is avascular there may also be total or partial collapse of the femoral head.

Clinically, after seemingly normal progress at first, the patient begins to complain of renewed pain. Often there is sudden deterioration with acute pain, lateral rotation of the limb, shortening, and inability to walk. This disaster may take place at any time from a few weeks to three years from the time of the nailing operation: it commonly occurs at about two to six months.

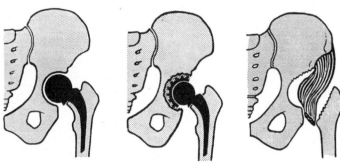

Fig. 217   Fig. 218   Fig. 219

Reconstructive operations for non-union of fractures of femoral neck. Figure 217—Half-joint replacement arthroplasty (prosthetic replacement of femoral head). Figure 218—Total replacement arthroplasty (prosthetic replacement of femoral head and acetabulum). Figure 219—Excision arthroplasty (Girdlestone pseudarthrosis).

Treatment. Non-union almost inevitably necessitates further operation, and this is especially true if it is associated with avascular necrosis and collapse of the femoral head. Methods of treatment have undergone re-appraisal in the past decade, and operations that formerly had wide support, such as displacement osteotomy (McMurray 1935), abduction osteotomy (Dickson 1947) and arthrodesis have been almost if not entirely discarded. At the present time the choice generally lies in one of the following methods: 1) simple removal of the nail without further treatment; 2) prosthetic replacement of femoral head (half-joint replacement arthroplasty, Fig. 217); 3) prosthetic replacement of femoral head and acetabulum (total replacement arthroplasty, Fig. 218); 4) excision arthroplasty (Fig. 219). In general, there is a strong preponderance of opinion in favour of replacement arthroplasty—usually by prosthetic replacement of the femoral head alone if the acetabulum appears healthy.

Removal of nail. This eliminates any local symptoms from protrusion of the nail in the thigh, but it has little effect in improving function. Nevertheless some patients manage to get about to a limited extent without further treatment, and in patients who are old, frail and perhaps in consequence confined to one or two rooms, there may be no indication for more drastic measures.

Half-joint replacement arthroplasty. Prosthetic replacement of the femoral head (Moore 1957; Thompson 1952; 1954) has become the mainstay of treatment for non-union of fractures of the neck of the femur. It is applicable almost to every type of case, whether or not there is associated avascular necrosis of the femoral head. The operation consists in removal of the head and neck of the femur and

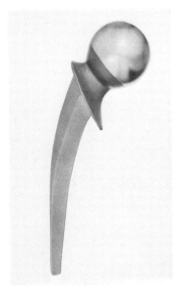

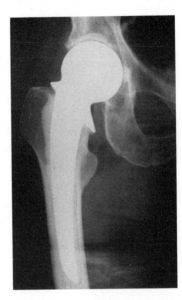

Fig. 220   Fig. 221

Figure 220—Femoral head prosthesis (Thompson pattern). Figure 221—Radiograph after half-joint replacement arthroplasty for femoral neck fracture. Acrylic cement, used to stabilise the prosthesis in the femur, is seen round the stem of the prosthesis. (The cement had been made radio-opaque by the addition of barium salts.)

their replacement by a metal prosthesis, the stem of which enters the medullary canal of the femoral shaft (Figs. 217, 220 and 221). To ensure more certain fixation of the prosthesis most surgeons now embed its stem in acrylic filling compound or 'cement' pressed into the medullary canal of the upper end of the femur. The patient may usually be encouraged to begin walking, at first with the partial support of crutches, within a few days after the operation.

Total replacement arthroplasty. In late cases with disorganisation of the acetabulum as well as of the femoral head, total replacement arthroplasty—that is, insertion of an artificial socket as well as of a femoral head prosthesis—is to be preferred to replacement of the femoral head alone. Indeed many surgeons prefer to undertake this more radical operation even when the acetabulum appears healthy, on the grounds that it offers more certain relief of pain. It also forestalls an important complication sometimes seen after replacement of the femoral head alone—namely erosion of the acetabulum with consequent upward and medial migration of the prosthetic femoral head.

Excision arthroplasty (Girdlestone pseudarthrosis). The head and neck of the femur are excised and the side wall of the pelvis is smoothed by removing the upper margin of the acetabulum (Adams 1976) (Fig. 219). A flap of muscle or other soft tissue is interposed between the shaft of the femur and the pelvis. The effect is to create a false joint which is painless and has a reasonable range of movement, but with some shortening and instability. This method is seldom used as a first-choice operation, but it is useful as a salvage operation especially in the occasional case in which replacement arthroplasty proves unsuccessful in restoring painless function.

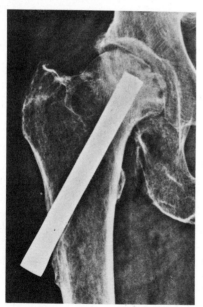

Fig. 222
Avascular necrosis of a large seg-ment of the femoral head two years after fracture of the femoral neck. Although the fracture appears to have united the ischaemic changes adjacent to the joint margin are caus-ing osteoarthritis. Pain necessitated operation, at which the femoral head was replaced by a metal prosthesis.

OSTEOARTHRITIS. Even when a fracture of the neck of the femur unites by bone there is a risk of the later development of osteo-arthritis. Arthritis may arise 1) from mechanical damage to the articular cartilage at the time of injury or operation; 2) from impairment of the blood supply to the basal layers of the cartilage, which are probably nourished largely from the vessels in the underlying bone (Fig. 222); or 3) from union in faulty alignment. It may develop within months of the original injury, as is usually the case after avascular necrosis of the femoral head; or the onset may be delayed for as long as twenty years or more, as in cases of mal-alignment. Treatment is along the usual lines for osteoarthritis from other causes.

FATIGUE FRACTURE OF NECK OF FEMUR

Fatigue or stress fracture of the neck of the femur is well recognised, though uncommon. The fracture develops insidiously, with increasing pain in the region of the hip. Unlike stress fractures of the metatarsal bones, it is liable eventually to lead to displacement of the fragments,

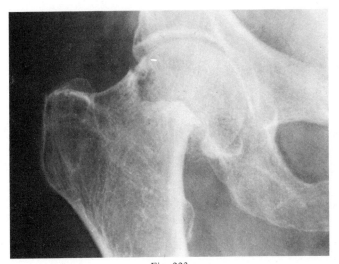

Fig. 223

Fatigue fracture of femoral neck. The radiograph shows the fracture two months after the spontaneous onset of pain. There is marked displacement of the fragments.

with almost total loss of function of the hip. A similar fracture is sometimes observed after irradiation therapy for neoplastic lesions in or about the pelvis (Fig. 223). Treatment should generally be by internal fixation, as for ordinary displaced fracture of the neck of the femur, or in appropriate circumstances by replacement arthroplasty.

FRACTURE OF THE TROCHANTERIC REGION

The term trochanteric fracture[1] may be used to describe any fracture in the region that lies approximately between the greater and the lesser trochanter (Fig. 210). It is unnecessary to retain such terms as 'intertrochanteric' and 'pertrochanteric', which only lead to confusion.

A trochanteric fracture is a much more benign injury than a fracture of the neck of the femur, because it unites readily no matter how it is treated, and it is immune from the serious complications for which femoral neck fractures are notorious.

Trochanteric fractures are common in the old—especially in women, who form the bulk of the aged population. If anything, they have a higher average age incidence than femoral neck fractures. Thus they are seen very often in persons of 75 to 85. The cause is nearly always a fall.

Clinical features. The history is much the same as that in cases of fracture of the neck of the femur. After being knocked down or falling the patient is unable to pick herself up without assistance, and is unable to put weight on the limb. On examination the findings resemble those of a femoral neck fracture in that the limb is shortened and rotated laterally. But pain is most marked over the trochanteric region, and after a day or two a visible ecchymosis often appears at the back of the upper thigh—a feature not seen in cases of femoral neck fracture because extravasated blood is retained within the joint capsule.

Radiographic examination. In most cases the fracture is obvious (Fig. 224), but a minor fracture without displacement may easily be overlooked. Careful scrutiny of good antero-posterior and lateral radiographs is required.

Treatment. Since trochanteric fractures unite readily the main objects of treatment are to ensure that the fragments are held in good position, and to encourage the patient in regaining perfect function. These objects can be achieved by conservative treatment, but since most of these patients are old the advantage of earlier mobility that can be gained by operative fixation generally outweighs the disadvantages of operation.

Standard method. Internal fixation by a nail-plate (Figs. 213 and 225) is the routine method of treatment at most centres. A nail-plate is more effective in holding the fragments than a plain nail, because there is not enough width of bone in the shaft fragment to afford a firm

---

[1] See footnote on page 202.

grip to a nail. With the nail-plate a rigid grip on the shaft fragment is obtained by means of screws.

Technique of internal fixation for trochanteric fracture. With the patient on an orthopaedic table the fracture is reduced by traction and medial rotation, and the foot is bandaged to the sole-plate with the limb in a neutral position as regards rotation. Through a lateral incision in the upper part of the thigh

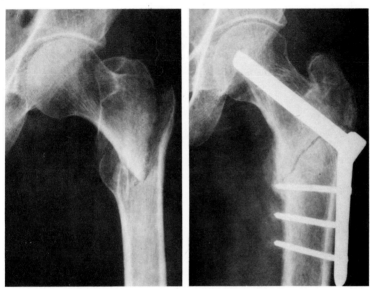

Fig. 224   Fig. 225
A typical trochanteric fracture before and after internal
fixation with a nail-plate.

the femur is exposed for about ten centimetres below the greater trochanter. A guide wire is entered a little below the trochanter and passed along the neck into the head of the femur. The position of the wire is checked by radiographs in two planes. When a wire has been placed centrally in the neck a nail-plate of the correct size and angle is driven home along the guide wire and secured to the femoral shaft by screws (Fig. 225).

After operation the patient is nursed free in bed, active hip and knee exercises being practised from the beginning. Usually, walking with the partial support of crutches is begun within a day or two of the operation. Early walking is especially important in the aged, for old people tolerate inactivity badly. Conversely, for a relatively young patient it is reasonable to allow a longer period of rest in bed to insure against bending or fracture of the nail-plate.

Alternative methods for special cases. Continuous traction. In young patients, or in those who refuse operation, it is reasonable to rely on conservative treatment by rest in bed with continuous weight traction. The method of traction devised by Russell[1] is very suitable for these cases (Fig. 226). Traction must be maintained until the fracture is soundly united—usually a matter of ten or twelve weeks.

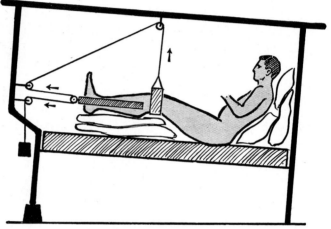

Fig. 226

Continuous traction by the Russell technique. In this method a splint is not used. The traction grip on the leg may be obtained by adhesive skin strapping (as shown here) or alternatively by a pin through the tibia (as in Figures 229 and 230). A canvas sling gives support under the knee from the overhead beam, and the lower leg rests upon two pillows. By the simple mechanical system shown a single weight serves the double purpose of supporting the limb and exerting continuous traction. Because of the system of pulleys the distalward pull is twice the upward pull (friction being discounted); so the resultant pull is approximately in the line of the femur. The foot of the bed is raised on blocks so that the patient's own weight provides counter-traction. Russell traction, or one of the several modifications of it, is useful for any condition about the hip or trochanteric region for which continuous traction is desired. It is not suitable for fractures of the shaft of the femur because there is nothing to give support under the fracture to prevent sagging.

Plaster spica. There is an occasional place for treatment by reduction and immobilisation in a plaster hip spica, especially in children. This method is seldom used in adults because it is less comfortable for the patient than the methods just described.

[1] Hamilton Russell, a British surgeon who worked under Lister and who later settled in Melbourne, Australia, described the technique that bears his name in 1923.

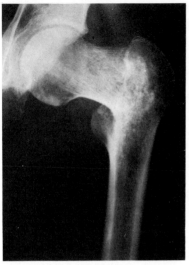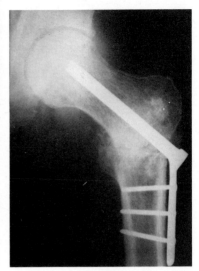

| Fig. 227 | Fig. 228 |

Figure 227—Mal-union of a trochanteric fracture in a young man. Note that the neck-shaft angle, normally 130 degrees, has been reduced to about 90 degrees. Figure 228—After corrective osteotomy and fixation by nail-plate. (In old persons, who are the usual victims of this injury, a deformity such as this would usually be accepted.)

Complications. Unlike fractures of the neck of the femur, trochanteric fractures are almost free from serious complications.

MAL-UNION. The only complication that is frequent is mal-union, and this is seldom of severe degree. Despite the greatest care in treatment, many trochanteric fractures unite with a slightly reduced neck-shaft angle (coxa vara). This may occur through bending or breakage of the nail-plate, or simply through compression of the soft cancellous bone in contact with the metal. Coxa vara is associated with shortening, but this seldom exceeds two or three centimetres.

In neglected or untreated cases mal-union may be more troublesome, for the fracture may unite with marked lateral rotation of the shaft fragment as well as with severe coxa vara.

Treatment. In most cases mal-union can be accepted without treatment other than perhaps building up the shoe on the affected side to compensate for shortening. Occasionally a severe deformity may demand correction, especially if it occurs in a young person. The bone is divided in the trochanteric region and the fragments are secured in the correct position by a nail-plate, as in the treatment of a fresh fracture (Figs. 227 and 228).

FRACTURE OF THE SHAFT OF THE FEMUR

Fracture of the shaft of the femur occurs at any age, usually from severe violence such as may be caused by a road accident or aeroplane crash. It may occur at any site, and is almost equally common in the uppermost, middle, and lowest thirds of the shaft. Likewise the pattern of the fracture is variable, for it may be transverse, oblique, spiral, comminuted, or (in children) of the greenstick type. More often than not there is marked displacement of the fragments, in the form of angulation and overlap.

The femur is a common site for pathological fractures from carcinomatous metastases. Fractures from this cause generally occur in the upper half of the bone (Fig. 231).

Treatment. The well tried method of conservative treatment by sustained weight traction with the limb supported in a Thomas's splint is still often the method of choice. Though the period of disability is usually lengthy the results are nearly always excellent. It is true that the indications for internal fixation by a long intra-medullary nail have widened in recent years; and it is likely that, with modern refinements in the technique of femoral nailing, operation will be used increasingly in the future. Even now, in Britain, operation is probably used more often than conservative treatment. Nevertheless it must be remembered that by no means every fracture of the femoral shaft lends itself well to intramedullary nailing: many comminuted fractures and fractures close to the upper or lower end are unsuitable. And it has to be emphasised that when nailing is done by the open method, with wide exposure of the fracture site—the method generally used—the complications of infection and of knee stiffness are disconcertingly prevalent: sufficiently prevalent, in fact, to deter the conscientious surgeon and to tip the balance against operation unless some special indication for it exists.

Conservative treatment by sustained traction. The principles of this method are to reduce the fracture (if necessary) by traction and manipulation, to support the limb in a Thomas's splint, and to maintain continuous traction by means of a weight in order to preserve correct length (Fig. 229). Rehabilitation by exercises is begun at an early stage.

Reduction. An anaesthetic is not always required. Traction is applied to the lower leg either by adhesive skin strapping or by a Steinmann pin through the upper end of the tibia (Fig. 230). A Thomas's splint with Pearson knee flexion attachment (Fig. 40) is fitted. By a combination of traction and manipulation an attempt is made to bring the fragments into correct apposition and alignment, radiographs being taken as required to check the position.

Splintage. When satisfactory reduction has been achieved, canvas strips slung between the bars of the Thomas's splint are adjusted for tension, the splint with contained limb is suspended from an overhead beam by the balance-weight technique shown in Figure 229, and a

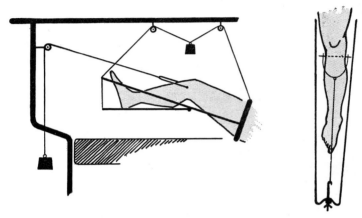

Fig. 229

Continuous traction with balanced suspension, using a Thomas's splint with Pearson knee flexion attachment. This is the standard technique of traction for fractures of the shaft of the femur. The larger diagram shows the general layout of the cords and pulleys. The traction grip on the leg may be obtained by adhesive skin strapping (as in Figure 226) or by a pin through the tibia (as shown here and in Figure 230). There are two systems of cords and weights. The purpose of one system is to support the splint and the contained limb from the overhead beam. This weight is adjusted until the limb is nicely balanced. The purpose of the other system is to exert continuous traction in the line of the femur. Counter-traction is through the cords that suspend the splint from the beam—particularly the cord that is attached to the distal end of the splint; so it is unnecessary to raise the foot of the bed on blocks. Many modifications of this method of traction are in use but the basic principles are the same. One modification is shown in the smaller diagram: here a screw traction device attached to the end of the splint is used instead of the traction weight. This technique is termed 'fixed traction' as distinct from the 'sliding traction' shown in the larger diagram.

suitable weight (usually 10 to 15 pounds, according to the build of the patient) is attached to the traction cord. The knee is flexed 15 or 20 degrees to permit control of rotation. Repeated check radiographs are advisable in the first two weeks, and appropriate adjustments to the slings or weights are made as required.

Rehabilitation. Exercises for the lower leg and foot are important in preserving muscle tone and in preventing deformity—especially that of equinus—and they should be begun immediately. As soon as the initial pain of the fracture begins to settle—usually about a week after the injury—active quadriceps and knee exercises are begun. Knee flexion through about 60 degrees may be allowed, but more important

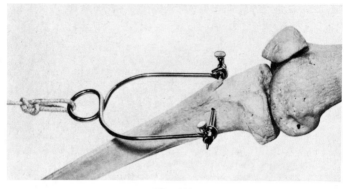

Fig. 230

Model showing correct site for transfixion of tibia by a Steinmann pin for purposes of traction. The stirrup slips over the ends of the pin. Sometimes a length of piano wire (Kirschner wire) held taut between the limbs of a 'horse shoe' is used instead of the rigid steel pin.

than flexion is the ability to extend the knee fully by quadriceps action. These activities do not interfere with union of the fracture and may be encouraged without fear.

The duration of splintage varies from case to case. Except in children, few fractures of the femoral shaft are firmly joined in twelve weeks: most take sixteen weeks or even longer. When the stage of sound union is reached the splint is removed and the patient is allowed to exercise freely in bed before walking is begun. Thereafter rehabilitation is continued in the gymnasium until adequate function is restored. The use of a walking caliper—often prescribed in the past to protect the newly-healed bone—is not recommended: a caliper is not a reliable safeguard against refracture and in fact is no more than an encumbrance.

Operative treatment: *Internal fixation.* Internal fixation, usually by a long intramedullary nail, is indicated in the following circumstances. 1) When satisfactory reduction cannot be secured and maintained by manipulation and traction—as, for instance, when a large mass of muscle has become wedged between the fragments. 2) In old or frail persons who would be likely to respond unfavourably to a long period of rest in bed with relative immobility. 3) In cases of severe multiple injuries to the lower limbs, to facilitate the management of the other injuries. 4) In patients with pathological fractures—especially those from metastatic deposits (Figs. 231 and 232)—in order to facilitate nursing and to allow some restoration of function even if the fracture

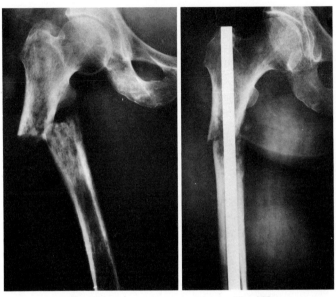

Fig. 231   Fig. 232

Figure 231—Pathological fracture of femur from carcinomatous metastasis. This is a common site. Figure 232—The same fracture after internal fixation with a long intramedullary nail.

fails to unite. 5) Intramedullary nailing—especially by the closed technique—may also be justified in certain other cases when the fracture is particularly suitable for nailing and when special economic or social factors make it important that the patient be got home with the least possible delay. In Britain, shortage of hospital beds and the patient's domestic or economic circumstances often place cases in this category, even though on general grounds the surgeon might have preferred to treat the patient conservatively.

Technique of intramedullary nailing for femoral fracture. Whenever possible, nailing should be done by the closed technique—that is, without exposing the fracture itself. The patient is placed in the lateral position, lying upon the sound side, with the knee and lower leg of the affected side supported upon a bridge or platform. To secure and maintain reduction of the fracture it may be necessary to apply strong traction upon the leg through a Steinmann pin inserted through the tibial tubercle or through the lower end of the femur. Through a lateral incision over the trochanteric region a long guide wire is introduced near the tip of the greater trochanter and passed down the shaft of the femur until its tip reaches the level of the fracture. The fragments are manipulated into correct apposition and alignment under radiographic control (an image-intensifier x-ray unit with

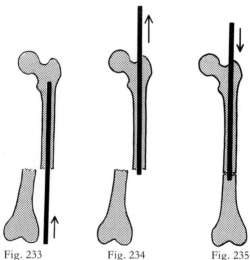

Fig. 233   Fig. 234   Fig. 235

In open nailing of the femur the nail is first driven into the proximal fragment from the fracture site (Fig. 233) and out through the greater trochanter (Fig. 234). After reduction of the fracture the nail is then engaged in the distal fragment (Fig. 235) and driven home.

television monitor is useful for this purpose), whereupon the guide wire is passed on into the distal fragment of the femur, well into the condylar region. With special power-operated cannulated reamers the medullary canal is enlarged to the diameter of the nail that has been selected— usually about 12 to 16 millimetres. A nail of the correct length is then threaded over the guide wire and driven home, the final position being checked again by radiographs.

When closed nailing is impracticable the open method may have to be used. The fracture is exposed, preferably through a postero-lateral incision. The medullary canal of the proximal fragment is reamed out to the desired calibre by a drill or reamer introduced at the site of fracture and driven proximally. The medullary canal of the lower fragment is then similarly enlarged. The selected nail is introduced into the proximal fragment at the site of the fracture (Fig. 233) and is driven backwards (that is, proximally) until its tip is level with the fracture, the proximal end of the nail being allowed to protrude through the greater trochanter and through the overlying skin (Fig. 234). The upper and lower fragments of the femur are now lined up and correctly apposed, and the nail is driven home from above into the lower fragment (Fig. 235).

Post-operative treatment. If it has been possible to secure rigid fixation with a strong nail of adequate diameter there is no need to immobilise the thigh in plaster or in a splint. The patient may lie free in bed and practise exercises for the hip and knee joints and for the related muscles. He may begin walking with the partial support of crutches two or three weeks after operation but should be discouraged from taking the full weight of the body upon the limb until there is radiographic evidence that bone union is occurring.

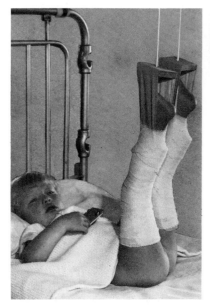

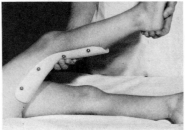

Fig. 237

'Gallows' or Bryant's traction for fractures of the femoral shaft in children of up to 4 years old. The cords are attached to an overhead beam. Note that the buttocks are suspended just clear of the mattress, so that the weight of the lower part of the trunk and pelvis exerts continuous traction on the limbs. The knees should be held slightly flexed by the simple plastic splint shown in Figure 237, included beneath the crepe bandages.

Fig. 236

Treatment in young children: 'Gallows' or Bryant's traction. This method of traction is convenient and satisfactory for children up to the age of 4 years. By means of adhesive skin strapping applied direct to the skin of the legs the child's lower limbs are suspended from an overhead beam. The cords are tightened just enough to raise the child's buttocks clear of the mattress (Fig. 236). The weight of the pelvis and lower trunk is sufficient to maintain full length of the fractured femur, and the vertical position of the limb, together with the continuous traction, automatically ensures good alignment. Small children tolerate this rather grotesque position without complaint. Since fractures unite rapidly in early childhood it is seldom necessary to maintain the traction for more than four weeks.

Caution. In children suspended in 'gallows' traction the knees should be kept slightly flexed by simple back-splints (Fig. 237) held in position with crepe bandages. Neglect of this precaution has led, very rarely, to spasm of the major artery of the limb and consequent ischaemia. It is also important that the strips of adhesive strapping used to support the limbs be applied direct to the skin, and not over encircling bandages: otherwise the limb may be constricted, with serious detriment to the circulation. As after all injuries to the limbs, the state of the circulation should be watched carefully, especially in the first three days.

Complications. The following complications of femoral shaft fractures will be considered: 1) infection; 2) injury to major artery; 3) injury to nerve; 4) delayed union; 5) non-union; 6) mal-union; and 7) stiffness of the knee.

INFECTION. In cases of open (compound) fracture contamination with consequent infection of the bone is an important potential complication. Clearly the risk of infection increases proportionately to the severity of the trauma and the degree of contamination. Thus in fractures that are 'compound from within', in which the skin is merely pierced from inside by a sharp fragment of bone, contamination may be negligible and the risk of osteomyelitis very slight. At the other extreme is the gunshot or bomb wound in which there is always heavy contamination and extensive tissue damage, and in these cases risk of infection is very high indeed. *Treatment* is along the lines suggested on page 48. It must be re-emphasised here that in the management of a heavily contaminated wound such as a gunshot wound it is not permissible ever to close the wound by primary suture: such closure courts disaster. The correct treatment is to leave the wound open after initial cleansing and then, if the wound appears healthy and free from major infection, to undertake delayed primary suture after a few days.

INJURY TO MAJOR ARTERY. Rarely, a sharp edge of the fractured bone may penetrate the soft tissues and damage the femoral artery. The vessel may be severed or it may be severely contused and occluded. In either case the outlook for the viability of the limb is grave unless continuity of the vessel can be restored by operation.

INJURY TO NERVE. Just as a major artery may be damaged, so a nerve trunk may be struck by a sharp fragment of bone at the time of the initial injury. The severity of the damage can vary from transient neurapraxia to complete severance of the nerve. The sciatic nerve is obviously the most significant in this type of injury. As the nerve is broad and may divide into tibial and common peroneal components high up in the thigh, one or other of these subdivisions may be injured while the other escapes. The management of peripheral nerve injuries was discussed on page 64.

DELAYED UNION. Four months is a fair average time for union of a fractured femoral shaft in an adult. There is no hard-and-fast time limit beyond which union is said to be delayed. But if union is still insufficient to allow unprotected weight bearing after five months' support in a splint additional methods of treatment must be considered.

Treatment. When callus is forming satisfactorily but is building up very slowly it is often wise to apply a full-length plaster hip spica and to allow the patient to walk. This method will often obviate the need for operation, but it is appropriate to the young and active patient rather than to the elderly. In other cases some form of bone grafting operation may offer the best solution to the problem, as for non-union.

A walking caliper cannot be relied upon to protect the femoral shaft adequately, and in the author's opinion a caliper has no place in the treatment of this fracture.

NON-UNION. If union fails to occur and the fracture surfaces are becoming rounded and sclerotic operation should be advised. The bone ends are freshened and bone grafts are applied. One of two techniques may be used: a strong cortical slab graft may be secured to the fragments with screws to serve the double purpose of internal fixation and provision of a bone 'scaffold' (Fig. 57); or internal fixation may be secured by a long intramedullary nail and the bone supplied in the form of slivers or chips of cancellous bone packed firmly about the site of fracture (Figs. 58 and 59).

MAL-UNION. Without constant supervision the fragments may suffer redisplacement in the form of angulation or overlap, and unless this is recognised the fracture will unite in the position of deformity. The commonest examples of mal-union are overlap with consequent shortening, and lateral bowing. Lateral bowing is especially common when the fracture is in the upper half of the femur. An angular deformity may have secondary effects years later in the form of osteoarthritis of the knee (Figs. 75 and 76, p. 72).

Treatment. In most cases mal-union of slight or moderate degree is best accepted, the shoe being built up if necessary to correct shortening. It is a formidable undertaking to reproduce the fracture by osteotomy, to re-align the fragments, and to fix them with an intra-medullary nail; but some such procedure may be advisable occasionally for mal-union of severe degree, especially if the patient is a young adult.

STIFFNESS OF KNEE. After a fracture of the femoral shaft the patient nearly always has some difficulty in regaining a full range of knee movement, but it is seldom that troublesome stiffness persists permanently. In most such cases stiffness is due not to a disturbance of the knee itself (for the joint is usually uninjured), but to periarticular and intramuscular adhesions which prevent free gliding of the muscle fibres one upon another, and to adhesions between the muscles and the femur.

Treatment. In most cases knee stiffness from a femoral shaft fracture responds well to treatment by active exercises if they are carried out intensively and for a long enough time. Many months may elapse before full recovery is gained. If the knee is uninjured and is therefore free from intra-articular adhesions dramatic improvement cannot be expected from manipulation, and the temptation to force movement passively should be resisted.

In the rare cases in which knee stiffness is severe and is resistant to conscientious treatment by exercises the range of movement may be increased by the operation of quadricepsplasty, in which all adhesions are divided and the quadriceps expansion may be freed further by division of its vastus medialis and vastus lateralis components. Quadricepsplasty demands prolonged and intensive after-treatment and is suitable only for robust adult patients.

SUPRACONDYLAR FRACTURE OF THE FEMUR

Although there is no strict line of demarcation between a low fracture of the femoral shaft and a supracondylar fracture, it is well to consider supracondylar fractures as a separate group because their treatment differs in certain respects from that of femoral shaft fractures.

Typically the fracture occurs just proximal to the point where the medial and lateral cortices of the femur flare out to form the condyles (Fig. 238). A vertical extension of the fracture may split the two condyles apart, and sometimes there is more extensive comminution. Usually the main fracture is more or less transverse, and commonly the distal fragment is tilted anteriorly upon the shaft, without serious loss of end-to-end apposition (Fig. 239).

Treatment. *Standard method.* Most supracondylar fractures of the femur may be treated successfully by supporting the limb on a Thomas's splint with a knee flexion attachment, with continuous weight traction, as for fractures of the femoral shaft (Fig. 229). But whereas in fractures of the femoral shaft the position of the knee is unimportant and is dictated mainly by considerations of comfort and convenience, in displaced supracondylar fractures the angle of knee flexion is often the key to the problem of reduction and stabilisation of the fracture. This point is illustrated in Figures 239 and 240 where it is seen that forward tilting of the distal fragment may be corrected by increasing the angle of knee flexion. The appropriate position for the knee is determined in the light of successive radiographs obtained during the first few days after the injury.

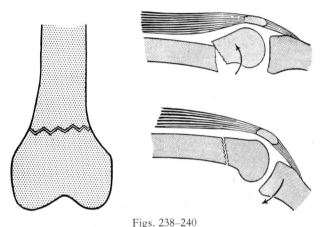

Figs. 238–240
Figure 238—Typical site of supracondylar fracture of the femur. Figure 239—A common displacement. Figure 240— A method of correction by increasing the angle of knee flexion.

In supracondylar fractures, unlike fractures of the femoral shaft proper, it is unwise to begin knee movements in the early days of treatment because the position of the fragments may be disturbed. For the first few weeks physiotherapy for the injured limb should be restricted to active ankle, foot and toe exercises, and static contractions of the quadriceps and gluteal muscles. Knee movements should be deferred until the fracture is becoming stable—usually about four weeks after the injury.

Alternative methods for special cases. Plaster spica. Supracondylar fractures without displacement may be treated by immobilising the limb in a plaster hip spica (or even in a long leg plaster if the patient is thin), and encouraging the patient to walk with sticks or crutches. This method is appropriate also for children.

Operative reduction and internal fixation. Operative fixation offers advantages when displacement cannot be well reduced by conservative means or when reduction cannot be maintained. As in fractures of the shaft of the femur, operative fixation may also be favoured in elderly patients in order to avoid prolonged recumbency, and occasionally in younger patients for the same reason. The problems of operation are mainly technical: the distal fragment is short, often comminuted, and not well controlled by an intramedullary nail. The best fixation device is probably a combined one-piece nail and plate (Brown and D'Arcy 1973): the nail is driven horizontally across the lower fragment and the plate, at right angles to the nail, is screwed to the side of the main upper fragment (Fig. 241).

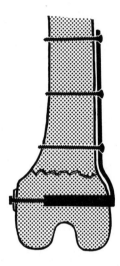

Fig. 241
Diagram to show use of nail-plate for fixation of supracondylar fracture of femur.

Complications. Most supracondylar fractures unite readily: delayed union and non-union are infrequent. Otherwise the common complications are the same as those of fractures of the femoral shaft—namely mal-union and stiffness of the knee. These were discussed on page 224. Rarely, a badly displaced supracondylar fracture may be complicated by injury to the popliteal artery or to a major nerve trunk.

FRACTURES OF THE FEMORAL CONDYLES
Condylar fractures of the femur are uncommon injuries, usually caused by direct violence to the region of the knee. Two patterns of fracture are illustrated in Figures 242 and 243. The fracture may be no more than a crack without displacement, or there may be complete separation of a condyle with marked displacement.

Treatment. This depends upon the degree of displacement.

Undisplaced fractures may be treated by immobilisation in a long leg plaster (Fig. 261) for about eight weeks, walking being allowed from an early stage.

DISPLACED FRACTURES demand accurate reduction because persistent displacement must inevitably disturb the mechanics of the knee and may lead to the later development of osteoarthritis. Reduction should be attempted by traction and manipulation: if these are successful the limb is supported in a Thomas's splint with continuous weight traction, or in a full length plaster.

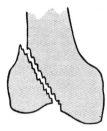 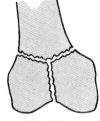

Fig. 242   Fig. 243

Two examples of condylar fractures of femur. Figure 242—Oblique fracture shearing the lateral condyle, which is here shown displaced upwards. Figure 243— T-shaped fracture separating both condyles.

If perfect reduction cannot be secured by traction and manipulation operative reduction and internal fixation should be advised. The method of fixation to be used will depend upon the nature of the individual fracture: in most cases a separated condyle can best be held in position by a long bolt or screw.

Complications. STIFFNESS OF KNEE. Most patients have difficulty in regaining a full range of knee movements. Stiffness is caused partly by intra-articular adhesions and partly by peri-articular and intramuscular adhesions. *Treatment* is mainly by active exercises. Gentle manipulation may be permissible later if steady progress is not being made with exercises alone.

OSTEOARTHRITIS OF KNEE. Osteoarthritis may develop months or years after the injury if the joint surface is left roughened or if the femoral condyles are out of alignment. Hence the importance of accurate reduction in the primary treatment of the fracture.

INJURY TO ARTERY OR NERVE. In violent injuries with marked displacement of a condylar fragment there may be direct mechanical injury to the popliteal artery or to one of the main nerve trunks. These are rare complications, but it is important that they be recognised promptly. This emphasises again the necessity of looking routinely for signs of arterial or nerve injury at the first examination of every patient with a limb injury. The treatment of arterial injuries was described on page 62, and of nerve injuries on page 64.

INJURIES OF THE KNEE

FRACTURES OF THE PATELLA

Fractures of the patella may be caused by two types of injury: 1) a sudden violent contraction of the quadriceps muscle—as in attempting to preserve the balance after stumbling; and 2) a fall or blow directly on the knee cap. Muscular violence usually causes a clean break with separation of the fragments, whereas a direct blow causes a crack fracture or a comminuted fracture. Pain is severe and well localised, and haemarthrosis is to be expected. Radiographically the fracture is shown best by a postero-anterior and a lateral projection.

Diagnosis from congenitally bipartite patella. The clinical and radiographic features usually make the diagnosis obvious. Nevertheless one must not jump too hastily to the diagnosis of fracture on the radiological evidence alone, because the radiographic appearance of a congenitally bipartite patella may be confused with that of a fracture. A congenitally bipartite patella ossifies from two bony centres instead of from the usual single centre, and the centres fail to coalesce. In postero-anterior radiographs a small part of the bone—nearly always the supero-lateral corner—appears separate from the main body of the patella, though in fact it is united by fibro-cartilage. The following features distinguish the gap in a bipartite patella from a fracture. 1) The margins of the gap are smooth, not jagged like those of a fracture. 2) Each side of the gap is bordered by a layer of cortical bone. 3) The site of the gap, at the supero-lateral corner of the patella, is not a common site for fracture. 4) Radiographs of the other knee will often show a similar congenital anomaly there. 5) The defect is not tender on direct palpation over it, whereas a recent fracture is always exquisitely tender.

Treatment. The treatment depends upon the type of fracture and in some cases upon the age of the patient. Three groups must be considered, as shown in Figure 244.

CRACK FRACTURE. In undisplaced crack fractures there is no fear of separation occurring later because the aponeurosis clothing the patella on its anterior and lateral aspects is intact and holds the fragments in position. Treatment is required only to relieve pain and to preserve and restore function. If there is a painfully tense haemarthrosis the blood should be aspirated. A plaster extending from groin to malleoli, with the knee in a position just short of full extension, should be worn for three weeks. Thereafter active exercises are practised under the supervision of a physiotherapist until full function is restored.

CLEAN BREAK WITH SEPARATION OF FRAGMENTS. Operation is required. Its nature should depend upon the age of the patient. If the patient is under 40 the fragments should be coapted accurately and fixed together rigidly by a bolt or screw driven vertically upwards through the two fragments (Fig. 244). Reduction must be perfect and the fragments in intimate contact: otherwise the irregular articular surface will surely cause osteoarthritis later. Indeed, if it proves impossible to restore the fragments so accurately that the articular surface is perfectly smooth it is better to excise the patella.

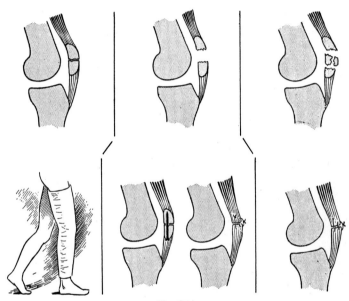

Fig. 244

Fractures of the patella and their treatment. The diagrams in the upper row show the three types of fracture, and those below depict the treatment for each type. 1. Crack without displacement. *Treatment:* Protection in walking plaster. 2. Clean break with separation of fragments. *Treatment:* Patient under 40—Fix fragments with screw. Patient over 40—Excise patella. 3. Comminuted fracture with displacement. *Treatment:* Excise patella irrespective of age.

After internal fixation of a fractured patella the knee should be protected in plaster for two months. Thereafter exercises are practised to mobilise the knee and to redevelop the quadriceps muscle.

If the patient is over 40 it is preferable to excise the patella rather than to undertake internal fixation, because with increasing age there is increasing difficulty in regaining a full range of knee movement after internal fixation, with the prolonged immobilisation that it entails. In excision of the patella the bone is dissected from the aponeurosis of the quadriceps, which closely invests it, and the aponeurosis is reconstructed by cat-gut sutures, tension being relaxed by holding the knee fully extended. After operation the knee is protected in plaster in almost full extension for three weeks, in the latter half of which active quadriceps exercises and leg raising exercises are encouraged. After removal of the plaster exercises are continued to restore movement and to redevelop the quadriceps muscle.

COMMINUTED FRACTURE. In comminuted fractures with displacement it is impossible to restore a perfectly smooth articular surface; so it is best to excise the patella, irrespective of the age of the patient. Only thus can the risk of troublesome osteoarthritis be avoided.

Results of excision of patella. Excision of the patella gives excellent results provided the operation and the after-treatment are carried out efficiently. The function of the knee is not quite so perfect as that of the normal knee: the power of full extension is slightly impaired because the mechanical advantage that the patella affords by holding the tendon away from the axis of movement is lost. If any disability is noticed by these patients it is usually in climbing or descending ladders or stairs.

OTHER INJURIES OF THE EXTENSOR MECHANISM OF THE KNEE

In injuries from sudden muscular violence the quadriceps apparatus may give way at one of three points, as shown in Figure 245: 1) at the point of

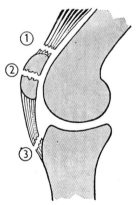

Fig. 245
The three points at which the quadriceps apparatus may rupture. 1. At insertion of quadriceps into patella. 2. Through the patella. 3. At insertion of patellar tendon into tibial tubercle.

attachment of the quadriceps tendon to the upper pole of the patella; 2) through the patella and surrounding quadriceps expansion (fractured patella); or 3) at the attachment of the patellar tendon to the tibial tubercle.

AVULSION FROM PATELLA. Avulsion of the quadriceps tendon from the upper pole of the patella occurs mainly in elderly men, in whom the tendon is often degenerate. The tendon should be reattached to the bone by sutures of stainless steel wire.

AVULSION AT TIBIAL TUBERCLE. This is the least common injury, occurring mainly in children or young adults. A fragment of bone may be pulled off with the tendon. The rupture should be repaired by sutures of stainless steel wire.

DISLOCATION OF THE KNEE

Despite its rather flat articular surfaces the knee is dislocated less often than the other major joints: indeed a dislocated knee must be regarded as a rare injury. This is fortunate, because dislocation of the knee is frequently complicated by injury to the popliteal artery or to one of the major nerve trunks.

Normally the knee is held stable by its strong ligaments (the two cruciate ligaments, the medial and lateral ligaments and the joint capsule) and by the protective control of the powerful quadriceps muscle. Dislocation is possible only if some or all of the ligaments are ruptured. The tibia may be displaced backwards, forwards, laterally or medially upon the femur.

Treatment. The dislocation should be reduced by traction and manipulation or, failing that, by operation. Thereafter the knee should be supported in a full-length lower limb plaster (Fig. 261) for eight or ten weeks before mobilising and muscle-strengthening exercises are begun.

Complications. The complications most to be feared are injuries of the popliteal artery and of the major nerve trunks behind the knee, all of which are especially vulnerable when the tibia is displaced backwards upon the femur. Less serious complications include persistent instability of the knee and late osteoarthritis.

LATERAL DISLOCATION OF THE PATELLA

Lateral dislocation of the patella is recognised in three types: 1) acute dislocation, a single isolated injury; 2) recurrent dislocation; and 3) habitual dislocation, in which the patella dislocates every time the knee is flexed. In recurrent dislocation and in habitual dislocation the knee shows abnormalities—often developmental—that render the patella unstable.

ACUTE DISLOCATION

As a result of an injury while the knee is flexed or semi-flexed the patella is displaced laterally over the lateral femoral condyle and lies at the outer side of the knee. *Clinically*, the patient is unable to straighten the knee unless reduction occurs spontaneously or the patella is pushed back into position. Later the knee swells from an effusion of fluid, which may be blood-stained if the medial part of the capsule is torn. There is well marked local tenderness antero-medially from strain or rupture of the capsule.

Treatment. The dislocation is easily reduced by applying medial-ward pressure upon the patella while the knee is gradually straightened. After a few days' rest with firm bandaging a course of quadriceps exercises should be arranged.

RECURRENT DISLOCATION

Recurrent dislocation of the patella is seen most commonly in girls. The first dislocation generally occurs during adolescence. Thereafter dislocations tend to recur with increasing ease, usually when the knee is being straightened from a flexed or semi-flexed position. The patient often shows generalised congenital joint laxity and may regard herself as 'double-jointed'. In addition, one or more of the following abnormalities may make the patella unstable: 1) a shallow inter-condylar groove of the femur with underdeveloped lateral condyle; 2) a high-lying patella, which therefore rests in the shallow upper part of the intercondylar groove; 3) genu valgum, in consequence of which the line of pull of the quadriceps muscle is shifted farther laterally than normal.

Treatment. If frequently recurring dislocations cause trouble-some disability operation should be advised. A reliable method is to detach the bony insertion of the patellar tendon and transpose it to a new bed in the tibia, medial and distal to the original insertion. In this way the patella is drawn lower into the intercondylar groove of the femur, and the line of pull of the quadriceps is transferred more to the medial side.

An alternative method is to excise the patella. It has been claimed that this may give better long-term results because the liability to late osteoarthritis is reduced, but the claim is not yet proved.

HABITUAL DISLOCATION

Habitual dislocation is uncommon. It occurs at a much younger age than recurrent dislocation—often in early childhood. The underlying cause is shortening of the quadriceps muscle—particularly its vastus lateralis component—possibly from fibrosis following intra-muscular injections in infancy. Sometimes there is an abnormal fibrous band tethering the vastus lateralis to the ilio-tibial tract (Jeffreys 1963). In consequence of the shortening or tethering of the muscle the patella is pulled laterally out of its groove every time the knee is flexed. In the absence of treatment the patella may eventually become permanently dislocated. *Treatment* is by releasing the tight muscle or band by dividing as much of it as is necessary to permit full flexion of the knee without displacement of the patella.

TEARS OF THE LIGAMENTS OF THE KNEE

Rupture of one or more of the ligaments of the knee, with momentary subluxation, is much more common than complete dislocation of the knee. These injuries may be classified into three groups: 1) tear of the medial ligament (with or without the cruciate ligaments); 2) tear of the lateral ligament (with or without the cruciate ligaments); and 3) tears of the cruciate ligaments alone.

TEAR OF MEDIAL LIGAMENT

This is caused by an injury that abducts the tibia upon the femur (Fig. 246). The joint is momentarily subluxated, as shown in the diagram, but when the patient is seen the subluxation has nearly

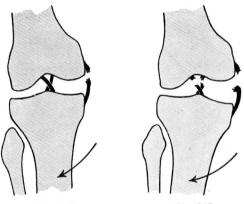

Fig. 246   Fig. 247

Rupture of the medial ligament allows the tibia to be abducted upon the femur so that a gap is opened up between the joint surfaces on the medial side (Fig. 246). If a wide gap is opened up it is almost certain that the cruciate ligaments and the capsule have been torn as well as the medial ligament (Fig. 247).

always been reduced spontaneously. Wide abduction of the tibia upon the femur cannot occur unless the cruciate ligaments and the capsule are torn as well as the medial ligament (Fig. 247). The medial meniscus may be torn at the same time, but it often escapes injury.

Clinical features. The knee is often distended with blood-stained fluid. The point of greatest tenderness is along the course of the medial ligament, usually at its upper end.

Diagnosis. Whether or not the rupture is complete can best be determined by taking antero-posterior radiographs while an abduction stress is applied to the tibia, with the patient anaesthetised. If there is complete rupture of the ligament the joint will be shown to open up at the medial side (Fig. 246). If the joint opens up widely (Fig. 247) it is likely that the cruciate ligaments and capsule are torn as well as the medial ligament.

Treatment. Treatment may be non-operative or operative. Some surgeons prefer the one method, some the other; and good results have been claimed for both. In relatively minor injuries with only slight abduction of the tibia upon the femur when examined under anaesthesia conservative treatment is probably adequate, for the capsular rent is unlikely to be extensive or the ends of the ligament widely separated. But when the subluxation has been severe, indicating a broad capsular tear and injury to the cruciate ligaments as well, operation should be advised.

Conservative treatment. If there is a tense and painful haemarthrosis the fluid should be withdrawn by aspiration. The knee is then supported in a long-leg plaster, which may or may not include the foot, according to individual preference. The plaster is moulded closely about the limb to prevent abduction of the tibia on the femur. The patient is allowed to walk in the plaster, which is retained for six weeks. Thereafter intensive exercises are carried out to mobilise the knee and to redevelop the quadriceps muscle.

Operative treatment. The knee is explored through a medial or antero-medial incision to determine the extent of the tear and to ascertain whether the medial meniscus and the cruciate ligaments are intact. If the meniscus is torn it should be removed. A torn cruciate ligament is generally best left alone unless repair is easily practicable, but any loose tags should be removed. Finally the rent in the capsule and in the medial ligament itself is sutured. After operation the knee is supported in plaster for six weeks, and the subsequent treatment is the same as for patients treated without operation.

TEAR OF LATERAL LIGAMENT

Tear of the lateral ligament is much less common than that of the medial. It is caused by a force adducting the tibia upon the femur. In some injuries of this type the ligament withstands the stress but the bony insertion of the ligament into the head of the fibula is avulsed with a fragment of bone. In other respects the injury is almost a mirror-image of a medial ligament tear, and the clinical features and treatment are comparable.

Complications. If the tibia is markedly adducted in relation to the femur at the time of injury—even though the displacement be momentary—there is a serious risk of injury to the common peroneal nerve from stretching. The effects of a severe stretch injury of the nerve are often irrecoverable.

TEARS OF THE CRUCIATE LIGAMENTS

The cruciate ligaments are sometimes torn with the medial or the lateral ligament, as has been mentioned already. Isolated tears of one or other of the cruciate ligaments may also occur. The anterior ligament is torn by a force driving the upper end of the tibia forwards relative to the femur, or by hyperextension of the knee; the posterior ligament is torn by a force driving the upper end of the tibia backwards.

Treatment. Treatment should usually be conservative because the results of attempted operative repair or reconstruction are seldom better than those of non-intervention. After a preliminary period of rest in plaster intensive physiotherapy should be arranged, to redevelop the quadriceps muscle. If a powerful muscle can be restored a ruptured cruciate ligament may cause little disability despite considerable laxity of the joint.

AVULSION OF TIBIAL SPINE

Rarely, a force acting through a cruciate ligament pulls a fragment of bone from the intercondylar ridge of the upper surface of the tibia, the ligament itself remaining intact. The bone fragment may be displaced slightly upwards, away from its bed. In most cases satisfactory reduction is achieved simply by extending the knee fully, and it is sufficient thereafter to immobilise the limb in a plaster for six weeks. If the bone fragment is more widely displaced and cannot be reduced by manipulation, it may have to be replaced at open operation and fixed in position by a small screw.

STRAIN OF THE MEDIAL OR LATERAL LIGAMENT

A force that is insufficient to tear a ligament completely may cause a partial tear or strain. Either the medial or the lateral ligament (with the adjacent part of the capsule) may be affected. The medial ligament is strained by a force that abducts the tibia upon the femur, whereas the lateral ligament is strained by an adduction force. Strain of the medial ligament is much the more common—indeed it is one of the commonest of all knee injuries.

Clinical features. There is a history of an abduction or of an adduction injury. The knee is painful at the site of the injured ligament and may be noticed to be swollen. On examination there is localised tenderness on palpation over the affected ligament, either in its course or at its upper or lower attachment. Applying stress to the ligament may cause pain, but the knee is stable. The quadriceps muscle may be slightly wasted, but this is not a striking feature (compare torn meniscus). Flexion and extension of the knee are restricted by a few degrees due to pain when the ligament becomes taut.

Diagnosis. Strain of the medial ligament cannot always be differentiated with certainty from a tear of the medial meniscus at the first examination (indeed the two injuries may coexist); but the diagnosis becomes clear if the knee is observed at intervals over a few weeks. After a strain the fluid effusion (if any) is usually absorbed within two or three weeks, and full movement is regained in a similar time. If effusion and painful limitation of extension persist for more than three weeks the diagnosis of strained ligament may have to be revised in favour of one of torn meniscus.

Course. Strains of the medial (or lateral) ligament tend to heal slowly. It is common for pain to persist in decreasing degree for eight or ten weeks.

Treatment. If pain and tenderness are severe a preliminary period of two weeks' rest in plaster (from groin to malleoli) should be advised. Thereafter treatment should be by active exercises to redevelop the quadriceps muscle.

PELLEGRINI-STIEDA'S DISEASE

In a few cases of incomplete avulsion of the medial ligament from the medial condyle of the femur ossification occurs in the small haematoma that forms between the ligament and the femoral condyle. This condition is sometimes referred to as Pellegrini-Stieda's disease.

Clinically there is persistent discomfort at the medial side of the knee after an injury to the medial ligament. There are thickening and slight tenderness over the site of attachment of the ligament to the medial femoral condyle. Radiographs show a thin plaque of new bone close to the medial condyle.

Treatment is by active mobilising and muscle-strengthening exercises.

TEARS OF THE MENISCI OF THE KNEE

Injuries of the menisci [semilunar cartilages] are common in men under the age of 45. A tear is usually caused by a twisting force with the knee semi-flexed or flexed. It is usually a football injury, but it is also common among men who work in a squatting position, such as coal miners. The medial meniscus is torn much more often than the lateral.

Pathology. There are three types of tear (Figs. 250 to 252). All begin as a longitudinal split (Fig. 248). If this extends throughout the length of the meniscus it becomes a *'bucket-handle' tear*, in which the fragments remain attached at both ends (Fig. 250). This is much the most common type. The 'bucket handle' (that is, the central fragment) is displaced towards the middle of the joint, so that the condyle of the femur rolls upon the tibia through the rent in the meniscus. Since the femoral condyle is so shaped that it requires most space when the knee is straight, the chief effect of a displaced 'bucket handle' is that it limits full extension (= 'locking').

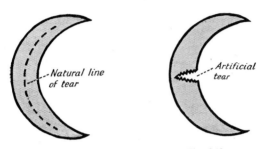

Fig. 248   Fig. 249

Figure 248—Direction of tear in a meniscus of the knee. Figure 249—Transverse tears do not occur naturally; a tear such as this is always an artefact.

ANTERIOR

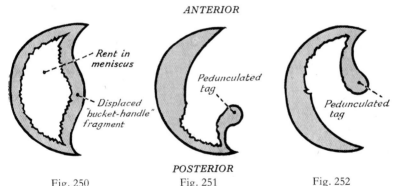

POSTERIOR

Fig. 250   Fig. 251   Fig. 252

The three types of meniscal tear. Figure 250—'Bucket-handle' tear, the commonest type. Figure 251—Posterior horn tear. Figure 252—Anterior horn tear.

If the initial longitudinal tear emerges at the concave border of the meniscus a pedunculated tag is formed. In *posterior horn tear* the fragment remains attached at its posterior horn (Fig. 251); in *anterior horn tear* it remains attached at its anterior horn (Fig. 252). A transverse tear through the meniscus is always an artefact, produced at the time of operation (Fig. 249).

The menisci of the knee are almost avascular: so when they are torn there is not an effusion of blood into the joint. But there is an effusion of synovial fluid, secreted in response to the injury. Major tears of the menisci do not heal spontaneously.

Clinical features of torn medial meniscus. The patient is 18 to 50 years old. The history is characteristic, especially with 'bucket-handle' tears. In consequence of a twisting injury the patient falls and has pain at the antero-medial aspect of the joint. He is unable to continue what he was doing, or does so only with difficulty. He is unable to straighten the knee fully. The next day he notices that the whole knee is swollen. He rests the knee. After about two weeks the swelling lessens, the knee seems to go straight again, and he resumes his activities. Within weeks or months the knee suddenly gives way again during a twisting movement; there are pain and subsequent swelling as before. Similar incidents occur repeatedly.

Locking. By 'locking' is meant inability to extend the knee fully. It is not a true jamming of the joint because there is a free range of flexion. Locking is a common feature of torn medial meniscus, but the limitation of extension is often so slight that it is not noticed by the patient and may indeed be overlooked by the surgeon. Persistent locking can occur only in 'bucket-handle' tears: tag tears cause momentary catching but not true locking in the accepted sense.

On examination in the recent stage of a meniscus injury the typical features are effusion of fluid, wasting of the quadriceps, local tenderness at the level of the joint antero-medially, and (characteristically in 'bucket-handle' tears) limitation of the *last few degrees* of extension by a springy resistance, with sharp antero-medial pain if passive extension is forced.

In the 'silent' phase between attacks there are often no signs other than wasting of the quadriceps muscle.

Clinical features of torn lateral meniscus. The features are broadly similar, but the clinical picture is often less clearly defined. The history may be vague, but a precipitating injury is always recalled. Pain is at the lateral rather than the medial side of the joint, but it is often poorly localised.

Radiographs are normal, whether the tear be of the medial or of the lateral meniscus.

Diagnosis. In the 'silent' phase diagnosis often depends largely upon the history. The surgeon should be very cautious in diagnosing a torn meniscus unless there is a clear history of injury and unless there have been recurrent incidents, each followed by synovial effusion. Often a period of observation is required before the diagnosis becomes reasonably certain. In doubtful cases arthrography or arthroscopy may help to establish the nature of the lesion.

Late effects. Long continued internal derangement from a torn meniscus predisposes to the later development of osteoarthritis. Arthritis may also develop years after a meniscus has been removed.

Treatment. Once the diagnosis is established the correct treatment is to excise the whole meniscus or, in appropriate cases, the displaced 'bucket handle' fragment alone.

Treatment of the locked knee. Manipulation under anaesthesia is the standard practice when there is a marked block to extension. But it cannot be expected that manipulation will restore the displaced 'bucket handle' to its normal position: it merely extends the tear longitudinally and thereby allows the 'bucket-handle' fragment to move farther towards the middle of the joint—that is, to the inter-condylar region. In this position the displaced fragment allows greater freedom of joint movement, but completely full extension is seldom restored. Manipulation is therefore worth while only in so far as it increases the patient's comfort while he is awaiting admission for operation.

HORIZONTAL TEAR OF DEGENERATE MEDIAL MENISCUS

The meniscal tears described above are uncommon in patients over the age of 50, when the menisci begin to show degenerative changes. But a degenerate meniscus is liable to suffer a different type of lesion. The medial meniscus in particular may split horizontally at a point near its attachment to the medial ligament of the knee. Such a split is usually of small dimensions, and since there is no separation of the fragments natural healing can occur.

Clinically there is troublesome and persistent pain at the medial aspect of the knee at the joint level. The pain may be noticed after a minor injury, but often it seems to come on spontaneously, without any preceding incident. In the early stages there is usually a small effusion of fluid into the joint.

Treatment should be expectant at first, by bandaging and quadriceps exercises. In most cases the symptoms resolve in the course of several months. In the occasional case in which they fail to do so, excision of the meniscus should be advised.

TRAUMATIC EFFUSIONS IN THE KNEE

The knee commonly becomes distended with fluid after an injury. The fluid may be a clear serous effusion, blood, or pus. A purulent effusion is easily distinguished by pyrexia and general constitutional disturbance associated with local signs of inflammation. The problem that usually arises is to distinguish clinically between a clear serous effusion and a haemarthrosis.

A serous effusion occurs after an injury that damages some part of the synovial tissues but does not tear any vascular structure. It occurs regularly after tears of the menisci and often after strains or contusions of the capsule or ligaments. The characteristics of a clear serous effusion are that it forms slowly over a period of twenty-four hours or so, and seldom becomes very tense.

A haemarthrosis, on the other hand, is caused by an injury that tears the vascular tissues of the joint, and it is observed therefore after complete ruptures of the ligaments or capsule, after fractures of the patella or of the articular surfaces of the femur or tibia, and after avulsion of the quadriceps tendon. The features of a haemarthrosis are that it forms rapidly, reaching a maximum within a few hours of the injury; and that the effusion is tense. The overlying skin is warmer than normal. Probably because of the greater tension, a haemarthrosis causes more severe pain than a clear serous effusion.

Treatment. Clear serous effusions should usually be allowed to absorb spontaneously. Blood effusions that are tense and causing severe pain should be reduced by aspiration, and controlled thereafter by firm bandaging and immobilisation.

References and bibliography, page 291.

CHAPTER 13

Leg, ankle and foot

The commonest injuries to be encountered in this region are undoubtedly those about the ankle—often fractures of the lateral or medial malleolus or of both malleoli, or strain of the ligaments of the ankle—particularly the lateral ligament. Also prevalent in this region are fractures of the shafts of the tibia and fibula, and it is remarkable how often such injuries are caused by motor-cycling accidents. Indeed, it is likely that their incidence would closely parallel the popularity of motor-cycling in a community.

Classification

The injuries to be described may be classified as follows.

Fractures of the tibia and fibula
Fractures of the condyles of the tibia
Fractures of the shafts of the tibia and fibula
Fracture of the shaft of the tibia alone
Fracture of the fibula alone
Fractures and fracture-dislocations about the ankle

Soft-tissue injuries about the ankle
Rupture of the lateral ligaments of the ankle
Strain of the lateral ligaments
Rupture of the calcaneal tendon

Injuries of the tarsus
Fractures of the talus
Fractures of the calcaneus
Other injuries of the tarsal bones

Fractures of the metatarsal bones and phalanges of the toes
Fractures of the metatarsal bones
Fractures of the phalanges of the toes

FRACTURES OF THE TIBIA AND FIBULA

Classification

Fractures of the bones of the lower leg will be considered in three groups (Fig. 253): 1) Fractures of the condyles of the tibia; 2) fractures of the shafts of the tibia and fibula, separately or together; and 3) fractures and fracture-dislocations about the ankle.

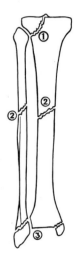

Fig. 253
Visual classification of fractures of the tibia and fibula. 1. Fracture of tibial condyle. 2. Fractures of shafts of tibia and fibula, separately or together. 3. Fractures and fracture-dislocations about the ankle.

FRACTURES OF THE CONDYLES OF THE TIBIA

Most fractures of the tibial condyles involve only the lateral condyle. Less often the medial condyle is fractured alone, and occasionally both condyles are fractured together.

FRACTURE OF THE LATERAL TIBIAL CONDYLE

The common fracture of the lateral condyle is caused by a force that abducts the tibia upon the femur while the foot is fixed on the ground[1] (Fig. 254). An example of this mechanism is seen when the bumper of a car strikes the outer side of the knee of a pedestrian. So often is this type of accident responsible that the injury has been called a bumper fracture.

[1] A force that abducts the tibia upon the femur is also the cause of injuries of the medial ligament of the knee (p. 235). In general, an abduction force will cause a condylar fracture rather than a ligamentous injury if the foot is bearing weight upon the ground at the time of the injury—especially in an old person with soft bones. A similar force applied when the foot is off the ground is more likely to injure the medial ligament. Occasionally the two injuries are associated.

The pattern of the fracture may be of three types, as follows: 1. *Compression fracture with fragmentation.* This is the commonest pattern. The lateral tibial condyle, including its articular surface, is crushed and fragmented by the impact of the lateral condyle of the femur which is driven down into it (Figs. 255 and 258). 2. *Depressed*

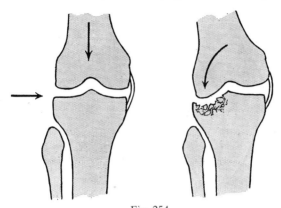

Fig. 254

Mechanism of fracture of lateral tibial condyle. Forcible abduction of the tibia upon the femur while the foot is on the ground causes the lateral condyle of the femur to be driven down into the upper end of the tibia.

plateau type. This is relatively uncommon. A large part of the articular surface of the lateral condyle is depressed into the shell of the bone but remains as a single piece, without fragmentation (Fig. 256). 3. *Oblique shearing fracture.* This is also uncommon. The whole or a large part of the condyle is sheared off in one piece through an oblique fracture (Fig. 257).

Treatment. The treatment depends largely upon the type of fracture as seen radiographically.

COMPRESSION FRACTURE WITH FRAGMENTATION. This forms by far the largest group. Since the articular surface of the condyle is broken into innumerable tiny pieces, many of which are crushed down into the underlying soft cancellous bone, it is impossible to restore the articular surface to its original smooth state. On the other hand further displacement is unlikely to occur because the forces acting through the knee under conditions of treatment will be small compared with the force that caused the injury. And the fracture, which is through spongy bone, will always unite readily. Accordingly the logical method of treatment, and the method now generally adopted for this type of fracture, is to accept the displacement, to avoid rigid immobilisation and to encourage active movements of the knee from the beginning. It may indeed be hoped that movement of the joint, at a stage when the granulation tissue covering the broken surfaces is still pliable, will help to restore a smooth articular surface.

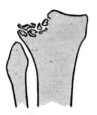 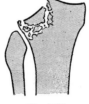 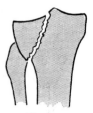

Fig. 255   Fig. 256   Fig. 257

Three types of fracture of lateral tibial condyle. Figure 255—Compression fracture with fragmentation. This is the common type. Figure 256—Depressed plateau fracture without severe fragmentation. A large piece of the articular surface has been driven down into the underlying bone. Figure 257—Oblique shearing fracture.

The patient is confined to bed, and if a tense haemarthrosis has formed the blood-stained fluid is aspirated. A removable plaster shell is constructed to protect the knee from unguarded and possibly painful lateral movements at night. During the day the plaster splint is removed to allow active exercises. These are carried out under the supervision of a physiotherapist; they include exercises to restore the tone of the quadriceps and hamstring muscles, and flexion and extension movements of the knee. After recumbency for from three to six weeks (according to the severity of the fracture) it is safe to allow walking with sticks without any external splintage. Thereafter rehabilitation may be continued daily in the gymnasium.

DEPRESSED PLATEAU FRACTURE WITHOUT FRAGMENTATION. In this small group it may be possible by operation to restore the articular surface of the tibial condyle to something approaching normal. A 'window' is cut in the antero-lateral cortex of the tibia a little below the level of the joint. Through this aperture the depressed fragment is pushed up from below until its articular surface is flush with the surrounding cartilage, as confirmed by inspection through an upward prolongation of the incision that opens the knee joint. The cavity in the lower part of the tibial condyle is then packed firmly with cancellous bone chips to hold the fragment in position.

OBLIQUE SHEARING FRACTURE (Fig. 257). This type of fracture lends itself to reduction by manipulation under anaesthesia, or occasionally by operation.

Manipulative reduction. The displaced condylar fragment may be restored to position by direct pressure upon its lateral side, forcing it upwards and medially. A method that sometimes works well is to apply a few turns of Esmarch rubber bandage as a protective covering round the upper end of the tibia, and then to drive the displaced condylar fragment home by light taps with a mallet.

After manipulative reduction it is necessary to enclose the limb in a full-length plaster to prevent redisplacement. The plaster should be retained for four weeks, and thereafter treatment is by active exercises, as for the common compression fracture.

Operative reduction and internal fixation. Operation may be justified if manipulation fails to restore a good position of the fragment, especially in a patient under 60. After the fragment has been replaced it can usually be held in position best by a long transfixion screw.

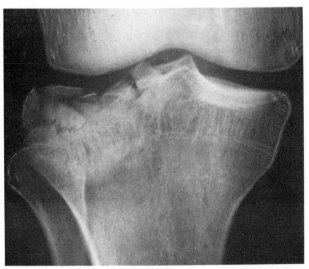

Fig. 258
A typical depressed fracture of the lateral tibial condyle with
fragmentation of the articular surface.

Comment. The opportunities for worth-while improvement of lateral tibial condylar fractures by operation are few, and the temptation to operate for the common compression fracture with fragmentation should be resisted. In this type the results of conservative treatment by immediate active exercises in recumbency fully justify the method.

Complications. These are: 1) genu valgum; 2) joint stiffness; and 3) late osteoarthritis.

GENU VALGUM. Since there is usually some residual and irremediable depression of the lateral tibial condyle a minor degree of genu valgum is often inevitable. In most cases it is insufficient to cause serious inconvenience and may therefore be accepted.

STIFFNESS OF KNEE. With treatment by early exercises it is surprising how quickly a good range of knee movement is regained, and indeed in the average case knee stiffness is not a serious problem. There are exceptions, however, and sometimes many months of physiotherapy by active exercises are required before reasonable movement is restored. Manipulation under anaesthesia may sometimes be helpful.

OSTEOARTHRITIS. Since the damaged articular surface of the tibial condyle often remains irregular there is, theoretically, a serious risk of later osteoarthritis. But when the articular damage is relatively slight arthritis may take many years to reach the stage of causing severe disability, and since many patients with this injury are beyond middle age the need for active treatment of the arthritis may never arise.

In cases of severe painful osteoarthritis operation may sometimes be justified: corrective osteotomy, by removal of a medial wedge from the upper end of the tibia, often gives adequate relief. Only exceptionally is a more radical operation required: this may take the form of arthroplasty or—more reliable—arthrodesis.

FRACTURE OF THE MEDIAL TIBIAL CONDYLE
This injury, which is relatively uncommon, is virtually the mirror-image of fracture of the lateral condyle. Its features and treatment are comparable to those of lateral condylar fractures, and no special description is required.

FRACTURES OF THE SHAFTS OF THE TIBIA AND FIBULA
Most fractures in this region involve both the tibia and the fibula, and the following description applies to such combined injuries. Fractures of the tibia alone and of the fibula alone will be considered in a later section.

Mechanism and displacement. Fractures of the shafts of the tibia and fibula may occur either from an angulatory force or from a rotational force. Fractures from an angulatory force tend to be transverse or of the short oblique type, and the fractures of tibia and fibula are at about the same level. Fractures from a rotational force are spiral, and at a different level in the two bones. Often the tibial fracture is at the junction of the middle and lowest thirds whereas

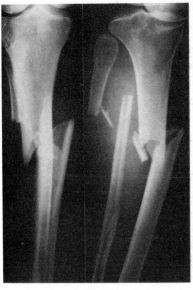
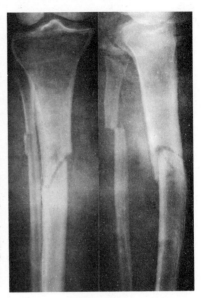

Fig. 259   Fig. 260

Typical fractures of shafts of tibia and fibula before and after manipulative
reduction and immobilisation in plaster.

the fibular fracture is near the junction of the middle and uppermost
thirds. As a rule there is considerable displacement of the fragments,
though undisplaced crack fractures are seen commonly in children.

Since the tibia is so close to the surface and so poorly protected by
muscles, many fractures of its shaft are of the open (compound) type;
indeed the tibial shaft is more often the site of an open fracture than
is any other bone.

In Britain motor-cycle accidents are by far the commonest single
cause of major fractures of the shafts of the tibia and fibula.

Treatment. In fresh fractures of both bones of the leg attention
should be concentrated solely on the fracture of the tibia. The fibular
fracture may be disregarded because it always unites readily, and in
any case the bone is of such secondary importance that the position
of the fragments is immaterial. In contrast the tibial fracture requires
close supervision to ensure normal length and correct alignment.
Imperfect end-to-end apposition of the fragments may be accepted
provided the displacement is not enough to cause ugly deformity (Fig.
30, p. 31).

As with fractures of the shaft of the femur, conservative treatment
should still be the method of choice whenever it is practicable. Indeed

there is less justification for abandoning conservative treatment in favour of operative fixation for these fractures than there is in the case of the femur, because during conservative treatment the patient is usually able to get about well in plaster, he need not remain in hospital for long, and he may often return to work while the leg is still in plaster. Nevertheless there should be no hesitation in advising operative fixation when the indications for it arise, and with the wider adoption of 'closed' intramedullary nailing the scope for operation is perhaps wider than it was a few years ago.

Standard method of conservative treatment. The accepted method of treatment is to reduce the fracture (when necessary) by closed manipulation and to immobilise the limb in a full-length plaster with the knee slightly flexed and the ankle at a right angle (Fig. 261). The plaster may later be 'wedged' if necessary to correct an imperfection of alignment, by dividing it round two-thirds of its circumference at the level of the fracture and angulating it in the required direction. The plaster may be changed from time to time if it should become loose or uncomfortable.

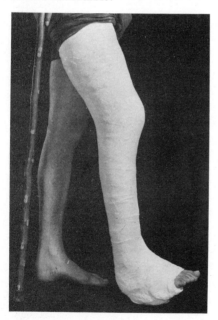

Fig. 261
Plaster used for fractures of the shafts of the tibia and fibula. The knee is held slightly flexed to help to prevent rotation of the limb within the plaster and to facilitate walking and sitting. The ankle is held at a right angle, and the toes are left free. A plaster rocker has been fitted under the sole for walking.

If the fracture seems stable against redisplacement (as, for example, a transverse fracture) walking should be encouraged after two or three weeks, when the acute local reaction to the injury has settled down. For this purpose a walking heel or rocker (made from plaster, wood, or rubber) is applied to the sole of the plaster, and a canvas overboot may be provided. But if the pattern of fracture suggests that it is liable to redisplacement, walking on the affected leg should be deferred for about six weeks, though walking with crutches may be allowed earlier.

The plaster is retained until the tibial fracture is firmly united as shown by clinical and radiographic examination (Figs. 26 and 27)— usually a matter of between three and four months. Thereafter active exercises are carried out under the supervision of a physiotherapist to restore a full range of knee, ankle and foot movements and to redevelop the muscles.

Operative treatment: internal fixation. Internal (operative) fixation is required mainly when the fracture cannot be reduced adequately by manipulation, or when plaster alone fails to maintain an acceptable position of the fragments. Operation is required much more often for oblique or spiral fractures, which always tend to be unstable, than for transverse fractures (Fig. 7, p. 7).

The method of internal fixation must be chosen to suit each individual fracture: there is no universal method. It is true that in recent years fixation by a long intramedullary nail has gained much favour. It is often a satisfactory method, especially for fractures near the middle of the tibial shaft without much comminution (Fig. 262). It is less satisfactory when the fracture is severely comminuted, and it has serious limitations in the treatment of fractures close to the upper or the lower end of the bone. For suitable fractures its popularity will probably prove to be justified, especially when the operation can be done by the closed technique (that is, without exposing the fracture itself), thus reducing the risk of infection to a minimum. When done by the open method, intramedullary nailing still offers the advantage of greater rigidity compared with other methods of internal fixation, including plating.

Technique of intramedullary nailing for tibial fractures. Whenever possible, the operation should be done by the closed technique, without exposing the fracture. Reduction may have to be aided by mechanical traction by screw or weight acting through a Steinmann pin in the lower end of the tibia. For this purpose the limb may be supported upon a special apparatus which holds the knee flexed about 120 degrees and allows for counter-traction upon the back of the thigh. A short incision medial to the patellar tendon exposes the intercondylar ridge of the upper surface of the tibia, and a long guide wire is introduced near the front of this ridge and pushed down the medullary canal as far as the fracture. When reduction has been secured and checked by radiographs the guide wire is driven on into the distal fragment, its position and the depth of penetration being again controlled by check radiographs. With the guide wire in position, the medullary canal is enlarged to the required size by cannulated reamers and the appropriate nail, usually about 12 millimetres in diameter, is driven home over the wire.

If rigid fixation is obtained there is no need to immobilise the limb in plaster; exercises for the muscles and joints may be begun within a few days of the operation, and walking, at first with crutches, may be permitted after two or three weeks. Function of the knee is not disturbed by entering the nail through the intercondylar ridge because this region of the tibia does not form part of the articular surface.

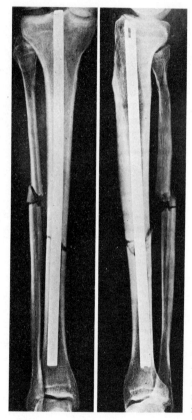

Fig. 262

Transverse fractures of the shafts of the tibia and fibula treated by intramedullary nailing of the tibia. This method is applicable mainly to fractures near the middle of the shaft.

Other methods of internal fixation still have their place in treatment. They include fixation by oblique transfixion screws, by circumferential wires, by metal plate held by screws, and by cortical bone graft held by screws.

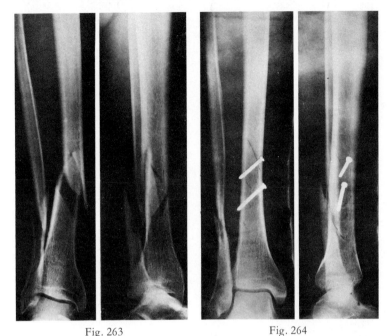

Fig. 263   Fig. 264

Figure 263—A spiral fracture of the tibial shaft of a type that is generally unstable and not well controlled by plaster alone. (The fibula is also fractured.) Figure 264—The same fracture after internal fixation by oblique transfixion screws.

Oblique transfixion screws. Transfixion of the tibial fragments by oblique screws is a simple method of maintaining reduction of long oblique or spiral fractures, which are notoriously difficult to control by plaster (Figs. 263 and 264). But it is not safe to rely upon the screws alone, and the additional support of a full-length plaster is required until bone union is well advanced.

Circumferential wires. For long oblique fractures an alternative to fixation by transfixion screws is to hold the fragments together by two or three wires each passed round the bone circumferentially and tightened by twisting. This method usually entails rather more stripping of periosteum and soft tissues from the bone than does the insertion of transfixion screws, and the technique, never widely used, fell into disfavour. Recently there has been a revival of interest with the development of less traumatic devices for passing the wire round the bone. At present circumferential wiring seems to have a small place in the treatment of long oblique or spiral fractures; it is also useful as an adjunct to intramedullary nailing, to hold in place a triangular or so-called 'butterfly' fragment split off from the main fragment.

Metal plate with screws. When the fracture is unsuitable for fixation by oblique screws another method that is widely used is to bridge the fracture by a metal plate held by screws. The plate should always be applied to a submuscular surface of the tibia—that is, to the lateral or the posterior surface—never to the subcutaneous surface, where it might cause local discomfort. Again the additional support of a plaster is advisable unless the fixation can be made extremely rigid. The use of compression plates was discussed on page 42.

Cortical bone graft. Yet another method is to bridge the fracture by a bone graft instead of a metal plate. The graft is easily obtained from the same tibia; so the operation is only slightly more extensive than that of simple plating, and it may well be more reliable in promoting union.

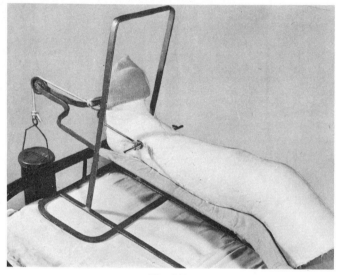

Fig. 265

Continuous weight traction through a lower tibial pin used with plaster to control unstable fractures of the tibia and fibula. This is a useful method for oblique or spiral fractures when internal fixation is inadvisable on account of unhealthy skin or wound infection.

Treatment by continuous traction. An unstable oblique fracture is sometimes unsuitable for internal fixation on account of an unhealthy soft-tissue wound or extensive blistering of the skin. In such a case continuous weight traction with the limb in plaster (Fig. 265) is a satisfactory alternative. The traction should be applied through a transfixion pin in the lower end of the tibia.[1] After traction for four or six weeks the fracture is usually stable enough to allow walking

---

[1] The use of a calcaneal pin for leg traction is to be condemned because the pin-track is more liable to troublesome infection or residual tenderness than is a pin-track through the tibia.

to be begun in a new close-fitting plaster. Thereafter the treatment is the same as in the standard method of conservative treatment already described.

External fixation. A modification of the last-mentioned technique is to insert dual transfixion pins above and below the fracture and to incorporate the ends of the pins in a plaster or in a special adjustable fixation device.

Complications. The common complications are 1) infection, and 2) delayed union or non-union. Rarely there may be 3) damage to an important artery or nerve, or 4) mal-union.

INFECTION. Because of the frequency with which tibial fractures are associated with a communicating skin wound, contamination and consequent osteomyelitis are more common than in any other bone. Nevertheless cases of serious infection are seen much less often now than they were some years ago, because contamination is reduced by prompt cleansing of the wound and excision of devitalised tissue (p. 48), and by the local and systemic administration of antibiotic drugs.

Established infection is indicated by persistent pyrexia and by a 'suppurative' odour over the wound. In that event the plaster must be split and free drainage provided (if it is not already established) by opening up the wound. Later, fragments of dead bone (sequestra) may have to be removed. When the infection has been overcome healing may be hastened by applying split-skin grafts to the granulating surface. In cases of serious infection union of the fracture is generally delayed or prevented (Fig. 54, p. 53).

DELAYED UNION AND NON-UNION. Whereas most tibial fractures unite readily (in the absence of infection), a small proportion may be very obstinate and may still be freely mobile three or four months after the injury. In that event surgical intervention is usually to be advised, provided the skin is healthy. In most cases a bone-grafting operation is recommended, and two methods of grafting are in common use. In the one, a cortical slab graft obtained from the same or from the opposite tibia is screwed to the submuscular (lateral) surface of the bone, the position of the fragments being adjusted as necessary to give accurate apposition and alignment. In the other method, which is applicable especially when the fragments are already in correct position and alignment, slivers of cancellous bone are inserted beneath the periosteum and the fracture itself is not disturbed (Phemister 1947). In suitable cases an intramedullary nail may be used in conjunction with cancellous bone grafting in order to provide adequate rigidity. There is no need to graft the fibula, which always unites readily: indeed it is usually necessary to divide the fibula before the tibial fragments can be brought into exact apposition.

Strut-like effect of intact fibula. In most cases of delayed union of the tibia the fibular fracture is soundly united. Although this might be thought an advantage, in practice an intact fibula may hinder union of the tibia; for if there has been slight absorption of the tibial fracture surfaces the fibula acts as a strut, holding the tibial fragments apart. If this factor is believed to be important it may be worth while to undertake the simple operation of excising a small length of the fibula. This allows the tibial fragments to come together, and the stimulus provided by walking in a plaster may cause the tibial fracture to unite. In this way the necessity for a bone grafting operation—a much more formidable procedure—may sometimes be avoided.

DAMAGE TO ARTERY OR NERVE. A displaced tibial fracture may damage a main branch of the popliteal artery or one of the major nerves—usually the tibial. Sometimes the arterial circulation has been impeded, not by any direct injury to the vessels, but by the constriction of over-tight dressings or plaster. It must be stressed once again that it is essential to examine for signs of circulatory impairment or peripheral nerve injury when the patient is first received for treatment. The condition of the circulation in the toes must be watched closely during the first two days after an injury or operation on the leg.

The general management of arterial injuries complicating fractures was discussed on page 62, and of nerve injuries on page 64.

MAL-UNION. With the general improvement in the standard of fracture treatment mal-union has become increasingly uncommon. Nevertheless cases are still seen in which union of a tibial fracture has occurred with overlap and consequent shortening, or with angulation, which may predispose to later osteoarthritis of the knee or ankle. In most cases it is wise to accept the disability if the deformity is slight, but if an angular deformity is severe it may be advisable to correct it by osteotomy of the tibia and fibula.

FRACTURE OF THE SHAFT OF THE TIBIA ALONE

Fracture of the tibial shaft without a fracture of the fibula is relatively uncommon. Displacement tends to be less severe than in fractures of both bones.

Treatment. The principles of treatment are the same as for fractures of the tibia and fibula together. In most cases the fragments can be held adequately by a full-length plaster (Fig. 261). Sometimes the intact fibula acts to the disadvantage of the tibial fracture, for it may prevent the fracture surfaces from coming together in close apposition, or hinder the restoration of normal alignment. If this strut-like effect of the intact fibula seems to be delaying union or leading to deformity a short length of the fibula should be excised.

FATIGUE FRACTURE OF TIBIA

Rarely, a crack fracture may occur through the shaft of the tibia from repeated minor stresses rather than from a major injury. This type of fracture—more common in the metatarsal bones—is termed a fatigue or stress fracture.

There is usually a history of unaccustomed activity, such as prolonged walking, running or dancing, preceding the onset of symptoms. The patient complains of pain over the tibia, and walking becomes difficult or impossible. There is local tenderness over the site of fracture, and radiographs show a faint transverse crack (Fig. 16, p. 17). Union occurs readily. Protection for a few weeks in a full-length walking plaster is advised.

PSEUDARTHROSIS OF TIBIA IN CHILDHOOD

Rarely, in infants or young children, a congenital abnormality of the bone of the lower half of the tibia leads to spontaneous fracture. This fracture is extraordinarily resistant to conservative treatment and to the usual methods of bone grafting: even when bone grafting has seemed to succeed refracture often occurs later. In these respects this clinical entity is quite unlike any ordinary childhood fracture, but the precise nature of the basic lesion that weakens the tibia is not fully understood. In many cases there is an association with neurofibromatosis. Unless the fracture can be made to heal the growth of the affected leg is seriously impaired, and in some cases amputation has been the eventual outcome.

Treatment. The best hope of promoting bone union with the least possible shortening lies in early rigid fixation by an intramedullary nail, with cancellous bone grafting. This method usually succeeds eventually, though repeat operations may be required for the insertion of larger nails as the limb grows.

FRACTURE OF THE FIBULA ALONE

The shaft of the fibula is seldom broken without the tibia, or without a simultaneous injury at the ankle. When an isolated fracture of the fibular shaft does occur it is usually caused by a direct blow over the bone. Displacement is seldom severe. There is marked local tenderness over the site of the fracture, but since the tibia is intact the patient is able to continue walking, and on this account the fracture may be overlooked.

No special treatment is required except to relieve pain. For this purpose protection in a below-knee walking plaster for three weeks is usually sufficient.

FRACTURE OF FIBULA WITH TIBIO-FIBULAR DIASTASIS

When a fracture of the fibular shaft is found without a fracture of the tibia the condition of the ankle should always be investigated. A fracture of the shaft of the fibula is a constant accompaniment of rupture of the inferior tibio-fibular ligament (tibio-fibular diastasis, p. 266).

FATIGUE FRACTURE OF FIBULA

Fatigue or stress fractures, though much more common in the metatarsals, are well recognised in the fibula. They usually affect the lowest third of the bone, but they may also occur at the middle or uppermost third. There is no history of sudden injury, and the patient seeks advice on account of spontaneous pain at the outer side of the leg, perhaps after an unusual amount of walking or running. Radiographs at first may show no more than a faint hair-line crack across the bone (Fig. 17, p. 17), but later the site of fracture is made evident by surrounding callus.

FRACTURES AND FRACTURE-DISLOCATIONS ABOUT THE ANKLE

The bones forming the ankle mortise are injured more often than any other bone except the lower end of the radius. Many distinct varieties of these fractures and fracture-dislocations are recognised, but they are often grouped together loosely under the general title 'Pott's[1] fracture'.

Mechanism of injury and patterns of fracture. Malleolar fractures with or without subluxation or dislocation of the talus may occur from three types of injury: 1) an abduction or lateral rotation force or a combination of both (the commonest type); 2) an adduction force; or 3) a vertical compression force. The patterns of fracture caused by each of these three types of violence are shown diagrammatically in Figure 266.

In practice it will be found that there are seven distinct groups of fracture or fracture-dislocation to be considered from the point of view of treatment, and these will be discussed individually in the following pages: 1) isolated fracture of the lateral malleolus; 2) isolated fracture of the medial malleolus; 3) fracture of the lateral malleolus with lateral shift of the talus; 4) fractures of both malleoli

[1]Percival Pott (1714–1788), a surgeon of St Bartholomew's Hospital, London, described in 1769 a fracture of the ankle region. The precise anatomical nature of the injury he described is uncertain, though it is clear from his description that he was referring to a fracture of the lower end of the fibula with lateral displacement of the talus. Pott himself suffered an open fracture of the lower leg, but this was almost certainly a fracture of the shaft of the tibia and had nothing to do with the ankle injury that bears his name.

with displacement of the talus; 5) tibio-fibular diastasis; 6) posterior marginal fracture of the tibia with posterior displacement of the talus; 7) vertical compression fracture of the lower articular surface of the tibia.

General principles of treatment. *In fractures without displacement* it is usually sufficient to protect the ankle in a below-knee walking plaster (Fig. 267) for three to six weeks, depending upon the nature of the injury.

In fractures with displacement the necessary action must be taken to ensure: 1) that the talus is restored to its normal relationship with the tibio-fibular mortise; and 2) that the tibia and the fibula are in normal relationship to one another at their lower ends. Reduction is effected by manipulation under anaesthesia, the talus and the displaced malleolar fragment or fragments being restored to position by firm pressure in a direction opposite to the direction of displacement. Thereafter the reduction must be maintained until union is well advanced—usually a matter of eight to ten weeks. In many cases sufficient immobilisation is afforded by a closely fitting plaster; but, since in these unstable fractures there is always a risk of redisplacement within the plaster, check radiographs should be obtained a week after the initial reduction to show whether or not a satisfactory position has been maintained.

When adequate reduction, with normal relationships between tibia and fibula and talus, cannot be maintained by plaster alone, operative fixation is required. The usual technique is to secure the fragments in perfect position by a screw or screws. The additional protection of a below-knee plaster for eight to ten weeks is nearly always advised.

Complications. The simpler types of ankle injury are almost free from complications, and perfect function should always be restored. The more serious fracture-dislocations may be complicated by: 1) stiffness of the ankle; and 2) later osteoarthritis. Both these complications are most likely to occur when the articular surface of the ankle mortise has been damaged by the fracture, or when there is persistent displacement of the talus.

STIFFNESS OF ANKLE. When the plaster is first removed there is a tendency to gravitational oedema, which may hinder the restoration of a full range of movement. Oedema may be controlled to some extent by crepe bandages or an elastic sock, but reliance should be placed mainly on exercises to restore muscle tone, with elevation of the limb when the patient is at rest. Oedema and stiffness are usually more troublesome in elderly patients than in the young.

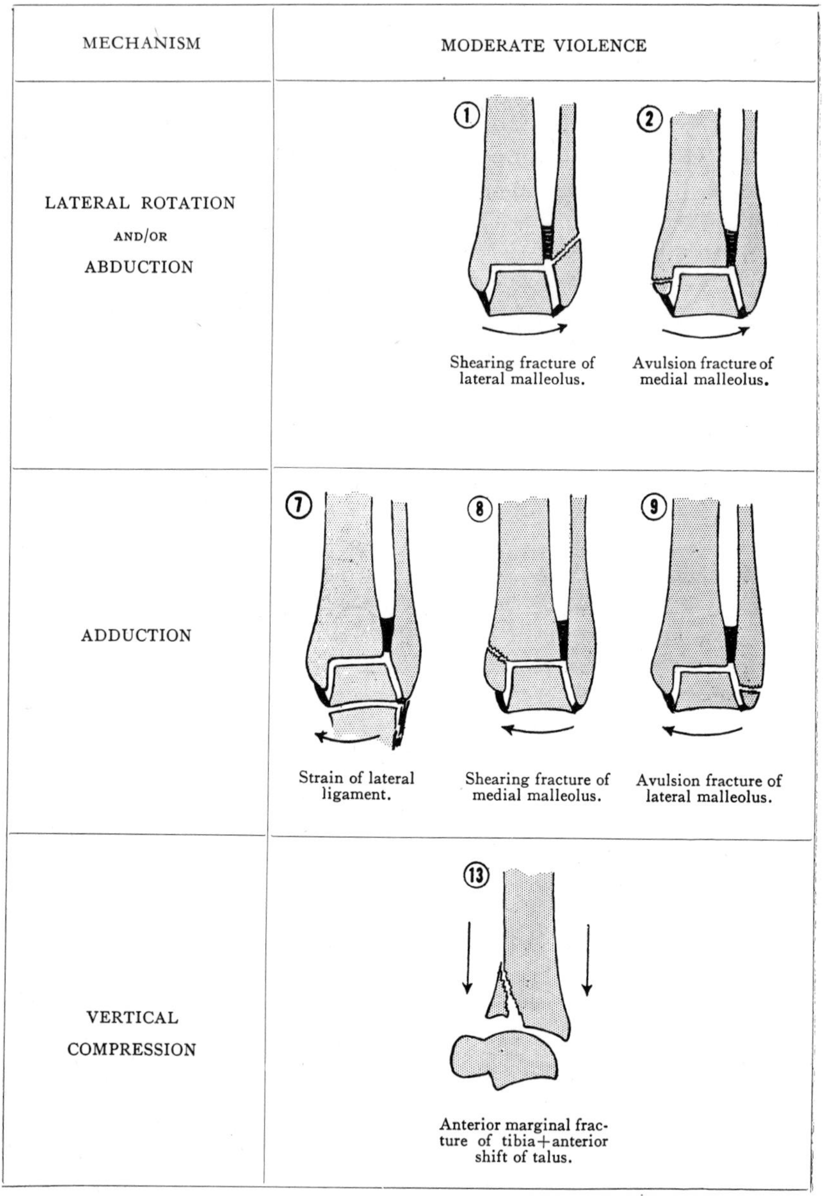

Fig. 266

Causative mechanisms and typical patterns of ligamentous injuries,
fractures and fracture-dislocations about the ankle.

SEVERE VIOLENCE			ADDITIONAL DISPLACEMENT IF MOMENTUM DRIVES TIBIA FORWARDS
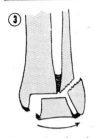 ③ Fracture lateral malleolus rupture medial ligament+lateral shift of talus.	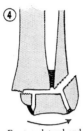 ④ Fracture lateral and medial malleoli+ lateral shift of talus.	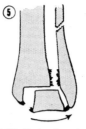 ⑤ Tibio-fibular diastasis. Rupture of tibio-fibular and medial ligaments +fracture shaft of fibula+lateral shift of talus.	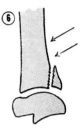 ⑥ Posterior marginal fracture of tibial articular surface+posterior shift of talus.
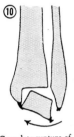 ⑩ Complete rupture of lateral ligament.	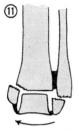 ⑪ Fracture medial and lateral malleoli+ medial shift of talus.		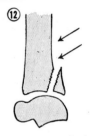 ⑫ Posterior marginal fracture of tibial articular surface+posterior shift of talus.
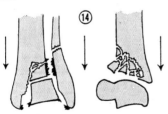 ⑭ Comminuted fracture of tibial articular surface+fracture of fibula+upward displacement of talus.			

Fig. 266

Causative mechanisms and typical patterns of ligamentous injuries, fractures and fracture-dislocations about the ankle.

OSTEOARTHRITIS. If a fracture involving the articular surface of the ankle mortise is not reduced perfectly so that the joint surfaces are smooth and congruous, wear-and-tear will be accelerated and osteoarthritis will develop months or years later (Fig. 74, p. 71). The greater the irregularity of the tibial articular surface, the more rapidly will the degenerative changes occur.

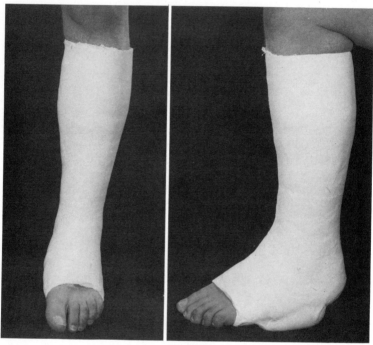

Fig. 267

Below-knee plaster as used for most ankle fractures and for certain fractures of the foot. The ankle is held at about a right angle, and the position of the foot is neutral between inversion and eversion. The toes are left free to allow active movement. In the example shown a plaster rocker has been applied beneath the sole to facilitate walking.

Once established, osteoarthritis of the ankle does not respond well to conservative treatment, and if the disability is severe the most satisfactory treatment is to eliminate the joint by arthrodesis. Replacement arthroplasty, by the insertion of tibial and talar components, has been undertaken but its long-term efficacy is unproven; and in view of the generally excellent results obtained from arthrodesis arthroplasty cannot yet be recommended.

ISOLATED FRACTURE OF LATERAL MALLEOLUS
(Diagrams 1 and 9 in Figure 266.)

The lateral malleolus may be sheared off by an abduction or lateral rotation force (the usual cause), or avulsed by an adduction force. In the group under consideration there is no displacement of the talus because the medial malleolus and the medial ligament are intact. Nor is there usually any significant displacement of the malleolar fragment (Fig. 268).

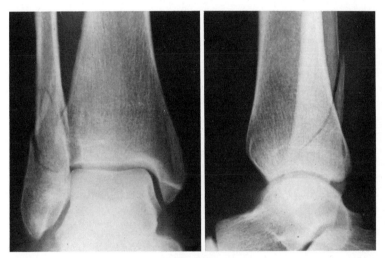

Fig. 268
Undisplaced fracture of lateral malleolus. (This injury
corresponds to diagram 1 in Figure 266.)

Treatment. Treatment is required mainly to relieve pain and to restore function. Immobilisation is not essential to union, but a period of three weeks or so in plaster is nevertheless usually desirable to relieve pain. Thereafter treatment is by active exercises to restore ankle and foot movements and muscle tone.

ISOLATED FRACTURE OF MEDIAL MALLEOLUS
(Diagrams 2 and 8 in Figure 266.)

This may be regarded as the 'mirror-image' of the injury just described. It is much less common. The malleolus may be sheared off by an adduction force or avulsed by an abduction force. The fracture is sometimes no more than a crack, but very often the malleolar fragment is displaced, with consequent loss of the smooth articular contour of the ankle mortise.

A notable feature of displaced fractures of the medial malleolus is that a fringe of periosteum may be turned in between the separated bone fragment and the main body of the bone, preventing accurate reduction by manipulation, and hindering union.

Treatment. The principle of treatment should be to rely upon conservative treatment by immobilisation in plaster if the malleolar fragment is not displaced, or if perfect reduction can be secured by manipulation; but to resort to operation if perfect reduction cannot be secured by manipulation. It is important that the fragment be replaced perfectly, to ensure a smooth articular contour. In practice most of these fractures—other than simple cracks—do require operative reduction and internal fixation, which is easily effected by a long transfixion screw driven upwards from the tip of the malleolus. After the operation the ankle is immobilised in a below-knee plaster until union is well advanced (usually about eight weeks), but walking in the plaster is allowed after the first two or three weeks.

FRACTURE OF LATERAL MALLEOLUS WITH LATERAL DISPLACEMENT OF TALUS
(Diagram 3 in Figure 266.)

The cause is an abduction or lateral rotation force. The medial malleolus is intact but the medial [deltoid] ligament is torn; otherwise lateral displacement of the talus could not occur. The shift of the

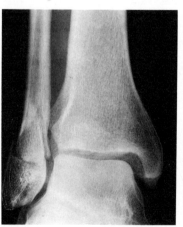
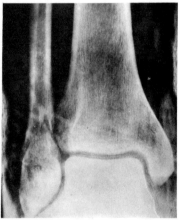

| Fig. 269 | Fig. 270 |

Figure 269—Fracture of lateral malleolus and lateral shift of the talus with the malleolar fragment. The widening of the joint space at the medial side indicates that the medial ligament is torn. The displacement is slight but it must nevertheless be corrected. Figure 270—Radiograph after reduction and immobilisation in plaster. (This injury corresponds to diagram 3 in Figure 266.)

talus is judged best from the width of the joint space between talus and medial malleolus. Normally this is equal to the space in the weight-bearing part of the joint; so if it is widened it follows that the talus must be displaced (Fig. 269).

Treatment. Accurate reduction is essential, to ensure congruous joint surfaces, and it can be achieved easily by strong inward pressure upon the lateral malleolus. In most cases the reduction can be held satisfactorily by a closely fitting plaster, in which walking may be permitted after the first few days (Figs. 267 and 270). The plaster should be retained for about eight weeks, after which rehabilitation is continued by active exercises.

If check radiographs show that redisplacement has occurred despite close moulding of the plaster about the malleoli, operation should be advised. The lateral malleolus is secured in position by a long screw driven obliquely upwards from its lateral surface into the tibia. After operation the ankle should be protected in a below-knee plaster for eight weeks, walking being encouraged after the first two weeks.

FRACTURES OF BOTH MALLEOLI WITH DISPLACEMENT OF TALUS
(Diagrams 4 and 11 in Figure 266.)

This injury is usually caused by an abduction or lateral rotation force, and is then merely a variation of the injury just described (Fig. 266 (4)), the medial malleolus being avulsed instead of the ligament torn.

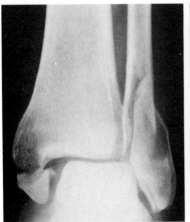 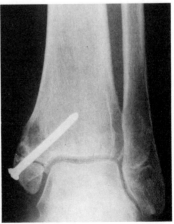

Fig. 271   Fig. 272

Fracture of both malleoli with lateral displacement of the talus. Figure 271—Before reduction. Figure 272—After reduction and fixation of medial malleolus with a screw. (This injury corresponds to that shown in diagram 4, Figure 266.)

In that case the malleolar fragments and the talus are displaced laterally (Fig. 271). The same type of injury, but with medial displacement, occurs less commonly from an adduction force (Fig. 266 (11)).

Treatment. These fractures are difficult to reduce accurately by manipulation, and even when well reduced they are difficult to hold in position by plaster alone. Hence operation is usually advised. In most cases it is sufficient to fix the medial malleolus back into position by a long transfixion screw (Fig. 272): this automatically holds the talus and the lateral malleolus in correct relationship because both the medial and the lateral ligaments are intact. (In effect, fixation of the medial malleolus converts the fracture to that shown in diagram 1 in Figure 266.) But there can be no objection to fixation of the lateral malleolus also by a second screw, and some surgeons prefer to do this to ensure greater stability.

After operation a plaster should be retained for about ten weeks to allow firm consolidation of the fractures, but walking in the plaster may be allowed after two or three weeks.

DIASTASIS OF INFERIOR TIBIO-FIBULAR JOINT
(Diagram 5 in Figure 266.)

If violence acting laterally in an abduction injury is withstood by the lateral malleolus the brunt of the force falls upon the inferior tibio-fibular ligament and may rupture it, with consequent tibio-fibular diastasis (Fig. 266 (5)). The talus is displaced laterally with the lower end of the fibula, the medial ligament being ruptured or the medial malleolus avulsed, and the fibula is fractured above the level of the inferior tibio-fibular ligament—often high up in the shaft (Fig. 273).

Diagnosis. Slight widening of the tibio-fibular mortise may be overlooked unless particular note is made of the joint space at the medial side of the talus, and the difficulty of diagnosis is increased by the fact that the fibular fracture may be too high in the shaft to be seen in the routine radiographs of the ankle. In tibio-fibular diastasis the talus is always carried laterally with the fibula; so the space between the medial malleolus and the talus is widened (Fig. 273). If widening of the space is observed without a fracture of the lateral malleolus a radiograph should always be obtained of the whole length of the fibula: this will invariably show a fracture of some part of the shaft—sometimes far above the ankle (Fig. 273). Even when the radiographs of the ankle region appear normal (as they may do if the displacement has been spontaneously reduced) the severe swelling and clinical disability should suggest the need for a more extensive radiographic examination.

Treatment. Although the displacement can nearly always be reduced by manipulation it is notoriously prone to recur within the plaster despite careful moulding. For this reason operation is advised. The tibio-fibular diastasis is reduced under direct vision and the fibula is secured to the tibia by a single long screw driven transversely across the two bones (Fig. 273). If the medial malleolus has been

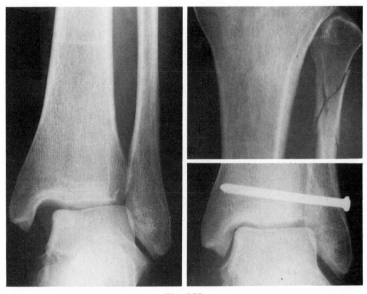

Fig. 273

Tibio-fibular diastasis. The inferior tibio-fibular ligament and the medial ligament of the ankle have been torn, allowing lateral displacement of the fibula and the talus. This injury is always accompanied by a fracture of the shaft of the fibula, which in this case was at its upper end (shown at top right). Radiograph at bottom right shows condition after reduction and fixation by a long screw. (This injury corresponds to diagram 5 in Figure 266.)

avulsed it should be fixed in position with a second screw. After operation the ankle is protected in a plaster for eight weeks to allow firm union of the tibio-fibular ligament, but walking in the plaster may be allowed after the first two weeks.

POSTERIOR MARGINAL FRACTURE OF TIBIA
(Diagrams 6 and 12 in Figure 266.)

When the momentum of the body carries the tibia forwards upon the foot at the time of the injury the posterior articular margin of the tibia may be sheared off. Radiographs may show the talus displaced backwards upon the tibia, but sometimes a momentary displacement has been reduced spontaneously by the time the patient is seen. This posterior marginal fracture of the tibia is additional to a fracture of one or both malleoli, and it may occur in conjunction either with an abduction-rotation injury or with an adduction injury (Fig. 266 (6) and (12)).

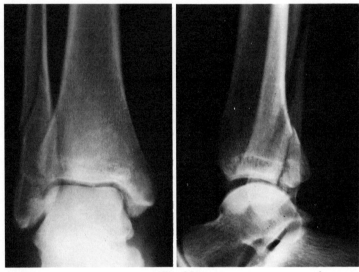

Fig. 274

Posterior marginal fracture of the tibia with associated spiral fracture of the lateral malleolus. There is slight posterior displacement of the talus, as evidenced by the fact that the opposed articular surfaces of the tibia and the talus are not congruous. (This injury corresponds to that shown in Figure 266, diagram 6.)

The separated posterior fragment of the tibia is nearly always displaced slightly upwards, forming a step in the articular surface. Fortunately the fragment is usually small and the greater part of the articular surface remains intact (Fig. 274). Occasionally, however, the fragment includes a large area of the articular surface, and unless it is restored perfectly to position the irregular step in the surface will lead inevitably to later osteoarthritis.

Treatment. When the posterior tibial fragment is small it may be ignored and attention directed solely to the other components of the injury, namely the associated malleolar fracture and the displacement of the talus. But when the posterior tibial fragment is large and includes a large area of the articular surface it must be replaced perfectly in position. It is seldom possible to obtain a satisfactory reduction by manipulation, and in practice it is necessary to resort to operative reduction and fixation by a screw. Thereafter the ankle is protected in plaster for ten weeks before mobilising exercises are begun.

VERTICAL COMPRESSION FRACTURE OF TIBIA
(Diagrams 13 and 14 in Figure 266.)

This injury is usually caused by a fall from a height. It is relatively uncommon, because most patients who fall from a height on to the foot sustain a fracture of the calcaneus rather than of the tibia.

A vertical force acting on the lower articular surface of the tibia may cause two types of injury, according to the severity of the violence. If the violence is only moderate, the front of the tibial articular surface is sheared off and the talus may be displaced slightly forwards (Fig. 266 (13)). If the violence is severe, there is a comminuted fracture involving the whole of the inferior articular surface of the tibia—and often also of the fibula—and the talus may be driven upwards between the two bones (Fig. 266 (14)).

Treatment. In the treatment of the less severe injuries the aim should be to secure accurate reduction of the articular fragments so that the joint surface is left perfectly smooth. This may sometimes be achieved by manipulation and immobilisation in plaster, but in most cases operative reduction and fixation by a screw are required.

In the severely comminuted fractures with upward displacement of the talus it is impossible to restore a smooth articular surface by any method, and it is pointless to attempt to do so. In active individuals the best results will be obtained by arthrodesis of the ankle as a primary measure, carried out within a few weeks of the injury; but in old persons it may be preferable to accept the inevitable disorganisation of the joint and to make the best of the ankle by rehabilitation after a few weeks' rest in plaster, arthrodesis being kept in reserve in case of persistent disabling pain.

SOFT-TISSUE INJURIES ABOUT THE ANKLE

RUPTURE OF THE LATERAL LIGAMENTS OF THE ANKLE

Rarely, a severe adduction force may cause complete rupture of the talo-fibular and calcaneo-fibular ligaments, with consequent subluxation of the talus in the tibio-fibular mortise (Fig. 266 (10)).

Clinical features. There is a history of a severe adduction injury, which is followed by rapid swelling about the lateral aspect of the ankle. Later, there is extensive visible bruising. Pain is severe, so that walking is difficult or impossible.

Diagnosis. Unless the special features of this injury are recognised it may be mistaken for a simple strain of the ligaments (p. 271). The extent of the swelling and bruising, the severe pain, and the marked disability should suggest the possibility of a complete tear of the ligaments, and the diagnosis should be settled by obtaining antero-posterior radiographs while an adduction stress is applied to the heel. (An anaesthetic is necessary if the injury is recent.) If the ligaments are torn, the talus will be shown tilted medially in the tibio-fibular mortise (Fig. 275). A tilt of less than 20 degrees is not necessarily abnormal: in doubtful cases the uninjured ankle should be radiographed in the same way for comparison.

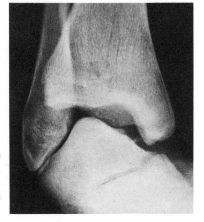

Fig. 275
Tilting of the talus in the ankle mortise under adduction stress, an indication of torn lateral ligaments. (This injury corresponds to diagram 10 in Figure 266.)

Treatment. If the injury is treated as a simple strain, with early exercises and activity, the torn ligaments may fail to heal and recurrent subluxation of the ankle may ensue. If conservative treatment is to be adopted it is essential that the ligaments be protected by a below-knee plaster for not less than six weeks. This method is usually successful, but some surgeons prefer to suture the torn capsule and ligaments at operation to ensure that the frayed ends are correctly apposed. After operation the ankle should be protected in plaster for six weeks.

RECURRENT SUBLUXATION OF THE ANKLE

When the lateral ligaments of the ankle are torn and fail to heal there may be persistent instability, with recurrent attacks of 'giving way' in which the talus tilts medially in the ankle mortise.

Clinical features. The patient complains that, after an initial injury, the ankle goes over at frequent intervals, sometimes causing him to fall. Each incident is accompanied by pain at the lateral side of the ankle. *On examination* there is often some oedema about the ankle. There is tenderness over the site of the lateral ligaments. The normal ankle movements—dorsiflexion and plantarflexion—are unchanged, but abnormal mobility is present as shown by the fact that the heel can be inverted passively beyond the normal range permitted by the subtalar joint. Moreover, when the heel is fully inverted a dimple or depression of the skin may be visible in front of the lateral malleolus, where the soft tissues have been sucked into the gap created between tibia and talus. *Radiographic examination:* Routine radiographs do not show any abnormality. Antero-posterior films must be taken while the heel is held fully inverted. If the lateral ligaments are torn the talus will be shown tilted away from the tibio-fibular mortise through 20 degrees or more (Fig. 275).

Treatment. If the disability is slight it may be sufficient to strengthen the evertor muscles (mainly the peronei) by exercises, to enable them to control the ankle more efficiently. At the same time the heel of the shoe may be splayed laterally, or 'floated out,' to reduce the tendency to going over.

If the disability is severe operation is required. A new lateral ligament is constructed from the peroneus brevis tendon.

STRAIN OF THE LATERAL LIGAMENTS OF THE ANKLE

When adduction violence is insufficient to rupture the lateral ligaments of the ankle completely one or more of the ligaments may be strained. Such strains are much more common than complete rupture of the ligaments. The injury corresponds to diagram 7 in Figure 266.

Clinical features. There are pain and swelling at the lateral aspect of the ankle, with difficulty in walking. The greatest tenderness is immediately below and in front of the lateral malleolus. There is a good range of plantarflexion and dorsiflexion at the ankle, but attempted adduction increases the pain.

Diagnosis. The possibility of a fracture must always be excluded by radiographic examination. If pain and swelling are severe, and especially if there is extensive bruising, the possibility of complete rupture of the lateral ligaments must be investigated by taking antero-posterior radiographs while an adduction stress is applied to the heel (p. 269).

Treatment. In the ordinary case little or no treatment is required. The usual practice is to support the ankle for two weeks with a crepe bandage. If pain and swelling are unusually severe it may be wise to protect the ankle in a walking plaster for two or three weeks.

STRAIN OF LATERAL LIGAMENT OF SUBTALAR JOINT

In many instances a 'sprained ankle' is in fact a strain of the lateral ligament of the subtalar (talo-calcaneal) joint rather than of the ankle joint proper. This injury is caused by excessive inversion-adduction of the foot in much the same way as a strain of the ankle ligaments, but the inversion-adduction movement is often associated with forced plantarflexion. The point of greatest tenderness is lower and farther forward than in strains of the ankle ligaments, and the pain is exacerbated not so much by pure adduction as by combined adduction and plantarflexion. The treatment is the same as for strains of the ankle ligaments.

RUPTURE OF THE CALCANEAL TENDON

Surprising as it may seem, a ruptured tendo calcaneus (tendo achillis) is often overlooked, the symptoms being wrongly ascribed to a strained muscle or a ruptured plantaris tendon.

Pathology. The rupture is always complete. It occurs about five centimetres above the insertion of the tendon. If it is left untreated the tendon unites spontaneously, but with lengthening.

Clinical features. While running or jumping the patient feels a sudden severe pain at the back of the ankle. He may believe that something has struck him. He is able to walk, but with a limp. *On examination* there is tenderness at the site of rupture. There is general thickening from effusion of blood and from oedema of the paratenon, but a gap can usually be felt in the course of the tendon. The power of plantarflexion at the ankle is greatly weakened, though some power remains through the action of the tibialis posterior, the peronei, and the toe flexors.

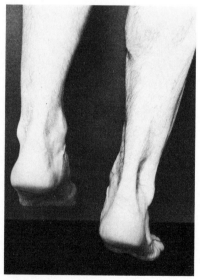

Fig. 276
The crucial test of intact calf function is to ask the patient to raise the heel from the ground while standing only on the affected leg. Inability to do this after an injury to the calcaneal tendon is diagnostic of complete rupture.

Diagnosis. The retention of some power of plantarflexion may deflect the unwary from the correct diagnosis. The crucial test is to ask the patient to lift the heel from the ground while standing only upon the affected leg (Fig. 276). This is impossible if the tendon is ruptured.

Treatment. Non-operative treatment is usually by immobilisation in plaster for five weeks, with the foot in slight equinus to relax the tendon and thus to help to prevent lengthening. Operative treatment entails repair of the tendon, preferably by sutures of stainless steel wire, tension on the suture line being relaxed by immobilising the limb with right-angled knee flexion and moderate ankle planta-flexion for two weeks. For the next four weeks a below-knee plaster with the ankle at 90 degrees is worn. Whether treatment is by plaster alone or by operation, it must be completed after removal of the plaster by increasingly vigorous exercises for the calf muscles, practised until full strength is restored.

COMMENT

Whereas formerly a fresh rupture was regularly repaired by operation, more recently the trend has been towards non-operative treatment. Probably there is still a place for operation in athletic persons, to reduce the risk of lengthening of the tendon and consequent loss of 'spring-off', non-operative treatment being preferred for older patients. If rupture has been overlooked or neglected for more than four weeks conservative treatment by graduated exercises is to be preferred.

STRAINED CALF MUSCLE

Occasionally the calf muscle is strained or 'pulled', especially during athletic pursuits. The essential pathology is probably rupture of a few muscle fibres. There is sudden severe pain, well localised in the calf. The pain and tenderness are considerably higher in the calf than in a case of ruptured calcaneal tendon. Moreover there is no palpable gap, and the patient is able, despite pain, to raise himself on to the toes as in Figure 276. These diagnostic features distinguish strain of the calf muscle from rupture of the calcaneal tendon. The symptoms subside spontaneously and treatment is not required.

RUPTURE OF PLANTARIS MUSCLE

A diagnosis of rupture of the plantaris muscle must be made with caution: in many instances it has proved to be erroneous, the true condition being rupture of the calcaneal tendon itself. Rupture of the plantaris— usually near the junction of muscle and tendon—is a distinct entity, but it is very uncommon. It occurs with dramatic suddenness during running or leaping, as does rupture of the calcaneal tendon. There is sharp pain, often with later swelling and bruising. Pain and tenderness are higher in the calf than in a case of rupture of the calcaneal tendon, and a little towards the medial side, over the course of the plantaris muscle and tendon. The calcaneal tendon itself is felt to be intact, and the patient can lift the heel from the ground when standing on the affected leg (Fig. 276). Treatment is by firm elastic bandaging and curtailment of activities until the pain and swelling subside.

INJURIES OF THE TARSUS

FRACTURES OF THE TALUS

In most injuries caused by a fall from a height on to the feet it is the calcaneus that gives way under the stress, and fractures of the talus are uncommon. Most serious fractures of the talus occur through the neck of the bone; but minor fractures are also encountered in which a small chip or flake is detached, usually from the margin of one of the articular surfaces.

FRACTURE OF THE NECK OF THE TALUS

A typical cause of a major fracture of the talus is an aircraft crash in which the rudder-bar is driven forcibly up against the middle of the sole of the foot. The impact is transmitted to the head of the talus, and the bone gives way in the narrow neck immediately in front of the main body of the bone. In severe injuries the body of the talus may be dislocated backwards out of the ankle mortise: indeed it has sometimes been squeezed out through the skin and lost.

Treatment. The principles of treatment are to reduce the displacement (if any) by manipulation or, if that fails, by open operation. Thereafter the foot is immobilised in a below-knee plaster until the fracture is united, walking being allowed after the first few weeks. Sometimes the reduction is stable only when the foot is in equinus, and it may be necessary to immobilise the foot in that position for the first three weeks.

Complications. NON-UNION AND AVASCULAR NECROSIS. Fractures through the neck of the talus are prone to non-union, which is often associated with avascular necrosis of the proximal (body) fragment from damage to the nutrient vessels at the time of the injury. In its proclivity to avascular changes the fractured talus closely resembles the fractured scaphoid bone in the wrist, and the effects are alike: the avascular fragment often fails to unite with the rest of the bone, it gradually collapses, and the overlying articular cartilage may be shed.

Diagnosis. As in the scaphoid bone, avascular necrosis of the talus may be recognised one or two months after the injury by a marked difference in the radiographic density of the affected fragment compared with the surrounding bones. The avascular bone does not share in the disuse osteoporosis that occurs in the foot as a whole; so it appears much denser than the neighbouring bones.

Treatment. If the fracture fails to unite and avascular necrosis is recognised operation is required. The aim should be to eliminate the peri-talar joints (the ankle, subtalar and talo-navicular joints) by arthrodesis. If avascular necrosis has led to marked collapse and disintegration of the body of the talus it may be necessary to excise the avascular remnants and to fuse the tibia to the upper surface of the calcaneus.

OsteoArthritis. Osteoarthritis of the ankle and subtalar joints is almost inevitable after avascular necrosis of the body of the talus. Arthritis may also follow injury to the articular surface. If arthritis becomes disabling the only satisfactory treatment is to eliminate the affected joints by arthrodesis.

MINOR FRACTURES OF THE TALUS
Minor fractures in which a small chip or flake of the talus is pulled off are more common than the serious fractures just described. There is seldom severe displacement. As a rule the only treatment required is to immobilise the foot in a below-knee walking plaster for three or four weeks.

FRACTURES OF THE CALCANEUS
A fracture of the calcaneus may take the form of an isolated crack or minor fracture without displacement—usually in the region of the tuberosity—or of a compression injury which crushes the bone from above downwards. The more serious compression type of injury is unfortunately the more common.

Mechanism of injury. Almost all fractures of the calcaneus are caused by a fall from a height on to the heels: thus both heels may be injured at the same time. The type of fracture depends mainly upon the severity of the force, and therefore to a large extent on the height of the fall. The weight thrust is transmitted through the talus to the upper articular surface of the calcaneus. If this surface holds, the force is transmitted through the bone towards the tuberosity, which may be split or cracked. More usually, however, the articular surface of the calcaneus fails to withstand the stress: it is shattered by the impact and driven downwards into the body of the bone, crushing the delicate trabeculae of cancellous bone into powder. In addition, fractures radiate from the subtalar region into the tuberosity, and often also to the front of the calcaneus, emerging at the surface of the calcaneo-cuboid joint.

MINOR FRACTURE WITHOUT COMPRESSION
Clinical features. There is a history of a fall on to the heel—not usually from more than a few feet. There is severe local pain, and the patient is unable to put weight on the heel. Examination reveals a little soft-tissue swelling about the heel, marked local tenderness over the tuberosity of the calcaneus, but no palpable deformity of the bone. Later, an ecchymosis may be observed in the sole of the foot at the sides of the plantar aponeurosis. Movements of the ankle, subtalar and midtarsal joints are not appreciably restricted.

Diagnosis. The fracture may be overlooked unless adequate radiographic examination is carried out. It is not sufficient to rely only upon the ordinary lateral projection of the heel, which may fail to show the fracture. An axial view is essential: the central ray is projected obliquely through the heel from the plantar surface while the ankle is held fully dorsiflexed (Fig. 277).

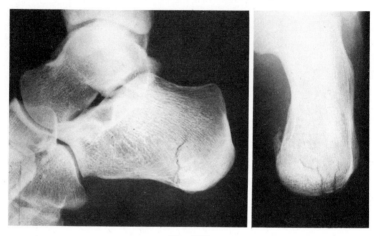

Fig. 277

Isolated fracture of tuberosity of calcaneus without displacement. The fracture is seen best in the axial radiograph (*right*). The subtalar joint surface is intact. Note the normal shape of the calcaneus, for comparison with that of the crushed calcaneus shown in Figure 279.

Treatment. Unlike the more serious compression fractures, isolated fractures of the calcaneus without displacement present little difficulty in treatment. All that is required is to protect the heel for four weeks or so by a below-knee plaster (Fig. 267), in which walking may be allowed almost from the beginning. Excellent results may be expected, and complications are exceptional.

COMPRESSION FRACTURE

A compression fracture of the calcaneus must be regarded as a serious injury which leads inevitably to permanent impairment of function despite the most careful treatment.

Clinical features. There is a history of a fall on to the heels, often from a considerable height. Both heels may be injured together. The patient is unable to bear weight on the affected foot or feet. On examination, the heel is palpably broadened out sideways, and careful measurements taken from the malleoli to the under surface of the

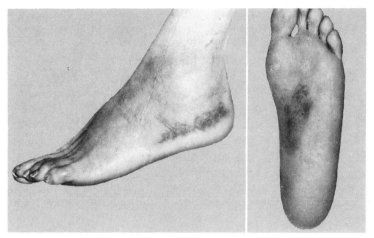

Fig. 278

Characteristic distribution of the visible bruising from fracture of the calcaneus. The tough central part of the plantar aponeurosis forms a barrier, preventing spread of the ecchymosis to the weight-bearing part of the sole. Discolouration therefore spreads towards the sides of the heel and the medial aspect of the instep.

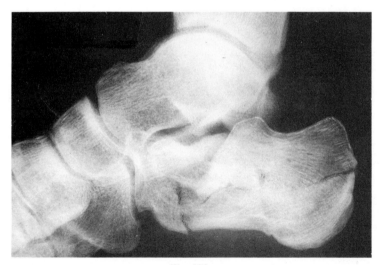

Fig. 279

Compression fracture of calcaneus. The subtalar joint surface—especially its posterior part—has been crushed down into the body of the bone. This is indicated by the flattened outline of the upper surface of the bone (compare with normal contour seen in Figure 277). The fracture line also enters the calcaneo-cuboid joint.

heel may show that it is reduced in height. There is marked local tenderness over the calcaneus. After a day or two a visible ecchymosis spreads into the sole of the foot at the sides of the plantar aponeurosis—a characteristic feature (Fig. 278). Movements of the ankle are not appreciably impaired, but there is marked restriction of inversion-eversion movement at the subtalar and midtarsal joints, which are nearly always damaged.

In many cases of crush fracture of the calcaneus there is also a compression fracture of a vertebral body, usually in the lower thoracic or upper lumbar region. This common association is explained by the fact that the two fractures are caused by the same type of injury, namely a fall from a height.

Diagnosis. Unlike a minor crack fracture, a compression fracture of the calcaneus is easily diagnosed from the lateral radiograph if the shape of the bone is compared with the normal (Figs. 277 and 279). The most striking feature is that the upper surface of the calcaneus is distinctly flattened, so that the line of the subtalar joint may form almost a straight line with the upper surface of the tuberosity. This 'tuberosity-joint angle' (normally about 35 to 40 degrees) has been used as an index of the severity of the compression: in a severe case the angle is reduced to zero or it may even be inverted.

Treatment. Many different methods of treatment have been advocated for this difficult fracture, but it has to be admitted that no method at present available is capable of restoring the foot to normal. The main difficulty of treatment arises from the fact that the articular facets of the subtalar joint are shattered into numerous fragments which are driven down into the underlying cancellous bone. Thus it is virtually impossible both to restore the general shape of the bone to normal and to refashion a perfectly smooth articular surface. In these respects a compression fracture of the calcaneus resembles a comminuted depressed fracture of the lateral tibial condyle ('bumper' fracture, p. 245), and, as in that injury, the most reliable method of treatment is to accept the displacement, to avoid immobilisation, and to encourage movement of the joints from the beginning. It is hoped that in this way the pliable granulations that form over the shattered joint surface in the process of healing will be moulded to a reasonably smooth contour, and that intra-articular adhesions will be minimised.

Standard method. The foot is elevated on a Braun's frame (Fig. 42) to reduce oedema. No attempt is made to correct the displacement. Active exercises are begun at once to encourage movement at the ankle, subtalar and midtarsal joints. Ankle movement (plantarflexion-dorsiflexion) is usually regained without difficulty because the joint surfaces are undamaged; but there is always considerable restriction of subtalar and midtarsal movement (inversion-eversion), which yields gradually to intensive exercises.

The patient should be confined to bed for three to four weeks; if walking is allowed earlier gravitational oedema may be troublesome and may hinder the restoration of useful movement. When walking is eventually resumed exercises should be continued daily in the gymnasium for many weeks.

In practice the results of this simple method of treatment compare favourably with those of the more elaborate techniques—such as mechanical traction through transfixion pins—that aim to restore the shape of the bone more nearly to normal.

Alternative methods for special cases. If it is clear that the subtalar joint surfaces are badly shattered there is an argument for immediate arthrodesis of the joint on the supposition that painful osteoarthritis will otherwise inevitably supervene. The indications for this method of primary arthrodesis are not clearly defined. Whereas some surgeons advocate it almost as a routine for all severe compression fractures, most prefer to rely entirely upon conservative treatment in the first instance, reserving arthrodesis for cases in which troublesome pain persists for more than three months after the injury.

Complications. STIFFNESS OF SUBTALAR AND MIDTARSAL JOINTS. Some impairment of inversion-eversion movement is an almost inevitable sequel of a compression fracture of the calcaneus, because the subtalar joint (and often also the midtarsal joint) is nearly always extensively damaged. Though stiffness cannot be prevented altogether it can be kept to a minimum by insisting upon elevation of the foot for several weeks after the injury to control oedema, and by encouraging early active exercises.

OSTEOARTHRITIS. The subtalar joint is left distorted and irregular after a compression fracture of the calcaneus, and, as would be expected, osteoarthritis is a common sequel; indeed the surprising fact is that it does not always become disabling. In some cases severe pain does cause serious disability at an early stage, and demands operative treatment; but in others the patient may be able to carry on indefinitely with only slight pain and with little disability. The symptoms are always aggravated by walking on rough ground.

Treatment. It is probable that the development of severe osteoarthritis may to some extent be prevented by mobilising exercises begun soon after the injury. When established arthritis becomes disabling the only satisfactory treatment is by arthrodesis of the subtalar joint and, if necessary, of the midtarsal joint.

LIMP. An effect of severe depression of the subtalar articular surface is that the calcaneal tuberosity—and with it the insertion of the calcaneal tendon—is displaced proximally. In consequence the calf muscles are unduly slack, and the power of raising the heel from the ground is impaired. This loss of 'spring' may cause a persistent slight limp. Treatment is by intensive exercises for the calf muscles, which may be able eventually to take up the slack.

ASSOCIATED FRACTURE OF SPINE. The frequent association between crush fracture of the calcaneus and compression fracture of a vertebral body has already been mentioned. The spinal column should be examined clinically and radiographically in every case of calcaneal fracture, whether or not there are any symptoms in the spine. Only thus can the risk of overlooking a spinal fracture be avoided.

OTHER INJURIES OF THE TARSAL BONES

Fractures of the other tarsal bones are uncommon and do not require detailed consideration here. Dislocation of the tarsal joints is also uncommon. It may occur at the subtalar joint, at the midtarsal joint or at the tarso-metatarsal joints, and at any of these sites dislocation may be associated with a fracture. The principles of treatment are to reduce the dislocation and thereafter to immobilise the foot in a below-knee walking plaster for six or eight weeks. When manipulative reduction is impossible operation may be required, and if the joint is badly shattered arthrodesis may have to be considered.

FRACTURES OF THE METATARSAL BONES AND PHALANGES OF THE TOES

FRACTURES OF THE METATARSAL BONES

Most metatarsal fractures are caused by direct violence from a heavy object falling upon the foot. A metatarsal may also be fractured by muscular violence in a twisting injury, or by repeated stress without any specific injury (stress or fatigue fractures).

FRACTURE OF THE BASE OF THE FIFTH METATARSAL

Fracture of the base of the fifth metatarsal bone is common. It is nearly always caused by a twisting injury in which the foot is forced into inversion and equinus. It is an avulsion fracture, the base of the metatarsal being pulled off by the tendon of the peroneus brevis muscle which is inserted into it.

Clinically, there is pain at the outer border of the foot, with difficulty in walking. There is marked local tenderness over the base of the metatarsal, and the diagnosis of fracture is easily confirmed by radiography (Fig. 280).

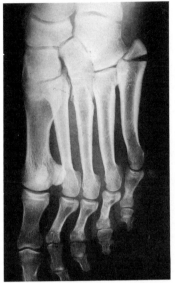 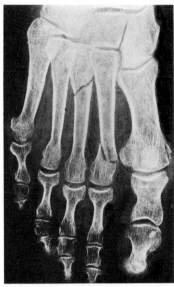

Fig. 280	Fig. 281
Avulsion fracture of the base of the fifth metatarsal bone caused by forcible inversion of the foot.	Fractures of the second and third metatarsal bones from a crushing injury.

Treatment. Although immobilisation is not essential to union of the fracture a plaster should usually be advised for the relief of pain. A below-knee walking plaster of standard type (Fig. 267) is used. The plaster need not be retained for longer than three weeks, and thereafter the only treatment required is a course of active exercises to restore movement and muscle tone.

OS VESALIANUM

In childhood the single epiphysis of the fifth metatarsal is normally at the distal end, as it is also in the second, third and fourth metatarsals. Occasionally an accessory ossicle, the os Vesalianum, is seen in relation to the base of the fifth metatarsal, and it may be mistaken for a fragment avulsed from the base of the metatarsal by injury. Differentiation is aided by the fact that these accessory ossicles are nearly always bilateral, and in cases of doubt the uninjured foot should be radiographed for comparison.

FRACTURES OF THE METATARSAL SHAFTS

One or more of the metatarsals may be fractured by a heavy object falling upon the foot. The fracture may occur at any point in the shaft—near the base, in the mid-shaft, or at the metatarsal neck. It is usually of the transverse or short oblique type, and displacement is seldom severe (Fig. 281).

Treatment. Here again immobilisation is required mainly for the relief of pain: union will occur readily whether or not the fracture is immobilised. As a rule a walking plaster should be worn for three or four weeks, and thereafter active exercises should be arranged.

FATIGUE OR STRESS FRACTURE OF A METATARSAL BONE
('March' fracture)

Fatigue fractures occur more commonly in the metatarsals than in any other bone. They differ from ordinary fractures in that there is no history of violence: the pain seems to arise spontaneously and the possibility of a fracture may be overlooked.

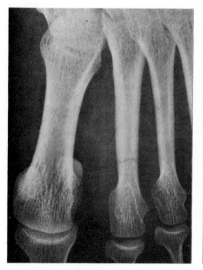
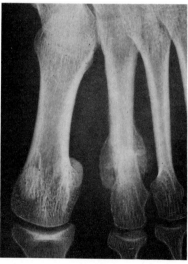

Fig. 282   Fig. 283

A typical march or fatigue fracture of the second metatarsal. In the initial radiograph (Fig. 282) taken soon after the onset of symptoms the fracture is seen only as a faint hair-line crack. Two weeks later the fracture is surrounded by abundant callus (Fig. 283).

Cause. The fracture is ascribed to long-continued or oft-repeated stress, particularly from prolonged walking, in those who are not accustomed to it. Thus it may occur in army recruits freshly committed to marching; hence the term 'march fracture'. It has been likened to the fatigue fractures that sometimes occur in metals.

Pathology. The fracture usually affects the shaft or neck of the second or third metatarsal bone. It is no more than a hair-line crack, and there is no displacement of the fragments. In the process of healing a large mass of callus may form around the bone at the site of fracture.

Clinical features. The complaint is of severe pain in the fore-foot on walking. The onset is rapid but the patient is usually unable to ascribe it to an obvious cause. Enquiry may reveal, however, that he has done an unusual amount of walking a day or two before the onset. Indeed sometimes the pain begins to come on during the march. *On examination* there is swelling on the dorsum of the foot, with well marked local tenderness over the affected metatarsal. *Radiographs* at first show only a faint hairline crack which may be easily overlooked (Fig. 282). But after a week or two the callus surrounding the fracture is clearly visible (Fig. 283).

Treatment. The fracture heals spontaneously, so treatment is purely symptomatic. In some cases no treatment is needed; but if pain is severe immobilisation in a below-knee walking plaster for four weeks is advised.

FRACTURES OF THE PHALANGES OF THE TOES

Most fractures of the toes are caused by crushing injuries, as from the fall of a heavy object. The great toe, being the most prominent, is the one most often affected. In many cases the phalanx is severely comminuted, but a satisfactory general alignment is preserved. Sometimes the fracture is associated with a bursting wound of the skin and soft tissues. Swelling and pain are often severe.

Treatment. Little or no treatment is required for these fractures. If there is much swelling, with severe pain, it is wise to elevate the foot for a few days, but otherwise the only treatment required is to protect the toe from accidental knocks by a soft woolly dressing.

Appendix I

SUMMARY OF THE TREATMENT OF UNCOMPLICATED FRACTURES OF THE EXTREMITIES

UPPER EXTREMITY

CLAVICLE (p. 114)

Figure-of-eight bandage for two weeks. Begin active shoulder exercises after the first week.

SCAPULA (p. 115)

Disregard the fracture and concentrate on restoring shoulder function by active exercises. Rarely, excision of acromion process is required for depressed comminuted fracture.

NECK OF HUMERUS (p. 127)

Old persons. Disregard the fracture and concentrate on restoring shoulder function by active and assisted exercises. *If fracture is impacted,* begin exercises from sling immediately. *If fracture is not impacted,* defer shoulder exercises until the fragments are 'sticky'— usually three weeks.
Young adults. If displacement is not severe, treat as above. If displacement is severe, attempt reduction by manipulation and immobilise shoulder in the most stable position for six weeks; then active mobilising exercises.

GREATER TUBEROSITY OF HUMERUS (p. 130)

If tuberosity fragment is not displaced, disregard the fracture and concentrate on restoring shoulder function by active and assisted exercises from a sling. If tuberosity fragment is displaced, reduce by abducting the arm to meet the elevated fragment, or if necessary by operation, and immobilise for three weeks, if necessary in abduction; then arrange mobilising exercises.

SHAFT OF HUMERUS (p. 131)

Reduce severe displacement by manipulation and support by plaster cylinder round upper arm, or by full-length arm plaster with elbow at a right angle. If fracture irreducible or unstable, undertake internal fixation by intramedullary nail introduced from below.

SUPRACONDYLAR REGION OF HUMERUS (p. 135)

Reduce by manipulation and immobilise in full-length arm plaster with elbow at a right angle or less. Correct lateral tilting of lower fragment, but slight loss of apposition may be accepted.

LATERAL CONDYLE OF HUMERUS (p. 140)

Attempt manipulative reduction and if successful immobilise in right-angled arm plaster. (Perfect reduction essential because articular surface is involved.) If manipulation fails, undertake operative reduction and internal fixation by a screw.

MEDIAL EPICONDYLE OF HUMERUS (p. 143)

Ignore displacement (except when the fragment is included in the joint). Rest in right-angled arm plaster for three weeks, then arrange mobilising exercises.

OLECRANON PROCESS (p. 149)

Crack fracture without displacement. Protect in right-angled arm plaster for three weeks. Then exercises.

Clean break with separation of fragments. Undertake operative reduction and fixation with screw.

Comminuted fracture. Excise olecranon fragments and suture triceps to stump of olecranon.

HEAD OF RADIUS (p. 151)

Fracture with slight or no displacement. Rest in right-angled arm plaster for three weeks, then arrange mobilising exercises.

Severely comminuted fracture. Excise head of radius. Rest in plaster for two weeks, then exercise.

UPPER SHAFT OF ULNA, WITH DISLOCATION OF HEAD OF RADIUS (p. 154)

Attempt reduction by manipulation. If successful, immobilise in right-angled arm plaster. If manipulation unsuccessful, undertake operative reduction and internal fixation of the fracture with plate or intramedullary nail, and reduction or excision of head of radius.

SHAFT OF RADIUS OR ULNA, OR BOTH BONES (p. 154)

Attempt manipulative reduction. If successful, immobilise arm in full length plaster with elbow at right angle. (Accurate reduction important, to preserve rotation and to ensure equal length of the two bones.) If manipulation unsuccessful, operative reduction and internal fixation (by plates and screws, or intramedullary nail).

SHAFT OF RADIUS, WITH DISLOCATION OF HEAD OF ULNA (p. 158)

Attempt manipulative reduction. If successful, immobilise arm in full length plaster with elbow at right angle. Closed reduction is often imperfect; so in most cases operative reduction and fixation of radius by plate are required. The dislocation is then usually reduced easily.

LOWER END OF RADIUS (p. 159)

Reduce by manipulation. Immobilise forearm and wrist in complete plaster or dorsal plaster slab for six weeks. In the exceptional case in which displacement of the distal fragment is forwards rather than backwards (Smith's fracture) operative fixation may be required.

SCAPHOID BONE (p. 173)

Generally, immobilise in close fitting plaster until fracture united. If union delayed beyond four to six months decide between bone-grafting operation (if persistently painful) and deliberate mobilisation with disregard of the fracture.

BASE OF FIRST METACARPAL BONE (p. 181)

Fracture not involving joint. Reduce and immobilise in plaster for eight weeks.

Fracture involving joint (Bennett's fracture). Attempt manipulative reduction and retention in plaster. (Accurate reduction essential because joint surface is involved.) If plaster immobilisation fails to hold adequate reduction undertake operative reduction and stabilisation, preferably by a screw.

OTHER METACARPALS (p. 182)

Fractures with slight or no displacement. Protect by dorsal plaster slab for three weeks. Maintain full finger movements by active use of the hand from the beginning.

Severely displaced fractures. Reduce by manipulation and protect by splint or plaster in most stable position for two weeks. If fracture irreducible or unstable despite splintage, undertake open reduction and internal fixation by intramedullary wire or, for those with unacceptable shortening, apply traction and transfix with wire through adjacent metacarpal necks.

PHALANGES (p. 185)

Undisplaced fractures. Disregard fracture or support lightly for two weeks.

Displaced fractures. Reduce by manipulation and splint for two or three weeks. If this is impracticable, fix internally by intramedullary wire. Begin mobilising exercises not later than three weeks after injury, irrespective of the state of the fracture.

LOWER EXTREMITY

PELVIS (p. 190)

Minor fractures. Confine patient to bed until severe pain subsides (about two weeks). Encourage exercises for the lower limbs from the beginning.

Major fractures with disruption of pelvic ring. If displacement is slight, confine patient to bed for four to six weeks to allow fractures to become stable. Encourage exercises for the lower limbs from the beginning. If displacement is severe, attempt reduction by limb traction and coapt the halves of the symphysis pubis.

NECK OF FEMUR (p. 203)

Unimpacted fracture (the usual type). Internal fixation by combination of three-flanged (Smith-Petersen) nail and Venable hip screw, or by suitable alternative device. Hip movements encouraged immediately. A limited amount of walking with sticks or crutches may be permitted when the wound is healed. In elderly patients primary replacement arthroplasty (femoral head alone, or femoral head and acetabular socket) is a commonly used·alternative method.

Impacted abduction fracture (relatively uncommon). Operation not required. Confine patient to bed for three weeks. Thereafter allow walking with crutches but not full weight-bearing for eight weeks.

TROCHANTERIC REGION OF FEMUR (p. 214)

Old persons. Undertake fixation by nail-plate. Encourage early weight-bearing.

Young adults. Choice of conservative treatment by continuous weight traction, or operative treatment by fixation by nail-plate.

SHAFT OF FEMUR (p. 218)

Reduce severe displacement by manipulation, and support limb in Thomas's or similar splint with continuous weight traction until fracture united (usually twelve to sixteen weeks). (Selected patients may be got up earlier, with the limb supported in a close-fitting plaster.) Encourage quadriceps and knee exercises almost from the beginning. If fracture irreducible or unstable, or patient elderly, undertake operative reduction and internal fixation by long intra-medullary nail.

SUPRACONDYLAR REGION OF FEMUR (p. 226)

Reduce displacement by manipulation, and support limb in Thomas's or similar splint with weight traction, as for fracture of femoral shaft. Control angulation of distal fragment by adjusting position of knee. Defer knee movements for six weeks. If fracture irreducible or unstable, undertake internal fixation by nail-plate.

CONDYLES OF FEMUR (p. 228)

Crack fracture. Protect in full-length lower limb plaster for eight weeks. Then active knee exercises.

Displaced fracture. Reduce displacement and protect limb in Thomas's splint or plaster. If fracture cannot be reduced by manipulation, undertake operative reduction and internal fixation by long trans-fixion screw.

PATELLA (p. 230)

Crack fracture without displacement. Protect in plaster for three weeks.

Clean break with separation of fragments. If patient is under 40, fix fragments together with screw or bolt. If patient is over 40, excise patella.

Comminuted fracture with displacement. Excise patella.

LATERAL CONDYLE OF TIBIA (p. 244)

Comminuted depressed fracture (the usual type). Accept displacement. Confine patient to bed for three to six weeks (according to severity of fracture) and encourage knee exercises from the beginning, but protect the knee in a removable plaster splint at night.

Depressed fracture of plateau without comminution (relatively uncommon). Undertake operative reduction, pushing the depressed fragment up from below and supporting it underneath with cancellous bone chips. Immobilise knee in plaster for four weeks before movements are begun.

Oblique shearing fracture (relatively uncommon). Reduce displacement of condyle by manipulation or, if that fails, by operation. Immobilise knee in plaster for four weeks before active movements are begun.

SHAFT OF TIBIA, WITH OR WITHOUT FIBULA (p. 248)

Attempt reduction by manipulation. If successful, immobilise limb in full-length plaster until fracture is united. Encourage walking in plaster after first few weeks. If manipulation unsuccessful or if redisplacement occurs in plaster, undertake operative reduction and internal fixation (by intramedullary nail, oblique transfixion screws, circumferential wires, metal plate or bone graft).

SHAFT OF FIBULA (p. 257)

Protect limb in below-knee walking plaster for three weeks. (Note possibility of coexisting diastasis at inferior tibio-fibular joint.)

LATERAL MALLEOLUS, WITHOUT DISPLACEMENT (p. 263)

Protect in below-knee walking plaster for three weeks, mainly for relief of pain.

MEDIAL MALLEOLUS (p. 263)

If no displacement, or if perfect reduction obtained by manipulation, protect in below-knee walking plaster for six or eight weeks. If displacement not fully corrected by manipulation periosteum probably interposed: therefore undertake operative reduction and internal fixation by a screw. Thereafter protect in plaster for eight weeks.

LATERAL MALLEOLUS, WITH LATERAL SHIFT OF TALUS (p. 264)

Reduce displacement by medial pressure over lateral malleolus, and immobilise in plaster for eight weeks. (Accurate reduction essential, to preserve congruity of articular surfaces.) If redisplacement occurs in plaster, undertake operative reduction and fixation of lateral malleolus to tibia by a long oblique screw. Thereafter keep in plaster for eight weeks.

LATERAL AND MEDIAL MALLEOLI, WITH DISPLACEMENT (p. 265)

Undertake operative reduction and internal fixation of medial malleolus, and also of lateral malleolus if necessary. (Accurate reduction essential.) Keep in plaster for ten weeks.

FIBULA, WITH INFERIOR TIBIO-FIBULAR DIASTASIS (p. 266)

Fix fibula to tibia by long transverse screw to prevent lateral shift of talus and lower end of fibula. Protect in plaster for eight weeks.

POSTERIOR ARTICULAR MARGIN OF TIBIA (p. 267)

If fragment is small, disregard it and treat only the other elements of the injury. If fragment is large, reduce by operation and fix by screw. (Perfect reduction essential, to preserve smooth articular surface.)

INFERIOR ARTICULAR SURFACE OF TIBIA (p. 269)

Shearing fracture without severe comminution. Reduce fracture and immobilise, usually by internal fixation.

Severely comminuted fracture. Accept the disorganisation of the joint as irreparable, and undertake primary arthrodesis of the ankle.

TALUS (p. 274)
Fracture through neck of talus. Reduce by manipulation or, if that fails, by operation. Immobilise ankle in below-knee plaster until fracture is united (usually about twelve weeks).
Minor fractures. Protect ankle in below-knee walking plaster for three or four weeks.

CALCANEUS (p. 275)
Undisplaced fracture (relatively uncommon). Protect foot in walking plaster for about four weeks.
Compression fracture (the usual type). Accept displacement. Confine patient to bed for three to four weeks, and encourage active movements of subtalar and midtarsal joints from the beginning. Prepare to arthrodese the subtalar joint (and possibly also the midtarsal joint) in the event of severe or persistent pain.

METATARSAL BONES (p. 280)
Protect foot in below-knee walking plaster for about three weeks, mainly for relief of pain.

PHALANGES OF TOES (p. 283)
Rigid splintage not required. Protect with soft dressing.

Appendix II

SUMMARY OF THE INJURIES THAT MAY BE CAUSED BY A FALL ON THE OUTSTRETCHED HAND

(The more common injuries are denoted by heavy type)

CHILDREN
Greenstick fracture of lower end of radius
Fracture-separation of lower radial epiphysis
Fractures of both bones of forearm
Fracture of head (or neck) of radius
Dislocation of elbow
Supracondylar fracture of humerus
Fracture-separation of upper humeral epiphysis
Fracture of clavicle

YOUNG ADULTS
Fracture of scaphoid bone
Fracture of lower end of radius
Fracture of shaft of radius and/or ulna
Fracture of head of radius
Dislocation of elbow
Dislocation of shoulder
Fracture of clavicle

OLD PERSONS
Fracture of lower end of radius
Dislocation of elbow
Fracture of neck of humerus
Dislocation of shoulder
Fracture of clavicle

References and bibliography, page 291.

References and Bibliography

This list is not intended as a comprehensive guide even to the more recent literature on fracture surgery: space does not permit the inclusion of more than a limited selection. The aim has been to choose books and papers that will be of the greatest service to those seeking detailed information on a given subject, and a paper has generally been selected for one or more of the following reasons: 1) it reports recent work: 2) it reports authoritative opinion: 3) it is of special intrinsic interest: 4) it contains a comprehensive list of references. An original description or a classic paper has not always been listed when reference to it is made in more recent works, because it can thereby be easily traced. In the main the references are to works in the English language which will be readily accessible to most readers.

The list is arranged in two parts, 'general' and 'specific.' The general list cites comprehensive works of reference on fracture surgery as a whole or on branches of it. The specific list refers to papers or chapters on a particular topic.

Titles printed in *italics* refer to books or monographs: those printed in roman type refer to papers in journals.

GENERAL WORKS

ADAMS, J. C. (1976): *Standard Orthopaedic Operations*. Edinburgh and London: Churchill Livingstone.

AITKEN, A. P. (ed.) (1965): Epiphysial injuries (symposium). Clinical Orthopaedics, **41**, 7.

AMERICAN ACADEMY OF ORTHOPAEDIC SURGEONS (1966): *Joint Motion: Method of Measuring and Recording*. Edinburgh: Livingstone.

APLEY, A. G. (1977): *A System of Orthopaedics and Fractures*, 5th ed. London: Butterworth.

BÖHLER, L.(1935): *The Treatment of Fractures*, 4th English ed. Bristol: John Wright and Sons.

BOURNE, G. H. (ed.) (1972): *The Biochemistry and Physiology of Bone*, 2nd ed. New York and London: Academic Press.

CAMPBELL, W. C. (1971): *Operative Orthopaedics*, 5th ed., ed. Crenshaw. London: Henry Kimpton.

CHARNLEY, J. (1970): *The Closed Treatment of Common Fractures*, 3rd ed. Edinburgh and London: Churchill Livingstone.

ELLIS, M. (1970): *The Casualty Officer's Handbook*, 3rd ed. London: Butterworth.

HENRY, A. K. (1957): *Extensile Exposure*, 2nd ed. Edinburgh: Livingstone.

HOWORTH, B. (1966): Skiing injuries. Clinical Orthopaedics, **43**, 171.

LONDON, P. S. (1967): *A Practical Guide to the Care of the Injured*. Edinburgh: Livingstone.

LONDON, P. S. (ed.) (1970): *Modern Trends in Accident Surgery and Medicine* (2). London: Butterworth.

PERKINS, G. (1958): *Fractures and Dislocations*. London: London University, Athlone Press.

PLEWES, L. W. (ed.) (1966): *Accident Service*. London: Pitman Medical.

RING, P. A. (1964): *The Care of the Injured*. Edinburgh: Livingstone.

ROCKWOOD, C. A., & GREEN, D. P. (1975): *Fractures*. Philadelphia and Toronto: J. B. Lippincott Co.

SEDDON, H. J. (1975): *Surgical Disorders of the Peripheral Nerves*, 2nd ed. Edinburgh and London: Churchill Livingstone.

SEVITT, S., & STONER, H. B. (eds.) (1970): *The Pathology of Trauma*. (Supplement 4 of Journal of Clinical Pathology.) London: British Medical Association.

SUNDERLAND, S. (1970): *Nerves and Nerve Injuries*. Edinburgh: Livingstone.

WATSON-JONES, R. (1976): *Fractures and Joint Injuries*, 5th ed. (ed. Wilson). Edinburgh and London: Churchill Livingstone.

WICKSTROM, J. (1966): Current concepts in management of trauma. Clinical Orthopaedics, **44,** 99.

WOODS, C. G. (1970): *Diagnostic Orthopaedic Pathology*. Oxford: Blackwell Scientific Publications.

SPECIFIC WORKS

INTRODUCTION

BÖHLER, L. (1929): *The Treatment of Fractures*. Vienna: Maudrich.

JONES, A. ROCYN (1956): A review of orthopaedic surgery in Britain. Journal of Bone and Joint Surgery, **38B,** 27.

LISTER, J. (1867): On a new method of treating compound fracture, abscess, etc., with observations on the conditions of suppuration. Lancet, **1,** 326.

LISTER, J. (1867): On the antiseptic principle in the practice of surgery. Lancet, **2,** 353.

MAYER, L. (1950): Orthopaedic surgery in the United States of America. Journal of Bone and Joint Surgery, **32B,** 461.

OSMOND-CLARKE, H. (1950): Half a century of orthopaedic progress in Great Britain. Journal of Bone and Joint Surgery, **32B,** 620.

PLATT, H. (1950): Orthopaedics in Continental Europe, 1900–50. Journal of Bone and Joint Surgery, **32B,** 570.

RÖNTGEN, W. C. (1896): On a new kind of rays. Nature, **53,** 274, 377.

CHAPTER ONE

Pathology of Fractures and Fracture Healing

Healing of Fractures

ATTENBOROUGH, G. C. (1953): Remodelling of the humerus after supracondylar fractures in childhood. Journal of Bone and Joint Surgery, **35B,** 386.

BOURNE, G. H. (1972): *The Biochemistry and Physiology of Bone*, 2nd ed. New York and London: Academic Press.

BRIDGES, J. B., & PRITCHARD, J. J. (1958): Bone and cartilage induction in the rabbit. Journal of Anatomy, **92,** 28.

BRIGHTON, C. T., FRIEDENBERG, Z. B., ZEMSKY, L. M., & POLLIS, P. R. (1975): Direct-current stimulation of non-union and congenital pseudarthrosis. Journal of Bone and Joint Surgery, **57A**, 368.

BURWELL, R. G. (1964): Studies in the transplantation of bone. Journal of Bone and Joint Surgery, **46B**, 110.

CHALMERS, J., GRAY, D. H., & RUSH, J. (1975): Observations on the induction of bone in soft tissues. Journal of Bone and Joint Surgery, **57B**, 36.

DANIS, A. (1957): Etude de l'ossification dans les greffes de moelle osseuse. Acta Chirurgica Belgica, Supplement **3**, 1.

FRIEDENBERG, Z. B., ZEMSKY, L. M., POLLIS, R. P., & BRIGHTON, C. T. (1974): The response of non-traumatised bone to direct current. Journal of Bone and Joint Surgery, **56A**, 1023.

HAM, A. W., & HARRIS, W. R. (1956): Repair and transplantation of bone. In *The Biochemistry and Physiology of Bone* (ed. Bourne). New York: Academic Press.

HOLDSWORTH, F. W. (1954): Natural remodelling after fractures of the lower end of the humerus. Journal of Bone and Joint Surgery, **36B**, 693.

KEITH, A. (1927): Concerning the origin and nature of osteoblasts. Proceedings of the Royal Society of Medicine, **21**, 301.

NADE, S., & BURWELL, R. G. (1977): Decalcified bone as a substrate for osteogenesis. Journal of Bone and Joint Surgery, **59B**, 189.

NORDIN, B. E. C. (ed.) (1976): *Calcium, Phosphate and Magnesium Metabolism.* Edinburgh and London: Churchill Livingstone.

SEVITT, S. (1971): The healing of fractures of the lower end of the radius. Journal of Bone and Joint Surgery, **53B**, 519.

TRUETA, J. (1963): The role of the vessels in osteogenesis. Journal of Bone and Joint Surgery, **45B**, 402.

VAUGHAN, J. (1975): *The Physiology of Bone.* London: Clarendon Press, Oxford University Press.

See also under Bone Grafting (Chapter 4).

Pathological Fractures

BAUZE, R. J., SMITH, R., & MARTIN, J. O. F. (1975): A new look at osteogenesis imperfecta. Journal of Bone and Joint Surgery, **57B**, 2.

DOUGLASS, H. O., SHUKLA, S. K., & MINDELL, E. (1976): Treatment of pathological fractures of long bones excluding those due to breast cancer. Journal of Bone and Joint Surgery, **58A**, 1055.

FALVO, K. A., ROOT, L., & BULLOUGH, P. G. (1974): Osteogenesis imperfecta: clinical evaluation and management. Journal of Bone and Joint Surgery, **56A**, 783.

JAFFE, H. L. (1958): *Tumors and Tumorous Conditions of the Bones and Joints.* London: Kimpton.

MICKELSON, M. R., & BONFIGLIO, M. (1976): Pathological fractures in the proximal part of the femur treated by Zickel-nail fixation. Journal of Bone and Joint Surgery, **58A**, 1067.

NORDIN, B. E. C. (1973): *Metabolic Bone and Stone Disease.* Edinburgh and London: Churchill Livingstone.

PARRISH, F. F., & MURRAY, J. A. (1970): Surgical treatment for secondary neoplastic fractures. Journal of Bone and Joint Surgery, **52A**, 665.

SIM, F. H., DAUGHERTY, T., & IVINS, J. C. (1974): The adjunctive use of methylmethacrylate in fixation of pathological fractures. Journal of Bone and Joint Surgery, **56A**, 40.

WYNNE-DAVIES, R., & FAIRBANK, T. J. (1976): *Fairbank's Atlas of General Affections of the Skeleton*, 2nd ed. Edinburgh and London: Churchill Livingstone.

ZICKEL, R. E., & MOURADIAN, W. H. (1976): Intramedullary fixation of pathological fractures and lesions of the subtrochanteric region of the femur. Journal of Bone and Joint Surgery, **58A**, 1061.

Stress or Fatigue Fractures

BICKENSTAFF, L. D., & MORRIS, J. M. (1966): Fatigue fracture of the femoral neck. Journal of Bone and Joint Surgery, **48A,** 1031.

BURROWS, H. J. (1948): Fatigue fractures of the fibula. Journal of Bone and Joint Surgery, **30B,** 266.

BURROWS, H. J. (1956): Fatigue infraction of the middle of the tibia in ballet dancers. Journal of Bone and Joint Surgery, **38B,** 83.

DEVAS, M. B. (1958): Stress fractures of the tibia in athletes or 'skin soreness.' Journal of Bone and Joint Surgery, **40B,** 227.

DEVAS, M. B. (1963): Stress fractures in children. Journal of Bone and Joint Surgery, **45B,** 528.

DEVAS, M. (1975): *Stress Fractures.* Edinburgh and London: Churchill Livingstone.

DEVAS, M. B., & SWEETNAM, R. (1956): Stress fractures of the fibula. Journal of Bone and Joint Surgery, **38B,** 818.

MORRIS, J. M. (1967): *Fatigue Fractures.* Springfield, Illinois: Charles C. Thomas.

CHAPTER TWO

Clinical and Radiological Features of Fractures

Radiology

GREENFIELD, G. B. (1975): *Radiology of Bone Diseases,* 2nd ed. Philadelphia: J. B. Lippincott. Oxford: Blackwell Scientific Publications.

SHANKS, S. C., & KERLEY, P. (eds.) (1971): *A Text-book of X-Ray Diagnosis,* 4th ed. *Vol. VI, Bones, Joints and Soft Tissues.* London: Lewis.

CHAPTER THREE

Principles of Fracture Treatment

Shock and Resuscitation

BROOKS, D. K. (1967): The mechanism of shock. British Journal of Surgery, **54,** 441.

CLARKE, R. (1959): Resuscitation and transfusion in severe injuries. In *Modern Trends in Accident Surgery and Medicine.* London: Butterworth.

DUDLEY, H. A. F. (1963): Surgical shock and electrolyte balance. In *Recent Advances in Surgery of Trauma.* London: Churchill.

JONES, E. S. (1970): Intensive therapy. Proceedings of the Royal Society of Medicine, **60,** 1203.

MONCRIEF, J. A. (1967): Shock in the multiple injury patient. (Instructional Course Lecture, American Academy of Orthopaedic Surgeons.) Journal of Bone and Joint Surgery, **49A,** 540.

NORRIS, W., & CAMPBELL, D. (1971): *Anaesthetics, Resuscitation and Intensive Care,* 3rd ed. Edinburgh: Livingstone.

Plaster Technique, Splints and Appliances

BLECK, E. E., DUCKWORTH, N., & HUNTER, N. (1974): *Atlas of Plaster Cast Techniques.* London: Lloyd-Luke (Medical Books) Ltd.

BRIGDEN, R. J. (1969): *Operating Theatre Technique.* Edinburgh: Livingstone.

NANGLE, E. J. (1951): *Instruments and Apparatus in Orthopaedic Surgery.* Oxford: Blackwell Scientific Publications.

STEWART, J. D. M. (1975): *Traction and Orthopaedic Appliances.* Edinburgh and London: Churchill Livingstone.

Internal Fixation

ADAMS, J. C. (1976): *Standard Orthopaedic Operations*. Edinburgh and London: Churchill Livingstone.

ANDERSON, L. D. (1965): Compression plate fixation and the effect of different types of internal fixation on fracture healing. (Instructional Course Lecture, American Academy of Orthopaedic Surgeons.) Journal of Bone and Joint Surgery, **47A,** 191.

BATTEN, R. L. (1969): The place of compression techniques in the management of long bone fractures in an industrial city. Journal of Bone and Joint Surgery, **51B,** 177.

HICKS, J. H. (1961): Fractures of the forearm treated by rigid fixation. Journal of Bone and Joint Surgery, **43B,** 680.

KÜNTSCHER, G. (1965): Intramedullary surgical technique and its place in orthopaedic surgery. (Instructional Course Lecture, American Academy of Orthopaedic Surgeons.) Journal of Bone and Joint Surgery, **47A,** 809.

KÜNTSCHER, G. (1967): *Practice of Intramedullary Nailing*. Springfield, Illinois: Charles C. Thomas.

MÜLLER, M. E., ALLGÖWER, M., & WILLENEGGER, H. (1970): *Manual of Internal Fixation*. Berlin-Heidelberg-New York: Springer Verlag.

PARRISH, F. F., & MURRAY, J. A. (1970): Surgical treatment for secondary neoplastic fractures. Journal of Bone and Joint Surgery, **52A,** 665.

Metals for Internal Fixation

HICKS, J. H., & CATER, W. H. (1962): Minor reactions due to modern metal. Journal of Bone and Joint Surgery, **44B,** 122.

SCALES, J. T., WINTER, G. D., & SHIRLEY, H. T. (1959): Corrosion of orthopaedic implants. Journal of Bone and Joint Surgery, **41B,** 811.

WILLIAMS, D. (ed.) (1976): *Biocompatibility of Implant Materials*. London: Sector Publishing Ltd. for Pitman Medical.

WILLIAMS, D. F., & ROAF, R. (1973): *Implants in Surgery*. London, Philadelphia, Toronto: W. B. Saunders.

Rehabilitation

BÖHLER, L. (1935): *The Treatment of Fractures*, 4th English edition. Bristol: John Wright & Sons.

PARRY, C. B. WYNN (1973): *Rehabilitation of the Hand*, 3rd ed. London: Butterworth.

PLEWES, L. W. (1963): Rehabilitation. In *Recent Advances in Surgery of Trauma*. London: Churchill.

STEWART, M. J. (1949): Aspects of physical reconditioning. Journal of Bone and Joint Surgery, **31A,** 394.

WATSON-JONES, R. (1943): *Fractures and Joint Injuries*, 3rd ed. Edinburgh: Livingstone.

Treatment of Open Fractures

CLARKE, R. (1959): Principles and technique of wound surgery. In *Modern Trends in Accident Surgery and Medicine*, ed. Clarke, Badger and Sevitt. London: Butterworth.

CLEVELAND, M., MANNING, J. G., & STEWART, W. J. (1951): Care of battle casualties and injuries involving bones and joints. Journal of Bone and Joint Surgery, **33A,** 517.

SAAD, M. N. (1970): Problems of traumatic skin loss of lower limbs, especially when associated with skeletal injury. British Journal of Surgery, **57,** 601.

CHAPTER FOUR

Complications of Fractures

Infection Complicating Fractures

COLWILL, M. R., & MAUDSLEY, R. H. (1968): The management of gas gangrene with hyperbaric oxygen therapy. Journal of Bone and Joint Surgery, **50B**, 732.

EVANS, E. M. (1968): Treatment of chronic osteomyelitis by skin grafting. Journal of Bone and Joint Surgery, **50B**, 887.

KELLY, R. P. (1946): Skin-grafting in the treatment of osteomyelitic war wounds. Journal of Bone and Joint Surgery, **28**, 681.

KNIGHT, M. P., & WOOD, G. O. (1945): Surgical obliteration of bone cavities following traumatic osteomyelitis. Journal of Bone and Joint Surgery, **27**, 547.

NICOLL, E. A. (1956): The treatment of gaps in long bones by cancellous insert grafts. Journal of Bone and Joint Surgery, **38B**, 70.

ROWLING, D. E. (1959): The positive approach to chronic osteomyelitis. Journal of Bone and Joint Surgery, **41B**, 681.

Delayed Union, Non-union and Avascular Necrosis

BOYD, H. B., WRAY, J. B., BRASHEAR, H. R., & HOHL, M. (1965): Treatment of ununited fractures of long bones (symposium). (Instructional Course Lectures, American Academy of Orthopaedic Surgeons.) Journal of Bone and Joint Surgery, **47A**, 167.

CHRISTENSEN, N. O. (1973): Küntscher intramedullary reaming and nail fixation for non-union of fracture of the femur and tibia. Journal of Bone and Joint Surgery, **55B**, 312.

DAVIDSON, J. K. (1976): *Aseptic Necrosis of Bone.* Amsterdam and Oxford: Excerpta Medica.

MARMOR, L. (ed.) (1966): Management of non-union (symposium). Clinical Orthopaedics, **43**, 6.

SMITH, J. E. M. (1959): Internal fixation in the treatment of fractures of the shafts of the radius and ulna in adults. Journal of Bone and Joint Surgery, **41B**, 122.

TRUETA, J. (1966): Non-union of fractures. Clinical Orthopaedics, **43**, 23.

Bone Grafting

ADAMS, J. C. (1976): *Standard Orthopaedic Operations.* Edinburgh and London: Churchill Livingstone.

BURWELL, R. G. (1966): Studies in the transplantation of bone. Journal of Bone and Joint Surgery, **48B**, 532.

BURWELL, R. G. (1969): The fate of bone grafts. In *Recent Advances in Orthopaedics* (ed. Apley). London: Churchill.

CHALMERS, J. (1959): Transplantation immunity in bone homografting. Journal of Bone and Joint Surgery, **41B**, 160.

FORBES, D. B. (1961): Subcortical iliac bone grafts in fracture of the tibia. Journal of Bone and Joint Surgery, **43B**, 672.

HALLEN, L. G. (1966): Heterologous transplantation with Kiel bone. Acta Orthopaedica Scandinavica, **37**, 1.

PHEMISTER, D. B. (1947): Treatment of ununited fractures by onlay bone grafts without screw or tie fixation and without breaking down of the fibrous union. Journal of Bone and Joint Surgery, **29**, 946.

SOUTER, W. A. (1969): Autogenous cancellous strip grafts in the treatment of delayed union of long bone fractures. Journal of Bone and Joint Surgery, **51B**, 63.

Injury to Blood Vessels
ASHTON, F., & SLANEY, G. (1970): Arterial injuries in civilian surgical practice. Injury, **1,** 303.
CONNOLLY, J. F., WHITTAKER, D., & WILLIAMS, E. (1971): Femoral and tibial fractures combined with injuries to the femoral or popliteal artery. Journal of Bone and Joint Surgery, **53A,** 56.
EASTCOTT, H. H. G. (1965): The management of arterial injuries. Journal of Bone and Joint Surgery, **47B,** 394.
EASTCOTT, H. H. G. (1973): *Arterial Surgery,* 2nd ed. London: Pitman Medical.
ISAACSON, J., LOUIS, D. S., & COSTENBADER, J. M. (1975): Arterial injury associated with closed femoral shaft fractures. Journal of Bone and Joint Surgery, **57A,** 1147.
NOLAN, B., & McQUILLAN, W. M. (1965): Acute traumatic limb ischaemia. British Journal of Surgery, **52,** 559.
PORTER, M. F. (1967): Arterial injuries in an accident unit. British Journal of Surgery, **54,** 100.
ROSENTAL, J. J., GASPAR, M. R., GJERDRUN, T. C., & NEWMAN, J. (1975): Vascular injuries associated with fractures of the femur. Archives of Surgery, **110,** 494.
SEDDON, H. J. (1956): Volkmann's contracture: treatment by excision of the infarct. Journal of Bone and Joint Surgery, **38B,** 152.
SEDDON, H. J. (1966): Volkmann's ischaemia in the lower limb. Journal of Bone and Joint Surgery, **48B,** 627.
WADDELL, J. P., & LENCZNER, E. M. (1974): Arterial injury associated with skeletal trauma. Injury, **6,** 28.

Injury to Nerves
LEFFERT, R. D., & SEDDON, H. (1965): Infraclavicular brachial plexus injuries. Journal of Bone and Joint Surgery, **47B,** 9.
MEDICAL RESEARCH COUNCIL (1976): *Aids to the Examination of the Peripheral Nervous System.* London: Her Majesty's Stationery Office.
SEDDON, H. J. (1942): Classification of nerve injuries. British Medical Journal, **2,** 237.
SEDDON, H. J. (1963): Nerve grafting. Journal of Bone and Joint Surgery, **45B,** 447.
SEDDON, H. J. (1975): *Surgical Disorders of the Peripheral Nerves,* 2nd ed. Edinburgh and London: Churchill Livingstone.
SUNDERLAND, S. (1968): *Nerves and Nerve Injuries.* Edinburgh: Livingstone.

Injury to Viscera
ANDERSON, J. C., HOLDSWORTH, F. W., & MITCHELL, J. P. (1963): Injuries to the urinary tract (symposium). Proceedings of the Royal Society of Medicine, **56,** 1041.
MITCHELL, J. P. (1971): Trauma to the abdomen: management of bladder and urethral injuries. Annals of Royal College of Surgeons of England, **48,** 13.

Sudeck's Atrophy
PLEWES, L. W. (1956): Sudeck's atrophy in the hand. Journal of Bone and Joint Surgery, **38B,** 195.
GRIFFITHS, D. Ll. (1950): Certain vascular lesions. In *Modern Trends in Orthopaedics.* London: Butterworth.

Fat Embolism
EVARTS, C. M. (1970): The fat embolism syndrome. Surgical Clinics of North America, **50,** 493.

Gossling, H. R., Ellison, L. H., & Degraff, A. C. (1974): Fat embolism: the role of respiratory failure and its treatment. Journal of Bone and Joint Surgery, **56A,** 1327.

Murray, D. G., & Racz, G. B. (1974): Fat embolism syndrome: a rationale for treatment. Journal of Bone and Joint Surgery, **56A,** 1338.

Ross, A. P. J. (1970): The fat embolism syndrome. Annals of Royal College of Surgeons of England, **46,** 159.

Tachakra, S. S., & Sevitt, S. (1975): Hypoxaemia after fractures. Journal of Bone and Joint Surgery, **57B,** 197.

Wrobel, L. J., Virgilio, R. W., & Trimble, C. (1974): Inapparent hypoxemia associated with skeletal injuries. Journal of Bone and Joint Surgery, **56A,** 346.

CHAPTER FIVE

Special Features of Fractures in Children

Akbarnia, B., Torg, J. S., Kilpatrick, J., & Sussman, S. (1974): Manifestations of the battered child syndrome. Journal of Bone and Joint Surgery, **56A,** 1159.

Blount, W. P. (1954): *Fractures in Children.* Baltimore: Williams and Wilkins.

Central Health Services Council (1970): *The Battered Baby.* London: Her Majesty's Stationery Office.

Devas, M. B. (1963): Stress fractures in children. Journal of Bone and Joint Surgery, **45B,** 528.

Edvardsen, P., & Syversen, S. N. (1976): Overgrowth of the femur after fracture of the shaft in childhood. Journal of Bone and Joint Surgery, **58B,** 339.

Emneus, H., & Wiberg, G. (1957): Influence of fracture on growth in length of shaft bones. Rapport de le Septième Congrès de la Société Internationale de Chirurgie Orthopédique et de Traumatologie.

Godfrey, J. D. (1964): Trauma in children. (Instructional Course Lecture, American Academy of Orthopaedic Surgeons.) Journal of Bone and Joint Surgery, **46A,** 422.

Lichtenberg, R. P. (1954): A study of 2,532 fractures in children. American Journal of Surgery, **87,** 330.

Lloyd-Roberts, G. C. (1971): *Orthopaedics in Infancy and Childhood.* London: Butterworth.

Pollen, A. G. (1973): *Fractures and Dislocations in Children.* Edinburgh and London: Churchill Livingstone.

Rang, M. (1974): *Children's Fractures.* Oxford: Blackwell Scientific Publications.

Sharrard, W. J. W. (1971): *Paediatric Orthopaedics and Fractures.* Oxford: Blackwell Scientific Publications.

Weston, W. J. (1957): Metaphysial fractures in infancy. Journal of Bone and Joint Surgery, **39B,** 694.

See also under individual regions.

CHAPTER SIX

Joint Injuries

Barnett, C. H., Davies, D. V., & MacConaill, M. A. (1961): *Synovial Joints.* London: Longmans Green.

Kellgren, J. H., & Samuel, E. P. (1950): The sensitivity and innervation of the articular capsule. Journal of Bone and Joint Surgery, **32B,** 84.

WYKE, B. (1967): The neurology of joints. Annals of the Royal College of Surgeons of England, **41**, 25.
See also under individual joints.

CHAPTER SEVEN

Cervical Spine

ANDERSON, L. D., & D'ALONZO, R. T. (1974): Fractures of the odontoid process of the axis. Journal of Bone and Joint Surgery, **56A**, 1663.

BEATSON, T. R. (1963): Fractures and dislocations of the cervical spine. Journal of Bone and Joint Surgery, **45B**, 21.

BRAAKMAN, R., & VINKEN, P. J. (1967): Unilateral facet interlocking in the lower cervical spine. Journal of Bone and Joint Surgery, **49B**, 249.

BRASHEAR, H. R., VENTERS, G. C., & PRESTON, E. T. (1975): Fractures of the neural arch of the axis. Journal of Bone and Joint Surgery, **57A**, 879.

BURKE, D. C., & BERRYMAN, D. (1971): The place of closed manipulation in the management of flexion-rotation dislocations of the cervical spine. Journal of Bone and Joint Surgery, **53B**, 165.

CONE, W., & TURNER, W. G. (1937): The treatment of fracture-dislocations of the cervical vertebrae by skeletal traction and fusion. Journal of Bone and Joint Surgery, **19**, 584.

EVANS, D. K. (1976): Anterior cervical subluxation. Journal of Bone and Joint Surgery, **58B**, 318.

FORSYTH, H. F., MACNAB, I., & PETRIE, J. G. (1964): Trauma of the cervical spine (symposium). (Instructional Course Lectures, American Academy of Orthopaedic Surgeons.) Journal of Bone and Joint Surgery, **46A**, 1792.

FRIED, L. C. (1973): Atlanto-axial fracture-dislocations. Journal of Bone and Joint Surgery, **55B**, 490.

HENTZER, L., & SCHALIMTZEK, M. (1971): Fractures and subluxations of the atlas and axis. Acta Orthopaedica Scandinavica, **42**, 251.

JEFFERSON, G. (1920): Fracture of atlas vertebra. British Journal of Surgery, **7**, 407.

MARAR, B. C. (1974): Hyperextension injuries of the cervical spine. Journal of Bone and Joint Surgery, **56A**, 1655.

ROAF, R. (1960): A study of the mechanics of spinal injuries. Journal of Bone and Joint Surgery, **42B**, 810.

SCHATZKER, J., RORABECK, C. H., & WADDELL, J. P. (1971): Fractures of the dens. Journal of Bone and Joint Surgery, **53B**, 392.

SHERK, H. H., & NICHOLSON, J. T. (1970): Fractures of the atlas. Journal of Bone and Joint Surgery, **52A**, 1017.

STAUFFER, E. S., & KELLY, E. G. (1977): Fracture-dislocations of the cervical spine. Journal of Bone and Joint Surgery, **59A**, 45.

WILLIAMS, T. G. (1975): Hangman's fracture. Journal of Bone and Joint Surgery, **57B**, 82.

CHAPTER EIGHT

Spine and Thorax

BURKE, D. C. (1971): Hyperextension injuries of the spine. Journal of Bone and Joint Surgery, **53B**, 3.

HARRIS, P. (ed.) (1966): *Spinal Injuries: A Symposium*. The Royal College of Surgeons of Edinburgh.

HOLDSWORTH, F. W. (1970): Fractures, dislocations and fracture-dislocations of the spine. Journal of Bone and Joint Surgery, **52A**, 1534.

NICOLL, E. A. (1948): Closed fractures of the spine. Journal of Bone and Joint Surgery, **30B**, 725.

NICOLL, E. A. (1949): Fractures of the dorso-lumbar spine. Journal of Bone and Joint Surgery, **31B**, 376.

NICOLL, E. A. (1962): Fractures and dislocations of the spine. In *Modern Trends in Orthopaedics* (3). London: Butterworth.

ROAF, R. (1960): A study of the mechanics of spinal injuries. Journal of Bone and Joint Surgery, **42B**, 810.

CHAPTER NINE

Paraplegia from Spinal Injuries

BARNES, R. (1948): Paraplegia in cervical spine injuries. Journal of Bone and Joint Surgery, **30B**, 234.

BARNES, R. (1951): Mechanism of cord injury without vertebral dislocation. Journal of Bone and Joint Surgery, **33B**, 494.

BURKE, D. C., & MURRAY, D. D. (1976): The management of thoracic and thoraco-lumbar injuries of the spine with neurological involvement. Journal of Bone and Joint Surgery, **58B**, 72.

GUTTMAN, L. (1959): Management of spinal cord injuries. In *Modern Trends in Diseases of the Vertebral Column*. London: Butterworth.

GUTTMAN, L. (1976): *Spinal Cord Injuries. Comprehensive Management and Research*. Oxford: Blackwell Scientific Publications.

HARDY, A. G., McSWEENEY, T., GIBSON, N. O. K., SILVER, J. R., & KERR, A. S. (1971): The immediate management of paraplegia (symposium). Annals of Royal College of Surgeons in England, **48**, 14.

HOLDSWORTH, F. W., & HARDY, A. (1953): Early treatment of paraplegia from fractures of the thoraco-lumbar spine. Journal of Bone and Joint Surgery, **35B**, 540.

LEWIS, J., & McKIBBIN, B. (1974): The treatment of unstable fracture-dislocations of the thoraco-lumbar spine accompanied by paraplegia. Journal of Bone and Joint Surgery, **56B**, 603.

TAYLOR, A. R. (1951): The mechanism of injury to the spinal cord in the neck without damage to the vertebral column. Journal of Bone and Joint Surgery, **33B**, 543.

TAYLOR, A. R., & BLACKWOOD, W. (1948): Paraplegia in hyperextension cervical injuries with normal radiographic appearances. Journal of Bone and Joint Surgery, **30B**, 245.

TRIBE, C. R. (1963): Causes of death in the early and late stages of paraplegia. International Journal of Paraplegia, **1**, 19.

Chest Injuries

BICKFORD, R. J. (1971): Chest injuries. Annals of Royal College of Surgeons of England, **48**, 8.

DREW, C. (1963): Chest injuries. In *Recent Advances in the Surgery of Trauma*. London: Churchill.

HOWAT, D. D. C. (1970): Vascular and respiratory emergencies. Annals of Royal College of Surgeons of England, **47**, 162.

WADDINGTON, J. K. B. (1971): Management of chest injuries. Annals of Royal College of Surgeons of England, **48**, 10.

WILLIAMS, W. G., & ZEITLIN, G. L. (1965): Flail chest. British Journal of Diseases of the Chest, **59**, 15.

CHAPTER TEN

Shoulder, Upper Arm and Elbow

Shoulder Girdle

ALLMAN, F. L. (1967): Fractures and ligamentous injuries of the clavicle and its articulation. (Instructional Course Lecture, American Academy of Orthopaedic Surgeons.) Journal of Bone and Joint Surgery, **49A,** 774.

BAKER, D. M., & STRYKER, W. S. (1965): Acute complete acromio-clavicular separation. Journal of American Medical Association, **192,** 689.

BANKART, A. S. B. (1938): An operation for recurrent dislocation (subluxation) of the sterno-clavicular joint. British Journal of Surgery, **26,** 230.

BURROWS, H. J. (1951): Tenodesis of subclavius in the treatment of recurrent dislocation of the sterno-clavicular joint. Journal of Bone and Joint Surgery, **33B,** 240.

JACOBS, B., & WADE, P. A. (1966): Acromioclavicular-joint injury. Journal of Bone and Joint Surgery, **48A,** 475.

LUNSETH, P. A., CHAPMAN, K. W., & FRANKEL, V. H. (1975): Surgical treatment of chronic dislocation of the sterno-clavicular joint. Journal of Bone and Joint Surgery, **57B,** 193.

TYER, H. D. D., STURROCK, W. D. S., & CALLOW, F. Mc. C. (1963): Retrosternal dislocation of the clavicle. Journal of Bone and Joint Surgery, **45B,** 132.

SCOTT, J. C., & ORR, M. M. (1973): Injuries to the acromio-clavicular joint. Injury, **5,** 13.

SIMMONS, E. H., & MARTIN, R. F. (1968): Acute dislocation of the acromio-clavicular joint. Canadian Journal of Surgery, **11,** 473.

Shoulder Joint

ADAMS, J. C. (1950): Recurrent dislocation of the shoulder. In *Techniques in British Surgery.* Philadelphia: Saunders.

ADAMS, J. C. (1948): Recurrent dislocation of the shoulder. Journal of Bone and Joint Surgery, **30B,** 26.

BANKART, A. S. B. (1923): Recurrent or habitual dislocation of the shoulder joint. British Medical Journal, **2,** 1132.

BANKART, A. S. B. (1938): The pathology and treatment of recurrent dislocation of the shoulder joint. British Journal of Surgery, **26,** 23.

BOYD, H. B., & SISK, T. D. (1972): Recurrent posterior dislocation of the shoulder. Journal of Bone and Joint Surgery, **54A,** 779.

CURR, J. F. (1970): Rupture of the axillary artery complicating dislocation of the shoulder. Journal of Bone and Joint Surgery, **52B,** 313.

DEBEYRE, J., PATTE, D., & ELMELIK, E. (1965): Repair of ruptures of the rotator cuff of the shoulder. Journal of Bone and Joint Surgery, **47B,** 36.

HOYT, W. A. (1967): Etiology of shoulder injuries in athletes. (Instructional Course Lecture, American Academy of Orthopaedic Surgeons.) Journal of Bone and Joint Surgery, **49A,** 755.

JOHNSTON, G. W., & LOWEY, J. H. (1962): Rupture of the axillary artery complicating anterior dislocation of the shoulder. Journal of Bone and Joint Surgery, **44B,** 116.

MOSELEY, H. F. (1969): *Shoulder Lesions.* Edinburgh: Livingstone.

OSMOND-CLARKE, H. (1948): Habitual dislocation of the shoulder. Journal of Bone and Joint Surgery, **30B,** 19.

REEVES, B. (1969): Acute anterior dislocation of the shoulder. Annals of Royal College of Surgeons of England, **44,** 255.

ROWE, C. R. (1962): Acute and recurrent dislocations of the shoulder. (Instructional Course Lecture, American Academy of Orthopaedic Surgeons.) Journal of Bone and Joint Surgery, **44A,** 998.

Humerus (Upper End and Shaft)

AITKEN, A. P. (1936): End results of fractures of the proximal humeral epiphysis. Journal of Bone and Joint Surgery, **18**, 1036.

CARROLL, S. E. (1963): A study of the nutrient foramina of the humeral diaphysis. Journal of Bone and Joint Surgery, **45B**, 176.

KENNEDY, J. C., & WYATT, J. K. (1957): An evaluation of the management of fractures through the middle third of the humerus. Canadian Journal of Surgery, **1**, 26.

KLENERMAN, L. (1966): Fractures of the shaft of the humerus. Journal of Bone and Joint Surgery, **48B**, 105.

MILLS, K. L. G. (1974): Severe injury of the upper end of the humerus. Injury, **6**, 13.

NEER, C. S. (1970): Displaced proximal humeral fractures. Journal of Bone and Joint Surgery, **52A**, 1077.

NEVIASER, J. S. (1962): Complicated fractures and dislocations about the shoulder joint. (Instructional Course Lecture, American Academy of Orthopaedic Surgeons.) Journal of Bone and Joint Surgery, **44A**, 984.

STEWART, M. J., & HUNDLEY, J. M. (1955): Fractures of the humerus: a comparative study in methods of treatment. Journal of Bone and Joint Surgery, **37A**, 681.

Humerus (Lower End)

ATTENBOROUGH, C. G. (1953): Remodelling of the humerus after supracondylar fractures in children. Journal of Bone and Joint Surgery, **35B**, 3.

CONNER, A. N., & SMITH, M. G. H. (1970): Displaced fractures of the lateral humeral condyle in children. Journal of Bone and Joint Surgery, **52B**, 460.

EL-AHWANY, M. D. (1974): Supracondylar fractures of the humerus in children. Injury, **6**, 45.

FLYNN, J. C., RICHARDS, J. F., & SALTZMAN, R. I. (1975): Prevention and treatment of non-union of slightly displaced fractures of the lateral humeral condyle in children. Journal of Bone and Joint Surgery, **57A**, 1087.

FOWLES, J. V., & KASSAB, M. T. (1974): Fracture of the capitulum humeri: treatment by excision. Journal of Bone and Joint Surgery, **56A**, 794.

HARDACRE, J. A., NAHIGIAN, S. H., FROIMSON, A. I., & BROWN, J. E. (1971): Fractures of the lateral condyle of the humerus in children. Journal of Bone and Joint Surgery, **53A**, 1083.

HENRIKSON, B. (1966): Supracondylar fracture of the humerus in children. Acta Chirurgica Scandinavica, Supplementum 369.

JAKOB, R., FOWLES, J. V., RANG, M., & KASSAB, M. T. (1975): Observations concerning fractures of the lateral humeral condyle in children. Journal of Bone and Joint Surgery, **57B**, 430.

JAKOBSSON, A. (1957): Fracture of the capitellum of the humerus in adults. Acta Orthopaedica Scandinavica, **3**, 184.

JEFFERISS, C. D. (1977): Straight lateral traction in selected supracondylar fractures of the humerus in children. Injury, **8**, 213.

JEFFERY, C. C. (1958): Non-union of the epiphysis of the lateral condyle of the humerus. Journal of Bone and Joint Surgery, **40B**, 396.

SEDDON, H. J. (1956): Volkmann's contracture: treatment by excision of the infarct. Journal of Bone and Joint Surgery, **38B**, 152.

Elbow Joint

HUME, A. C. (1957): Anterior dislocation of the head of the radius associated with undisplaced fracture of the olecranon in children. Journal of Bone and Joint Surgery, **39B**, 508.

KEON-COHEN, B. T. (1966): Fractures at the elbow. (Instructional Course Lecture, American Academy of Orthopaedic Surgeons.) Journal of Bone and Joint Surgery, **48A,** 1623.
LOUIS, D. S., RICCIARDI, J. E., & SPENGLER, D. M. (1974): Arterial injury: a complication of posterior elbow dislocation. Journal of Bone and Joint Surgery, **56A,** 1631.
SNELLMAN, O. (1959): Subluxation of the head of the radius in children. Acta Orthopaedica Scandinavica, **28,** 311.
STELLING, F. H. (1955): Traumatic dislocation of the head of the radius in children. Journal of Bone and Joint Surgery, **37A,** 1116.
WAINWRIGHT, D. (1962): Fractures involving the elbow joint. In *Modern Trends in Orthopaedics* (3). London: Butterworth.

CHAPTER ELEVEN

Forearm, Wrist and Hand

Forearm Bones
BACORN, R. W., & KURTZKE, J. F. (1953): Colles' fracture. Journal of Bone and Joint Surgery, **35A,** 643.
BRUCE, H. E., HARVEY, J. P., & WILSON, J. C. (1974): Monteggia fractures. Journal of Bone and Joint Surgery, **56A,** 1563.
BURWELL, H. N., & CHARNLEY, A. D. (1964): Treatment of forearm fractures in adults with particular reference to plate fixation. Journal of Bone and Joint Surgery, **46B,** 404.
COLTON, C. L. (1973): Fractures of the olecranon in adults. Injury, **5,** 121.
ELLIS, J. (1965): Smith's and Barton's fractures. Journal of Bone and Joint Surgery, **47B,** 724.
EVANS, E. M. (1949): Pronation injuries of the forearm. Journal of Bone and Joint Surgery, **31B,** 578.
EVANS, E. M. (1951): Fractures of the radius and ulna. Journal of Bone and Joint Surgery, **33B,** 548.
FALLON, M. (1972): *Abraham Colles 1773–1843 Surgeon of Ireland.* London: Wm. Heinemann Medical Books.
FULLER, D. I. (1973): The Ellis plate operation for Smith's fracture. Journal of Bone and Joint Surgery, **55B,** 173.
GIUSTRA, P. E., KILLORAN, P. J., FURMAN, R. S., & ROOT, J. A. (1974): Missed Monteggia fracture. Radiology, **110,** 45.
JEFFERY, C. C. (1950): Fractures of the head of the radius in children. Journal of Bone and Joint Surgery, **32B,** 314.
JESSING, P. (1975): Monteggia lesions and their complicating nerve damage. Acta Orthopaedica Scandinavica, **46,** 601.
McLAUGHLIN, H. L. (1966): Prevention and repair of nonunion of fractures in the adult forearm. Clinical Orthopaedics, **43,** 55.
MIKIC, Z. DJ. (1975): Galeazzi fracture-dislocations. Journal of Bone and Joint Surgery, **57A,** 1071.
OLIVEIRA, J. C. DE (1973): Barton's fractures. Journal of Bone and Joint Surgery, **55A,** 586.
PEIRO, A., ANDRES, F., & FERNANDEZ-ESTEVE, F. (1977): Acute Monteggia lesions in children. Journal of Bone and Joint Surgery, **59A,** 92.
POULSEN, J. O., & TOPHOJ, K. (1974): Fracture of the head and neck of the radius. Acta Orthopaedica Scandinavica, **45,** 66.
RADIN, E. L., & RISEBOROUGH, E. J. (1966): Fractures of the radial head. Journal of Bone and Joint Surgery, **48A,** 1055.

RECKLING, F. W., & PELTIER, L. F. (1965): Riccardo Galeazzi and Galeazzi's fracture. Surgery, **58**, 453.

SAGE, F. P. (1959): Medullary fixation of fractures of the forearm. Journal of Bone and Joint Surgery, **41A**, 1489.

SMAILL, G. B. (1965): Long-term follow-up of Colles's fracture. Journal of Bone and Joint Surgery, **47B**, 80.

SMITH, J. E. M. (1959): Internal fixation in the treatment of fractures of the shafts of the radius and ulna in adults. Journal of Bone and Joint Surgery, **41B**, 122.

TOMPKINS, D. G. (1971): The anterior Monteggia fracture. Journal of Bone and Joint Surgery, **53A**, 1109.

WOODYARD, J. E. (1969): A review of Smith's fractures. Journal of Bone and Joint Surgery, **51B**, 324.

Carpal Bones

AITKEN, A. P., & NALEBUFF, E. A. (1960): Volar transnavicular perilunar dislocation of the carpus. Journal of Bone and Joint Surgery, **42A**, 1051.

BORGESKOV, S., CHRISTIANSEN, B., KJAER, A., & BALSLEV, I. (1966): Fractures of the carpal bones. Acta Orthopaedica Scandinavica, **37**, 276.

CAMPBELL, R. D., LANCE, E. M., & YEOH, C. B. (1964): Lunate and perilunar dislocations. Journal of Bone and Joint Surgery, **46B**, 55.

DOOLEY, B. J. (1968): Inlay bone grafting for non-union of the scaphoid bone by the anterior approach. Journal of Bone and Joint Surgery, **50B**, 102.

LONDON, P. S. (1961): The broken scaphoid bone: the case against pessimism. Journal of Bone and Joint Surgery, **43B**, 237.

MULDER, J. D. (1968): The results of 100 cases of pseudarthrosis of the scaphoid bone treated by the Matti-Russe operation. Journal of Bone and Joint Surgery, **50B**, 110.

SCANDINAVIAN CLUB FOR SURGERY OF HAND (1962): Symposium on fractures of the scaphoid bone. Journal of Bone and Joint Surgery, **44B**, 245.

UNGER, H. S., & STRYKER, W. C. (1969): Non-union of the carpal navicular: analysis of 42 cases treated by the Russe procedure. Southern Medical Journal, **62**, 620.

Hand

BOYES, J. H. (1971): *Bunnell's Surgery of the Hand*. Oxford: Blackwell Scientific Publications.

BRITISH ORTHOPAEDIC ASSOCIATION (1960): Symposium on hand surgery. Journal of Bone and Joint Surgery, **42B**, 646.

FLATT, A. E. (1972): *The Care of Minor Hand Injuries*. London: Henry Kimpton.

FLYNN, J. E. (ed.) (1966): *Hand Surgery*. Baltimore: The Williams and Wilkins Co.

GRIFFITHS, J. C. (1964): Fractures at the base of the first metacarpal bone. Journal of Bone and Joint Surgery, **46B**, 712.

KINMONTH, M., BOLTON, H., ELLIS, J. S., WAINWRIGHT, D., & DANIEL, J. W. (1964): The injured hand (symposium). Proceedings of the Royal Society of Medicine, **57**, 595.

LEE, M. L. H. (1963): Intra-articular and peri-articular fractures of the phalanges. Journal of Bone and Joint Surgery, **45B**, 103.

PARRY, C. B. WYNN (1964): The management of the severely injured hand. Proceedings of the Royal Society of Medicine, **57**, 1071.

PARRY, C. B. WYNN (1973): *Rehabilitation of the Hand*, 3rd ed. London: Butterworth.

POLLEN, A. G. (1968): The conservative treatment of Bennett's fracture-subluxation of the thumb metacarpal. Journal of Bone and Joint Surgery, **50B**, 91.

PULVERTAFT, R. G. (ed.) (1966): *Clinical Surgery. Volume 7: The Hand*. London: Butterworth.

PULVERTAFT, R. G., & REID, D. A. C. (1963): Surgery of the hand in Great Britain. British Journal of Surgery, **50,** 673.

PULVERTAFT, R. G. (ed.) (1977): *The Hand*, 3rd ed. In *Operative Surgery* (eds. Rob and Smith). London: Butterworth.

RANK, B. K., WAKEFIELD, A. R., & HUESTON, J. T. (1973): *Surgery of Repair as Applied to Hand Injuries*, 4th ed. Edinburgh: Livingstone.

CHAPTER TWELVE

Pelvis, Thigh and Knee

Pelvis and Hip Joint

BATRA, H. C. (1976): Central fractures of the acetabulum. Injury, **7,** 171.

CARNESALE, P. G., STEWART, M. J., & BARNES, S. N. (1975): Acetabular disruption and central fracture-dislocation of the hip. Journal of Bone and Joint Surgery, **57A,** 1054.

CHARNLEY, J. (1952): Experiences in the evolution of a new operation for osteoarthritis of the hip joint. Journal of Bone and Joint Surgery, **34B,** 506.

EPSTEIN, H. C. (1974): Posterior fracture-dislocations of the hip: long-term follow-up. Journal of Bone and Joint Surgery, **56A,** 1103.

FROMAN, C., & STEIN, A. (1967): Complicated crushing injuries of the pelvis. Journal of Bone and Joint Surgery, **49B,** 24.

GÖTHLIN, G., & HINDMARSH, J. (1970): Central dislocation of the hip. Acta Orthopaedica Scandinavica, **41,** 476.

GUSTAFSSON, A. (1970): Operative adaptation with cerclage in traumatic rupture of the symphysis. Acta Orthopaedica Scandinavica, **41,** 446.

HOLDSWORTH, F. W. (1948): Dislocation and fracture-dislocation of the pelvis. Journal of Bone and Joint Surgery, **30B,** 461.

HORTON, R. E., & HAMILTON, S. G. I. (1968): Ligature of the internal iliac artery for massive haemorrhage complicating fracture of the pelvis. Journal of Bone and Joint Surgery, **50B,** 376.

HUNTER, G. A. (1969): Posterior dislocation and fracture-dislocation of the hip. Journal of Bone and Joint Surgery, **51B,** 38.

JUDET, R., JUDET, J., & LETOURNEL, E. (1964): Fractures of the acetabulum: classification and surgical approaches for open reduction. Journal of Bone and Joint Surgery, **46A,** 1615.

McMURRAY, T. P. (1935): Osteoarthritis of the hip joint. British Journal of Surgery, **22,** 716.

PELTIER, L. F. (1965): Complications associated with fractures of the pelvis. (Instructional Course Lecture, American Academy of Orthopaedic Surgeons.) Journal of Bone and Joint Surgery, **47A,** 1060.

PROCTOR, H. (1973): Dislocations of the hip (excluding central dislocations) and their complications. Injury, **5,** 1.

SHARP, I. K. (1973): Plate fixation of disrupted symphysis pubis. Journal of Bone and Joint Surgery, **55B,** 618.

STEWART, M. J., & MILFORD, L. W. (1954): Fracture-dislocation of the hip: an end-result study. Journal of Bone and Joint Surgery, **36A,** 315.

Femur (Upper End)

BARNES, R., BROWN, J. T., GARDEN, R. S., & NICOLL, E. A. (1976): Subcapital fractures of the femur. Journal of Bone and Joint Surgery, **58B,** 2.

BENTLEY, G. (1968): Impacted fractures of the neck of the femur. Journal of Bone and Joint Surgery, **50B,** 551.

BROWN, J. T., & ABRAMI, G. (1964): Transcervical femoral fracture. Journal of Bone and Joint Surgery, **46B,** 648.

CANALE, S. T., & BOURLAND, W. L. (1977): Fracture of the neck and inter-trochanteric region of the femur in children. Journal of Bone and Joint Surgery, **59A,** 431.

CATTO, M. (1965): A histological study of avascular necrosis of the femoral head after transcervical fracture. Journal of Bone and Joint Surgery, **47B,** 749.

CATTO, M. (1965): The histological appearances of late segmental collapse of the femoral head after transcervical fracture. Journal of Bone and Joint Surgery, **47B,** 777.

CRAWFORD, H. B. (1965): Experience with the non-operative treatment of impacted fractures of the neck of the femur. (Instructional Course Lecture, American Academy of Orthopaedic Surgeons.) Journal of Bone and Joint Surgery, **47A,** 830.

CUTHBERT, H., & HOWAT, T. W. (1976): The use of the Küntscher Y nail in the treatment of intertrochanteric and subtrochanteric fractures of the femur. Injury, **8,** 135.

D'ARCY, J., & DEVAS, M. (1976): Treatment of fractures of the femoral neck by replacement with a Thompson prosthesis. Journal of Bone and Joint Surgery, **58B,** 279.

DICKSON, J. A. (1947): The high geometric osteotomy with rotation and bone graft for ununited fractures of the neck of the femur. Journal of Bone and Joint Surgery, **29,** 1005.

FIELDING, J. W., WILSON, S. A., & RATZAN, S. (1974): A continuing end-result study of displaced intracapsular fractures of the neck of the femur treated with the Pugh nail. Journal of Bone and Joint Surgery, **56A,** 1464.

GARDEN, R. S. (1964): Stability and union in subcapital fractures of the femur. Journal of Bone and Joint Surgery, **46B,** 630.

GARDEN, R. S. (1971): Malreduction and avascular necrosis in subcapital fractures of the femur. Journal of Bone and Joint Surgery, **53B,** 183.

HARROLD, A. J. (1960): Failure of union in fracture of the neck of the femur. Journal of Bone and Joint Surgery, **42B,** 226.

HUNTER, G. A. (1974): A further comparison of the use of internal fixation and prosthetic replacement for fresh fractures of the neck of femur. British Journal of Surgery, **61,** 382.

JENKINS, D. H. R., ROBERTS, J. G., WEBSTER, D., & WILLIAMS, E. O. (1973): Osteomalacia in elderly patients with fracture of the femoral neck. Journal of Bone and Joint Surgery, **55B,** 575.

JENSEN, J. S., & HOLSTEIN, P. (1975): Long-term follow-up of Moore arthroplasty in femoral neck fractures. Acta Orthopaedica Scandinavica, **46,** 764.

KAUFER, H., MATTHEWS, L. S., & SONSTEGARD, D. (1974): Stable fixation of intertrochanteric fractures. Journal of Bone and Joint Surgery, **56A,** 899.

KAVLIE, H., & SUNDAL, B. (1974): Primary arthroplasty in femoral neck fractures. Acta Orthopaedica Scandinavica, **45,** 579.

KOLIND-SORENSEN, W. (1975): Mortality in intertrochanteric fracture of the femoral neck. Acta Orthopaedica Scandinavica, **46,** 654.

LAM, S. F. (1971): Fractures of the neck of the femur in children. Journal of Bone and Joint Surgery, **53A,** 1165.

MOORE, A. T. (1957): The self-locking metal hip prosthesis. Journal of Bone and Joint Surgery, **39A,** 811.

MUCKLE, D. S. (ed.) (1977): *Femoral Neck Fractures.* London: Chapman and Hall.

MURRAY, R. C., & FREW, J. F. M. (1949): Trochanteric fractures of the femur. Journal of Bone and Joint Surgery, **31B,** 204.

NIEMINEN, S. (1975): Early weight-bearing after classic internal fixation of medial fractures of the femoral neck. Acta Orthopaedica Scandinavica, **46,** 782.

PUGH, W. L. (1955): A self-adjusting nail-plate for fractures about the hip joint. Journal of Bone and Joint Surgery, **37A**, 1085.

RISKA, E. B. (1971): Prosthetic replacement in the treatment of subcapital fractures of the femur. Acta Orthopaedica Scandinavica, **42**, 281.

RUSSELL, R. H. (1923): Fracture of the femur: a clinical study. British Journal of Surgery, **11**, 491.

SARMIENTO, A. (1970): The unstable intertrochanteric fracture. Journal of Bone and Joint Surgery, **52A**, 1309.

SEVITT, S., & THOMPSON, R. G. (1965): The distribution and anastomoses of arteries supplying the head and neck of the femur. Journal of Bone and Joint Surgery, **47B**, 560.

SOLOMON, L. (1973): Fracture of the femoral neck in the elderly: bone ageing or disease? South African Journal of Surgery, **11**, 269.

TAYLOR, R. G. (1950): Pseudarthrosis of the hip joint. Journal of Bone and Joint Surgery, **32B**, 161.

THOMPSON, F. R. (1952): Vitallium intramedullary hip prosthesis: preliminary report. New York State Journal of Medicine, **52**, 3011.

THOMPSON, F. R. (1954): Two and a half years' experience with a Vitallium intramedullary hip prosthesis. Journal of Bone and Joint Surgery, **36A**, 489.

Femur (Shaft and Lower End)

ADAIR, I. V. (1976): The use of plaster casts in the treatment of fractures of the femoral shaft. Injury, **7**, 194.

BROWN, A., & D'ARCY, J. C. (1971): Internal fixation for supracondylar fractures of the femur in the elderly patient. Journal of Bone and Joint Surgery, **53B**, 420.

CHRISTENSEN, N. O. (1973): Küntscher intramedullary reaming and nail fixation for non-union of fracture of the femur and the tibia. Journal of Bone and Joint Surgery, **55B**, 312.

CLAWSON, D. K., SMITH, R. F., & HANSEN, S. T. (1971): Closed intramedullary nailing of the femur. Journal of Bone and Joint Surgery, **53A**, 681.

CONNOLLY, J. F., & KING, P. (1973): Closed reduction and early cast-brace ambulation in the treatment of femoral fractures. Journal of Bone and Joint Surgery, **55A**, 1559.

EDVARDSEN, P., & SYVERSEN, S. M. (1976): Overgrowth of the femur after fracture of the shaft in childhood. Journal of Bone and Joint Surgery, **58B**, 339.

FISK, G. R. (1962): Fractures involving the knee. In *Modern Trends in Orthopaedics* (3). London: Butterworth.

HELAL, B., & SKEVIS, X. (1967): Unrecognised dislocation of the hip in fractures of the femoral shaft. Journal of Bone and Joint Surgery, **49B**, 293.

KAMDAR, B. A., & ARDEN, G. P. (1974): Intramedullary nailing for fractures of the femoral shaft. Injury, **6**, 7.

KOOTSTRA, G. (1973): *Femoral Shaft Fractures in Adults*. Assen, Netherlands: Van Gorcum.

LIDGE, R. T. (1960): Complications following Bryant's traction. Archives of Surgery, **80**, 557.

NICHOLAS, J. A., & KILLORAN, P. (1965): Fracture of the femur in patients with Paget's disease. Journal of Bone and Joint Surgery, **47A**, 450.

NICHOLSON, J. T., FOSTER, R. M., & HEATH, R. D. (1955): Bryant's traction. Journal of American Medical Association, **157**, 415.

NICOLL, E. A. (1963): Quadricepsplasty. Journal of Bone and Joint Surgery, **45B**, 483.

OLERUD, S. (1972): Operative treatment of supracondylar-condylar fractures of the femur. Journal of Bone and Joint Surgery, **54A**, 1015.

Knee

CARGILL, A. O'R., & JACKSON, J. P. (1976): Bucket-handle tear of the medial meniscus: a case for conservative surgery. Journal of Bone and Joint Surgery, **58A**, 248.

ELSASSER, J. C., REYNOLDS, F. C., & OMOHUNDRO, J. R. (1974): The non-operative treatment of collateral ligament injuries of the knee in professional football players. Journal of Bone and Joint Surgery, **56A**, 1185.

GREEN, N. E., & ALLEN, B. L. (1977): Vascular injuries associated with dislocation of the knee. Journal of Bone and Joint Surgery, **59A**, 236.

HELFET, A. J. (1974): *Disorders of the Knee*. Oxford: Blackwell Scientific Publications.

HUGHSTON, J. C., ANDREWS, J. R., CROSS, M. J., & MOSCHI, A. (1976): Classification of knee ligament instabilities. Journal of Bone and Joint Surgery, **58A**, 159, 173.

HUGHSTON, J. C., & EILERS, A. F. (1973): The role of the posterior oblique ligament in repairs of acute medial (collateral) ligament tears of the knee. Journal of Bone and Joint Surgery, **55A**, 923.

JEFFERY, C. C. (1972): Quadricepsplasty. Injury, **4**, 131.

KENNEDY, J. C., HAWKINS, R. J., WILLIS, R. V., & DANYLCHUK, K. D. (1976): Tension studies of human knee ligaments. Journal of Bone and Joint Surgery, **58A**, 350.

MEYERS, M. H., & HARVEY, J. P. (1971): Traumatic dislocation of the knee joint. Journal of Bone and Joint Surgery, **53A**, 16.

NICHOLAS, J. A. (1973): The five-one reconstruction for antero-medial instability of the knee. Journal of Bone and Joint Surgery, **55A**, 899.

NOBLE, J. (1977): Lesions of the menisci: autopsy incidence. Journal of Bone and Joint Surgery, **59A**, 480.

O'DONOGHUE, D. H. (1973): Reconstruction for medial instability of the knee. Journal of Bone and Joint Surgery, **55A**, 941.

PICKETT, J. C., & ALTIZER, T. J. (1971): Injuries of the ligaments of the knee. Clinical Orthopaedics, **76**, 27.

RATLIFF, A. H. C. (1972): Quadricepsplasty. Injury **4**, 126.

SMILLIE, I. S. (1970): *Injuries of the Knee Joint*, 4th ed. Edinburgh: Livingstone.

STOUGARD, J. (1970): Patellectomy. Acta Orthopaedica Scandinavica, **41**, 110.

TAYLOR, A. R., ARDEN, G. P., & RAINEY, H. A. (1972): Traumatic dislocation of the knee. Journal of Bone and Joint Surgery, **54B**, 96.

WILKINSON, J. (1977): Fracture of the patella treated by total excision. Journal of Bone and Joint Surgery, **59B**, 352.

CHAPTER THIRTEEN

Leg, Ankle and Foot

Tibia and Fibula

BÖHLER, J. (1966): Treatment of non-union of the tibia with closed and semiclosed intramedullary nailing. Clinical Orthopaedics, **43**, 93.

BURWELL, H. N. (1971): Plate fixation of tibial shaft fractures. Journal of Bone and Joint Surgery, **53B**, 258.

CHRISTENSEN, N. O. (1973): Küntscher intramedullary reaming and nail fixation for non-union of fracture of the femur and the tibia. Journal of Bone and Joint Surgery, **55B**, 312.

FRIEDENBERG, Z. B. (1971): Fatigue fractures of the tibia. Clinical Orthopaedics, **76**, 111.

HAMZA, K. N., DUNKERLEY, G. E., & MURRAY, C. M. M. (1971): Fractures of the tibia. Journal of Bone and Joint Surgery, **53B**, 696.

JORGENSEN, T. E. (1974): The influence of the intact fibula on the compression of a tibial fracture or pseudarthrosis. Acta Orthopaedica Scandinavica, **45**, 119.

KARLSTRÖM, G., & OLERUD, S. (1975): Percutaneous pin fixation of open tibial fractures. Journal of Bone and Joint Surgery, **57A**, 915.

NICOLL, E. A. (1964): Fractures of the tibial shaft. Journal of Bone and Joint Surgery, **46B**, 373.

NICOLL, E. A. (1969): Infantile pseudarthrosis of the tibia. Journal of Bone and Joint Surgery, **51B**, 589.

PORTER, B. B. (1970): Crush fractures of the lateral tibial table. Journal of Bone and Joint Surgery, **52B**, 676.

RASMUSSEN, P. S., & SORENSEN, S. E. (1973): Tibial condylar fractures: non-operative treatment of lateral compression fractures without impairment of knee joint stability. Injury **4**, 265.

SMITH, J. E. M. (1974): Results of early and delayed internal fixation in tibial shaft fractures. Journal of Bone and Joint Surgery, **56B**, 469.

SOFIELD, H. A. (1971): Congenital pseudarthrosis of the tibia. Clinical Orthopaedics, **76**, 33.

SØRENSEN, K. H. (1969): Treatment of delayed union and non-union ·of tibia by fibular resection. Acta Orthopaedica Scandinavica, **40**, 92.

VAN NES, C. P. (1966): Congenital pseudarthrosis of the leg. Journal of Bone and Joint Surgery, **48A**, 1467.

WEBER, B. G. (1977): Fibrous interposition causing valgus deformity after fracture of the upper tibial metaphysis in children. Journal of Bone and Joint Surgery, **59B**, 290.

Calcaneal Tendon

GILLIES, H., & CHALMERS, J. (1970): The management of fresh ruptures of the tendo Achillis. Journal of Bone and Joint Surgery, **52A**, 337.

HOOKER, C. H. (1963): Rupture of the tendo calcaneus. Journal of Bone and Joint Surgery, **45B**, 360.

LEA, R. B., & SMITH, L. (1972): Non-surgical treatment of tendo Achillis rupture. Journal of Bone and Joint Surgery, **54A**, 1398.

Ankle

BONNIN, J. G. (1965): Injury to the ligaments of the ankle. Journal of Bone and Joint Surgery, **47B**, 609.

BRODIE, I. A. O. D., & DENHAM, R. A. (1974): The treatment of unstable ankle fractures. Journal of Bone and Joint Surgery, **56B**, 256.

BURWELL, H. N., & CHARNLEY, A. D. (1965): The treatment of displaced fractures at the ankle by rigid internal fixation and early joint movement. Journal of Bone and Joint Surgery, **47B**, 634.

COBB, N. (1965): Oblique radiography in the diagnosis of ankle injuries. Proceedings of the Royal Society of Medicine, **58**, 334.

COLTON, C. L. (1968): Fracture-diastasis of the inferior tibio-fibular joint. Journal of Bone and Joint Surgery, **50B**, 830.

COLTON, C. L. (1971): The treatment of Dupuytren's fracture-dislocation of the ankle. Journal of Bone and Joint Surgery, **53B**, 63.

HOOKER, C. H. (1963): Rupture of the tendo calcaneus. Journal of Bone and Joint Surgery, **45B**, 360.

INMAN, V. T. (1976): *The Joints of the Ankle*. Baltimore: The Williams and Wilkins Co.

JOY, G., PATZAKIS, M. J., & HARVEY, J. P. (1974): Precise evaluation of the reduction of severe ankle fractures. Journal of Bone and Joint Surgery, **56A**, 979.

MENDELSOHN, H. A. (ed.) (1965): Injuries to the ankle joint (symposium). Clinical Orthopaedics, **42**, 2.

MILLER, A. J. (1974): Posterior malleolar fractures. Journal of Bone and Joint Surgery, **56B,** 508.

MONK, C. J. E. (1969): Injuries of the tibio-fibular ligaments. Journal of Bone and Joint Surgery, **51B,** 330.

YABLON, I. G., HELLER, F. G., & SHOUSE, L. (1977): The key role of the lateral malleolus in displaced fractures of the ankle. Journal of Bone and Joint Surgery, **59A,** 169.

Foot

COLTART, W. D. (1952): Aviator's astragalus. Journal of Bone and Joint Surgery, **34B,** 545.

DEBURGE, A., NORDIN, J-Y., & TAUSSIG, G. (1975): Articular fractures of the calcaneus: therapeutic indications from a series of 105 cases. Revue de Chirurgie Ortopèdique, **61,** 233.

ISBISTER, J. F. St.C. (1974): Calcaneo-fibular abutment following crush fracture of the calcaneus. Journal of Bone and Joint Surgery, **56B,** 274.

JEFFREYS, T. E. (1963): Lisfranc's fracture-dislocation. Journal of Bone and Joint Surgery, **45B,** 546.

JONES, F. WOOD (1949): *Structure and Function as seen in the Foot.* London: Baillière, Tindall & Cox.

KENWRIGHT, J., & TAYLOR, R. G. (1970): Major injuries of the talus. Journal of Bone and Joint Surgery, **52B,** 36.

MAIN, B. J., & JOWETT, R. L. (1975): Injuries of the mid-tarsal joint. Journal of Bone and Joint Surgery, **57B,** 89.

NADE, S., & MONAHAN, P. R. W. (1973): Fractures of the calcaneum: a study of the long-term prognosis. Injury, **4,** 201.

THORÉN, O. (1964): Os calcis fractures. Acta Orthopaedica Scandinavica, Supplementum 76.

TRICKEY, E. L. (1975): Treatment of fractures of the calcaneus. Journal of Bone and Joint Surgery, **57B,** 411.

WILEY, J. J. (1971): The mechanism of tarso-metatarsal joint injuries. Journal of Bone and Joint Surgery, **53B,** 474.

Index

(Where bold type is used it indicates the main reference)